# Health Effects of Exposure to Environmental Pollutants

# Health Effects of Exposure to Environmental Pollutants

Guest Editors

**Guang Jia**
**Zhangjian Chen**

Basel • Beijing • Wuhan • Barcelona • Belgrade • Novi Sad • Cluj • Manchester

*Guest Editors*
Guang Jia
School of Public Health
Peking University
Beijing
China

Zhangjian Chen
School of Public Health
Peking University
Beijing
China

*Editorial Office*
MDPI AG
Grosspeteranlage 5
4052 Basel, Switzerland

This is a reprint of the Special Issue, published open access by the journal *Toxics* (ISSN 2305-6304), freely accessible at: https://www.mdpi.com/journal/toxics/special_issues/OT05NV8946.

For citation purposes, cite each article independently as indicated on the article page online and as indicated below:

| |
|---|
| Lastname, A.A.; Lastname, B.B. Article Title. *Journal Name* **Year**, *Volume Number*, Page Range. |

**ISBN 978-3-7258-4747-1 (Hbk)**
**ISBN 978-3-7258-4748-8 (PDF)**
**https://doi.org/10.3390/books978-3-7258-4748-8**

# Contents

toxics

MDPI

*Editorial*

# Health Effects of Exposure to Environmental Pollutants: The Combination of Traditional and Emerging Pollutants

**Zhangjian Chen [1,2,*] and Guang Jia [1,2,*]**

1 Department of Occupational and Environmental Health Sciences, School of Public Health, Peking University, Beijing 100191, China
2 Beijing Key Laboratory of Toxicological Research and Risk Assessment for Food Safety, School of Public Health, Peking University, Beijing 100191, China
* Correspondence: zhangjianchen@pku.edu.cn (Z.C.); jiaguangjia@bjmu.edu.cn (G.J.)

## 1. Introduction

This editorial introduces the Special Issue titled "Health Effects of Exposure to Environmental Pollutants". The health effects of environmental pollutants, including traditional pollutants (such as particulate matters and heavy metals) and emerging pollutants (such as nanoparticles), has received widespread attention [1]. These pollutants can have serious impacts on the environment and human health. Research on the potential toxic effects and mechanisms of environmental pollutants can provide a scientific basis for related prevention work.

This Special Issue contains 11 articles: 10 research papers and 1 communication. The research papers focus on the potential toxicity and mechanisms of environmental pollutants affecting humans or the environment. Some papers highlight the potential toxicity and mechanisms of emerging pollutants such as nanomaterials using novel methods, such as multi-omics approaches. Some papers still focus on traditional pollutants, such as particulate matter, heavy metals, arsenic, benzene and its homologues, but they explore novel aspects in terms of toxicity mechanisms or biomarkers, such as microRNAs or circular RNAs. The only communication explored the associations between uranium and radium in groundwater and incidence of colorectal cancer in Georgia counties, USA.

## 2. An Overview of Published Articles

This Special Issue focuses on the potential toxic effects and mechanisms of both emerging and traditional environmental pollutants. Emerging pollutants are represented by nanoparticles. Shi et al. (Contribution 1) explore the size-dependent hepatotoxicity of nano-silica. Through in vitro cell experiments combined with multi-omics methods, the authors try to clarify the early health effects and key toxicity pathways of nanoparticles. Gao et al. (Contribution 2) focus on the potential respiratory toxicity of nano-zinc oxide, using animal experiments to study the MRI morphological effects on the olfactory epithelium and olfactory bulb of rats after intranasal instillation. There are many types of nanoparticles, and these two contributions are representative. They take typical nanoparticles as the research object, using in vitro cell experiments and in vivo animal experiments, respectively, combined with innovative technologies such as multi-omics, to elucidate their potential negative health effects and mechanisms. The research paradigm is worthy of reference for future studies.

In this Special Issue, traditional environmental pollutants are represented by air pollutants. Sun et al. (Contribution 3) investigate the effect of ambient air pollutants on the severity of allergic rhinitis symptoms. A prospective follow-up study was conducted among

 https://doi.org/10.3390/toxics13080641

patients with allergic rhinitis, and they found an association between short-term exposure to air pollutants and exacerbation of nasal symptoms in patients with allergic rhinitis. Wang et al. (Contribution 4) elucidate the role of Glycoprotein A Repetition Predominant (GARP) protein in $PM_{2.5}$-induced epithelial–mesenchymal transition (EMT) through the TGF-β/SMAD pathway in pulmonary epithelial cells and discuss the therapeutic potential of lentinan. Yang et al. (Contribution 5) focus on the neurotoxicity of $PM_{2.5}$ and attempt to elucidate the related gut–brain axis mechanism using a multi-omics approach.

In real-world environments, human exposure is often not to a single pollutant but to a combination of multiple pollutants [2]. Therefore, studying the health effects and mechanisms of combined exposure to environmental pollutants is of great significance. Zhang et al. (Contribution 6) focus on various endocrine-disrupting chemicals (EDCs), including perchlorate, nitrate, and thiocyanate, exploring their association with female infertility and the mediation of obesity. Mascari et al. (Contribution 7) focus on the associations between environmental pollutant mixtures and red blood cell folate concentrations, finding that higher exposure to PFASs, metals, and PAHs is associated with lower red blood cell folate concentrations. Zheng et al. (Contribution 8) focus on the association between combined exposure to various heavy metals and the aging biomarker α-Klotho, finding that exposure to certain metals, particularly in combination, may reduce serum α-Klotho levels, potentially accelerating aging processes. Li et al. (Contribution 9) explore the effects of co-exposure to benzene, toluene, and xylene (BTX) on genetic damage, providing further support for the gene-environment interactions of BTX co-exposure and microRNA single-nucleotide substitutions (mirSNPs) in determining the severity of DNA strand breaks. Xu et al. (Contribution 10) also focus on the important role of non-coding RNA in toxic biomarkers and toxicity mechanisms, but unlike contribution 9, they focus on circular RNA. The authors found that Circ_0000284 is involved in arsenite-induced hepatic insulin resistance by blocking the plasma membrane translocation of GLUT4 in hepatocytes via IGF2BP2/PPAR-γ.

Rooney et al. (Contribution 11) contribute a communication exploring the carcinogenic effects of radioactive pollutants through an ecological study. The study found that radium in groundwater may be linked with an increased incidence of colorectal cancer (CRC).

## 3. Conclusions

The health effects of environmental pollutants require continuous attention, which serves as the foundation for establishing environmental standards and formulating environmental protection strategies. There is a wide range of environmental pollutants, and more research evidence is needed on the potential negative health effects and related mechanisms of traditional and emerging pollutants. The health effects of combined exposure to multiple pollutants on the human body are one of the important research topics in the field of environmental health. The environmental health effects are also diverse and complex, and new research methods, including high-throughput methods such as multi-omics, deserve attention.

**Author Contributions:** Conceptualization, Z.C. and G.J.; writing—original draft preparation, Z.C.; writing—review and editing, Z.C. and G.J.; supervision, G.J.; project administration, Z.C. and G.J.; funding acquisition, Z.C. and G.J. All authors have read and agreed to the published version of the manuscript.

**Funding:** This research was funded by the Open Project Fund from Key Laboratory of Environment & Health (Huazhong University of Science and Technology), Ministry of Education (No. 2024GWKFJJ01), the Open Project Fund from the Key Laboratory of Coal Environmental Pathogenicity and Prevention (Shanxi Medical University), Ministry of Education, China (No. MEKLCEPP/SXMU-

202402), the National Natural Science Foundation of China (81703257) and the National Key R&D Program of the Ministry of Science and Technology of China (2017YFC1600200).

**Conflicts of Interest:** The authors declare no conflicts of interest.

**List of Contributions:**

1. Shi, J.; Zhang, H.; Zhang, Y.; Ma, Y.; Yu, N.; Liu, W.; Liu, Y.; Nie, J.; Chen, Z.; Jia, G. Size-Dependent Cytotoxicity and Multi-Omic Changes Induced by Amorphous Silicon Nanoparticles in HepG2 Cells. *Toxics* **2025**, *13*, 232.
2. Gao, L.; Meng, Y.; Luo, X.; Chen, J.; Wang, X. ZnO Nanoparticles-Induced MRI Alterations to the Rat Olfactory Epithelium and Olfactory Bulb after Intranasal Instillation. *Toxics* **2024**, *12*, 724.
3. Sun, W.; Ding, C.; Jiang, Z.; Zheng, X.; Jiang, J.; Xu, H. The Impact of Ambient Air Pollution on Allergic Rhinitis Symptoms: A Prospective Follow-Up Study. *Toxics* **2024**, *12*, 663.
4. Wang, Z.; Xu, S.; Bian, B.; Hu, Z.; Wu, F.; Zhao, S.; Wang, X.; Wang, L.; Ma, T. Lentinan Alleviated PM2.5 Exposure-Induced Epithelial–Mesenchymal Transition in Pulmonary Epithelial Cells by Inhibiting the GARP/TGF-β/Smad Pathway. *Toxics* **2025**, *13*, 166.
5. Yang, Z.; Zhang, Y.; Ran, S.; Zhang, J.; Tian, F.; Shi, H.; Wei, S.; Li, X.; Li, X.; Gao, Y.; et al. A Multi-Omics Study of Neurodamage Induced by Growth-Stage Real-Time Air Pollution Exposure in Mice via the Microbiome–Gut–Brain Axis. *Toxics* **2025**, *13*, 260.
6. Zhang, L.; Peng, Y.; Song, Y.; Zhang, Y.; Qin, Q.; Ying, M.; Bi, Y.; Yin, P. Associations of Urinary Perchlorate, Nitrate, and Thiocyanate with Female Infertility and Mediation of Obesity: Insights from NHANES 2013–2018. *Toxics* **2025**, *13*, 15.
7. Mascari, M.; Reeves, K.; Balasubramanian, R.; Liu, Z.; Laouali, N.; Oulhote, Y. Associations of Environmental Pollutant Mixtures and Red Blood Cell Folate Concentrations: A Mixture Analysis of the U.S. Adult Population Based on NHANES Data, 2007–2016. *Toxics* **2025**, *13*, 200.
8. Zheng, X.; Zhou, W.; Jiang, Z.; Ding, C.; Feng, M.; Li, Y.; Kurniasari, F.; Xie, S.; Xu, H. Independent and Combined Associations of Urinary Heavy Metal Exposures with Serum α-Klotho in Middle-Aged and Older Adults. *Toxics* **2025**, *13*, 237.
9. Li, S.; Liao, X.; Ma, R.; Deng, N.; Wu, H.; Zhang, Z.; Chen, L., Wang, Q.; Liao, Q.; Li, Q.; et al. Effects of Co-Exposure to Benzene, Toluene, and Xylene, Polymorphisms of microRNA Genes, and Their Interactions on Genetic Damage in Chinese Petrochemical Workers. *Toxics* **2024**, *12*, 821.
10. Xu, S.; Hu, Z.; Wang, Y.; Zhang, Q.; Wang, Z.; Ma, T.; Wang, S.; Wang, X.; Wang, L. Circ_0000284 Is Involved in Arsenite-Induced Hepatic Insulin Resistance Through Blocking the Plasma Membrane Translocation of GLUT4 in Hepatocytes via IGF2BP2/PPAR-γ. *Toxics* **2024**, *12*, 883.
11. Rooney, T.; Soares, L.; Babalola, T.; Kensington, A.; Williams, J.; Meliker, J. Uranium and Radium in Groundwater and Incidence of Colorectal Cancer in Georgia Counties, USA: An Ecologic Study. *Toxics* **2024**, *12*, 705.

## References

1. Abd-Elhakim, Y.M.; Hashem, M.M.; Abo-El-Sooud, K.; Hassan, B.A.; Elbohi, K.M.; Al-Sagheer, A.A. Effects of Co-Exposure of Nanoparticles and Metals on Different Organisms: A Review. *Toxics* **2021**, *9*, 284. [CrossRef] [PubMed]
2. Vermeulen, R.; Schymanski, E.L.; Barabási, A.L.; Miller, G.W. The exposome and health: Where chemistry meets biology. *Science* **2020**, *367*, 392–396. [CrossRef] [PubMed]

toxics

MDPI

*Article*

# Size-Dependent Cytotoxicity and Multi-Omic Changes Induced by Amorphous Silicon Nanoparticles in HepG2 Cells

**Jiaqi Shi [1,2,†], Huifang Zhang [3,†], Yi Zhang [1,2], Ying Ma [1,2], Nairui Yu [1,2], Wenhao Liu [4], Ying Liu [4], Jisheng Nie [3,*], Zhangjian Chen [1,2,*] and Guang Jia [1,2]**

1 Department of Occupational and Environmental Health Sciences, School of Public Health, Peking University, Beijing 100191, China; 2311110200@bjmu.edu.cn (J.S.); 1710306142@pku.edu.cn (Y.Z.); mayingmmyy@163.com (Y.M.); 1810306112@bjmu.edu.cn (N.Y.); jiaguangjia@bjmu.edu.cn (G.J.)

2 Beijing Key Laboratory of Toxicological Research and Risk Assessment for Food Safety, School of Public Health, Peking University, Beijing 100191, China

3 Shanxi Key Laboratory of Environmental Health Impairment and Prevention, NHC Key Laboratory of Pneumoconiosis, MOE Key Laboratory of Coal Environmental Pathogenicity and Prevention, School of Public Health, Shanxi Medical University, Taiyuan 030001, China; zhf201101@sxmu.edu.cn

4 CAS Key Laboratory for Biomedical Effects of Nanomaterials and Nanosafety, CAS Center for Excellence in Nanoscience, National Center for Nanoscience and Technology, Beijing 100190, China; wenhaoliu2020@163.com (W.L.); liuy@nanoctr.cn (Y.L.)

* Correspondence: niejisheng@sxmu.edu.cn (J.N.); zhangjianchen@pku.edu.cn (Z.C.)

† These authors contributed equally to this work.

**Abstract:** (1) Background: Silica nanoparticles ($SiO_2$ NPs) have a high potential for human exposure and tend to accumulate in the liver. This study aimed to explore the size-dependent cytotoxicity induced by $SiO_2$ NPs and identify key molecular pathways at the in vitro level through proteomics, metabolomics, and a combination of multiple omics methods. (2) Methods: The human hepatoma cells (HepG2) cells were exposed to $SiO_2$ NPs of three different sizes (60, 250, and 400 nm) at doses of 0, 12.5, 25, 50, 100, and 200 μg/mL for 24 h. (3) Results: Exposure to 60 nm $SiO_2$ NPs induced more reduction in cell viability than the other two larger-scale particles. Changes in the metabolomic and proteomic profiles of HepG2 cells induced by $SiO_2$ NPs were also size-dependent. The main pathways that were significantly affected in the 60 nm $SiO_2$ NPs treatment group represented cholesterol metabolism in proteomics and central carbon metabolism in metabolomics. Moreover, common enrichment pathways between differential proteins and metabolites included protein digestion and absorption and vitamin digestion and absorption. (4) Conclusions: Exposure to $SiO_2$ NPs could induce size-dependent cytotoxicity and changes in proteomics and metabolomics, probably mainly by interfering with energy metabolism pathways.

**Keywords:** metabolomics; multi-omics; nanomaterials; proteomics; silica nanoparticles

## 1. Introduction

Silica particles are abundant in nature and mainly in two forms: crystalline and amorphous. The chemical formula for crystalline silica and amorphous silica is the same, yet their structures differ. Crystalline silica is arranged regularly, while amorphous silica is arranged in disorder. Crystalline silica includes tridymite, quartz, and cristobalite. Amorphous silica includes mesoporous silica and crystalline silica. There are three sources of amorphous silica: natural existence, the by-product of power stations or metallurgical processing, and synthesis [1]. Silicon dioxide is one of the most produced nanomaterials in the world [2]. Synthetic amorphous silica (known as E551 in the European Union) is widely used in processed foods, for example, to prevent powdered products from clumping and for thickening paste products [3]. $SiO_2$ NPs have some unique properties, such as larger specific surface area and pore volume, controllable particle size, easy-to-modify surfaces, excellent porosity, good biocompatibility, etc. Because of these characteristics, porous $SiO_2$ NPs are widely used in drug delivery and biomedicine [4,5], coatings [6,7], cosmetics [8], etc. Therefore, $SiO_2$ NPs have a high potential for human exposure through food, industrial, pharmaceutical, and cosmetic exposure, and they enter the body through oral, inhalation, intravenous, and skin-to-skin contact methods.

Many in vivo and in vitro experiments have shown that $SiO_2$ NPs may can cause harm to a variety of organs, including the liver and spleen [9], lungs, immune system [10], cardiovascular system [11], and intestines [12]. Hepatotoxicity was one of the target-organ effects of oral exposure to nanomaterials, including $SiO_2$ NPs [13–15]. Previous in vivo studies have found that $SiO_2$ NPs tend to accumulate in the liver and cause pathological changes after oral exposure [16,17]. Furthermore, other investigations demonstrated the transport of $SiO_2$ NPs to the liver in mice via intratracheal instillation [18] or intravenous exposure [9,19]. In several subchronic and chronic animal trials, $SiO_2$ NPs were shown to generate adverse hepatotoxicity results such as liver atrophy, fatty liver, and hepatic fibrosis [20,21]. For example, adult male Sprague–Dawley rats treated with 1000 ppm $SiO_2$ NPs for 28 days showed severe vacuolar degeneration of hepatocytes and focal coagulation necrosis of some hepatocytes [16]. In addition, smaller-sized $SiO_2$ NPs can cause liver damage even at a lower dose [22,23]. In vitro experiments have also shown that $SiO_2$ NPs can induce oxidative stress [24,25] and DNA damage [26] and increase mitochondrial-induced apoptosis [27] in human hepatoma cells. However, the key mechanism and toxic pathway of hepatotoxicity induced by $SiO_2$ NPs as well as its size dependence are still unclear and need further study. The human hepatoma cells (HepG2) are widely used to study hepatotoxicity experimental materials [28–32]. Although HepG2 cells are a type of liver cancer cells, they can perform many differentiated liver functions and are often used as an in vitro substitute for primary human hepatocytes. Therefore, the cytotoxicity of $SiO_2$ NPs of different sizes was carried out to provide ideas and clues for toxicity.

High-throughput technologies like proteomics and metabolomics have arisen and are still developing as a result of the ongoing advancements in biotechnology, which are aimed at determining the mechanism of toxicity [33–35]. Increasingly, in vitro cell studies and omics technologies are being used in nanotoxicology to investigate toxicity pathways and mechanisms [36–38]. Proteomics is the study of the whole complement of proteins in cells, their structure and function, and the identification of biomarkers that can forecast both qualitative and quantitative changes in cells upon exposure to harmful substances [39]. Compared to the transcriptome or proteome, metabolomics measures the total metabolites in living systems and concentrates on metabolic pathways, which are more representative of the cellular phenotype [40]. Multiple omics can integrate phenotypic changes at different levels to demonstrate a more comprehensive biological phenotype and better proof, whereas individual omics can indicate cellular phenotypic changes at separate molecular levels. The function of biomolecules can be thoroughly examined using multi-omics combination analysis, which can also screen important proteins, or metabolic pathways and provide coordination mechanisms for various biological layers.

Proteomics and metabolomics were employed in this study to investigate the fundamental toxic pathway and demonstrate the cytotoxicity of $SiO_2$ NPs in human hepatoma cells (HepG2). In order to investigate the size dependency of the cytotoxicity, three amorphous $SiO_2$ NPs with varying diameters (60, 250, and 400 nm) were chosen as the test nanoparticles. In order to properly screen for important proteins and metabolites linked to the liver cytotoxicity of $SiO_2$ NPs and associated hazardous pathways, a correlation study between proteomics and metabolomics was also conducted.

## 2. Materials and Methods

### 2.1. Characterization of $SiO_2$ NPs

Three different sizes (60, 250, and 400 nm) of silica nanoparticles ($SiO_2$ NPs) were synthesized by the National Center for Nanoscience and Technology (Beijing, China). The particle size and dispersity were measured by transmission electron microscope (TEM; JEOL JEM-200CX, Tokyo, Japan) and quantitatively analyzed by GMS 3.0 software. To evaluate the agglomeration and stabilization of nanoparticles in ultrapure water, dynamic light scattering (DLS) was used to detect the hydrodynamic diameters and zeta potential of $SiO_2$ NPs (at the concentration of 100 μg/mL) in ultrapure water using the ZetaSizer Nano ZS90 (Malvern Instruments Ltd., Malvern, UK).

### 2.2. Cell Culture and Exposure to $SiO_2$ NPs

Human hepatocellular carcinoma cells (HepG2) used in the study were purchased from the National Biomedical Experimental Cell Resource Library of China. HepG2 cells were grown in Minimum Essential Medium (MEM, Gibco, New York, NY, USA) supplemented with 10% fetal bovine serum (FBS, Hyclone, Thermo Scientific, New York, NY, USA), 1% MEM Non-Essential Amino Acids Solution (100×) (NEAA, Gibco, Thermo Scientific, New York, NY, USA), and 2% GlutaMAX-1 (Gibco, Thermo Scientific, New York, NY, USA) and maintained at 37 °C in a humidified atmosphere containing 5% $CO_2$. After reaching 80% confluence, the cells were digested by 0.25% trypsin and seeded to 96-well plates at a density of $1 \times 10^4$ cells per well or 60 × 15 MM plates with $5 \times 10^5$ cells per well. After a 36 h cultivation period, the medium was replaced by the fresh medium that contained different concentrations of $SiO_2$ NPs suspensions.

### 2.3. Cell Viability Assay

To determine the cytotoxicity of $SiO_2$ NPs, cell viability was assessed by the Cell Counting Kit-8 assay (CCK-8, Biotopped, Dojindo Laboratories, Kumamoto, Japan). After exposure to 0, 12.5, 25, 50, 100, and 200 μg/mL $SiO_2$ NPs (60, 250 and 400 nm) for 24 h, the cells in the 96-well plate were incubated with CCK-8 solution for 2 h. Then, the supernatants were collected, and a microplate reader was used to detect the value of optical density (OD) at 450 nm. The cell viability was assessed by the following formula: [(experimental wells − blank wells)/(control wells − blank wells)] × 100%.

### 2.4. Proteomics

#### 2.4.1. Protein Sample Preparation

HepG2 ($1 \times 10^7$/sample) was exposed to $SiO_2$ NPs (0 and 100 μg/mL) for 24 h and then lysed with lysate containing 1 mM PMSF. Three biological replicates were set up. Protein concentration was measured using the BCA assay kit (ThermoFisher, New York, NY, USA). Next, 50 μg of protein per sample was taken and different groups of samples diluted with lysate to the same concentration and volume. Then, 1/50 sample mass was added to 1 mg/mL pancreatic enzyme Trypsin-TPCK and digested overnight at 37 °C. After transferring the samples to a new tube, a labeling reaction was performed using a TMTpro reagent containing 20 μL of anhydrous acetonitrile (ThermoFisher, USA); then, it was incubated for 1 h at room temperature. The reaction was terminated with 5 μL 5% hydroxylamine for 15 min, and the aliquots were stored at −80 °C for later use.

#### 2.4.2. High-pH Reverse-Phase Separation and Mass Spectrometry (HPLC-MS) Assay

Reverse-phase separation was performed on an Agilent 1100 HPLC, and the gradient consisted of mobile phases A (H2O-FA (99.9:0.1, *v*/*v*)) and B (ACN-H2O-FA (80:19.9:0.1, *v*/*v*/*v*)). Samples were loaded at a flow rate of 2 μL/min to pre-column Acclaim PepMap100, 100 μm × 2 cm (RP-C18, ThermoFisher, New York, NY, USA), and then separated by Acclaim PepMap RSLC, 75 μm × 50 cm (RP-C18, ThermoFisher, New York, NY, USA), at the flow rate of 300 μL/ min. Samples were collected for 8–60 min. Samples were lyophilized for mass spectrometry (MS) using EASY-NLC 1200 liquid chromatography (ThermoFisher, New York, NY, USA). The mass range of the full MS scan was set at 350–1500 $m/z$, and the 20 highest peaks were MS/MS-scanned.

#### 2.4.3. Proteomic Data Analysis

All raw data were analyzed using Proteome Discover 2.4. Then, the trusted proteins were screened according to the Score Sequest HT > 0 and the unique peptide ≥ 1, and the blank values were removed. Differential proteins were screened on the condition that foldchange > 1.2 times and $p$-value < 0.05. The differential proteins were then analyzed for GO/KEGG enrichment to describe their functions.

### 2.5. Metabolomics

#### 2.5.1. Metabolomic Sample Preparation

HepG2 ($1 \times 10^7$/sample) was exposed to $SiO_2$ NPs (0 and 100 μg/mL) for 24 h. The sample was treated with 20 μL of internal standard (L-2-chlorophenyl alanine, 0.06 mg/mL, methanol configuration), pre-chilled methanol/water (V:V = 4:1), and 200 μL of chloroform and then sonicated in the ice water bath for 20 min and centrifuged for 10 min (13,000 rpm, 4 °C). The supernatant was evaporated with a centrifugal concentration dryer, i.e., 80 μL of methoxyamine hydrochloride pyridine solution (15 mg/mL), and then vortexed for 2 min. An oxime reaction was performed in a 37 °C shaking incubator for 90 min. The sample was treated with 50 μL of BSTFA (containing 1% TMCS) derivatization reagent, 20 μL of n-hexane, and 10 μL internal standards (C8/C9/C10/C12/C14/C16/C18/C20/C22/C24; all were configured with chloroform) at 70 °C for 60 min. At last, the sample was kept at room temperature for 30 min for GC-MS metabolomics analysis.

#### 2.5.2. Gas Chromatography–Mass Spectrometry (GC-MS) Analysis

Metabolic spectra were analyzed using gas chromatography–mass spectrometry (7890B-5977A, Agilent, Santa Clara, CA, USA). DB-5MS capillary columns (30 m × 0.25 mm × 0.25 μm, Agilent J&W Scientific, Folsom, CA, USA) were used; the carrier gas was high-purity helium (purity was not less than 99.999%), the flow rate was 1.0 mL/min, and the temperature of the inlet was 260 °C. Electron bombardment of the ion source (EI) was used at a temperature of 230 °C, with a four-stage rod temperature of 150 °C and electron energy of 70 eV. The scanning mode was the full-scan mode (SCAN), and the quality scanning range was 50–500 $m/z$.

#### 2.5.3. Metabolomic Data Analysis

Qualitative and relative quantitative analyses of the original non-targeted metabolomics data were conducted by the software of MS-DIAL 4.70. After standardization of the original data, unsupervised principal component analysis (PCA) and supervised orthogonal partial least squares analysis (OPLS-DA) were used to observe the overall distribution. The criteria for screening were the VIP value of the first principal component of the OPLS-DA model > 1 and the $p$-value value of the $t$-test < 0.05. Finally, based on the KEGG database, the differential metabolites were enriched by metabolic pathway enrichment.

### 2.6. Integrative Metabolomics and Proteomics Analysis

To determine their shared pathway information, the differential proteins and differential metabolites were concurrently mapped to the KEGG pathway database using the MetaboAnalyst 6.0 platform. The linkages between graphical objects in the KEGG pathway and details about the orthogenic genes in the KEGG GENES database are both contained in the KGML (KEGG Markup Language) file, a sub-library of the KEGG database. A more methodical investigation of the relationship between the proteome and the metabolome is made possible by the ability to determine the network relationship between proteins and metabolites.

### 2.7. Statistical Analysis

For statistical analysis, R software (version 4.1.1) was utilized. Additionally, all of the outcomes were mean ± SD. When necessary, one-way ANOVA with Tukey's correction and unpaired Student's *t*-test were employed. For all data, a *p*-value of less than 0.05 was deemed statistically significant.

## 3. Results

### 3.1. Characterization of $SiO_2$ NPs

$SiO_2$ NPs were characterized before use. Transmission electron microscopy (TEM) images showed that the 60 nm, 250 nm, and 400 nm $SiO_2$ NPs used in this study were all spherical and well dispersed (Figure 1a–c), with equivalent diameters of 73 ± 3.573 nm, 278.41 ± 10.324 nm, and 426.173 ± 27.428 nm, respectively. The hydrated particle sizes of these three $SiO_2$ NPs in ultrapure water were 173.8 ± 6.259 nm, 472.4 ± 14.81 nm, and 500.7 ± 14.16 nm, respectively, and zeta potentials were −28.4 ± 0.424 mV, −36.2 ± 0.696 mV, and −36.84 ± 0.865 mV, respectively. This indicates that $SiO_2$ NPs still had slight agglomeration in an aqueous solution, even if they were well dispersed.

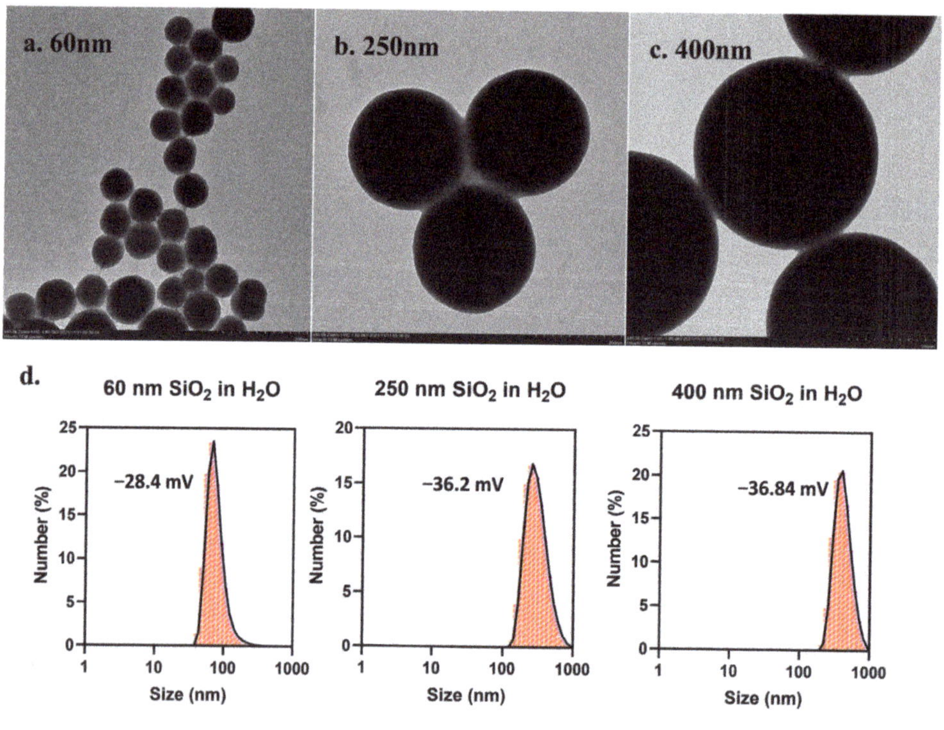


**Figure 1. Characterization of $SiO_2$ NPs.** The morphologies of $SiO_2$ NPs at 60 nm (**a**), 250 nm (**b**), and 400 nm (**c**) were observed under transmission electron microscopy (TEM). The hydrated particle size distribution and zeta potential of $SiO_2$ NPs of three different sizes in ultrapure water were detected by DLS (**d**).

### 3.2. Cytotoxicity of $SiO_2$ NPs in HepG2 Cells

The cell viability was measured using the CCK-8 kit after treatment of $SiO_2$ NPs with three different sizes at gradient concentrations for 24 h. As shown in Figure 2, cell viability was decreased after exposure to $SiO_2$ NPs, and 60 nm $SiO_2$ NPs induced more reduction in cell viability than the other two larger-scale particles. Compared with the control group (0 μg/mL), the 60 nm $SiO_2$ NPs treatment group at a dose of 100 μg/mL reduced the cell viability significantly. However, the result did not show a significant dose–response relationship. After exposure to 60 nm $SiO_2$ NPs, cell viability in the 12.5, 25, 50, 100, and 200 μg/mL groups was reduced to 89.30%, 77.56%, 76.11%, 80.81%, and 83.49%, respectively. Cell viability after exposure to the other two larger-scale $SiO_2$ NPs (250 and 400 nm) at these doses barely showed any cytotoxicity.

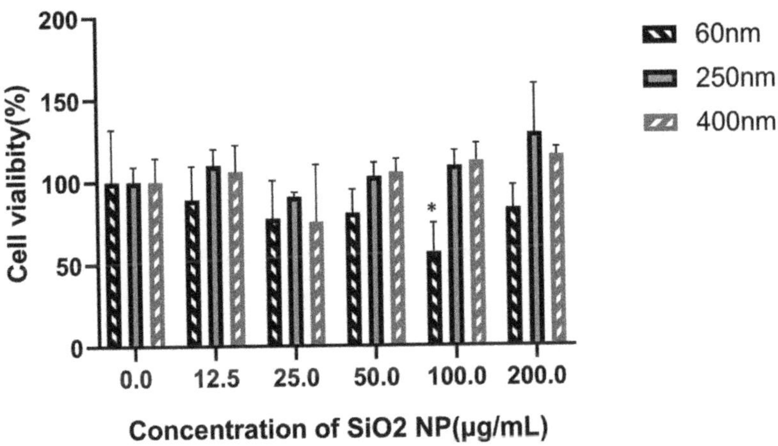


**Figure 2. Effect of $SiO_2$ NPs on the viability of HepG2 cells (mean ± SD, $n$ = 3).** HepG2 cells were treated with $SiO_2$ NPs (60, 250, and 400 nm) at 0, 12.5, 25, 50, 100, and 200 μg/mL for 24 h. The cell viability was significantly decreased in the 60 nm $SiO_2$ NPs treatment groups when the treatment concentration was 100 μg/mL, but no obvious change was found in the 250 nm and 400 nm $SiO_2$ NPs treatment groups. Cell viability did not decrease in a dose-dependent relationship. Significant difference from the control (* $p < 0.05$).

### 3.3. Proteomics

After being treated with 100 μg/mL $SiO_2$ NPs for 24 h, HepG2 cells were lysed, and proteins were extracted. Proteomics was performed in HPLC-MS. Through the processing of raw MS data, 67,388 peptides were extracted, and 6829 protein groups were identified. As shown in Figure 3, PCA scoring plots revealed a significant difference between the control group and the three $SiO_2$ NPs treatment groups, especially between the 60 nm or 250 nm $SiO_2$ NPs treatment group and control group, in which the difference was shown in proteomics characteristics.

Then, differentially expressed proteins between the $SiO_2$ NPs treatment groups and control groups were screened. It was found that there were 236, 120, and 48 differential proteins in the 60 nm, 250 nm, and 400 nm $SiO_2$ NPs treatment groups, respectively (Figure 4a). This suggests that the smaller the particle size of $SiO_2$ NPs, the more differential proteins affected, and the greater the effect on cells. Meanwhile, these differential proteins intersected with other size groups, but the proportion was less than 50%, which meant that SiO2 particles as small as 60 nm may induce many new effects on cell protein expression. Among 236 differential proteins between the 60 nm $SiO_2$ NPs treatment group and control group, 131 proteins were up-regulated, and 105 were down-regulated (Figure 4b). The cluster heat map of these differential proteins visually demonstrates the characteristic difference between $SiO_2$ NPs treatment groups and control groups (Figures 4c and A1a,b).

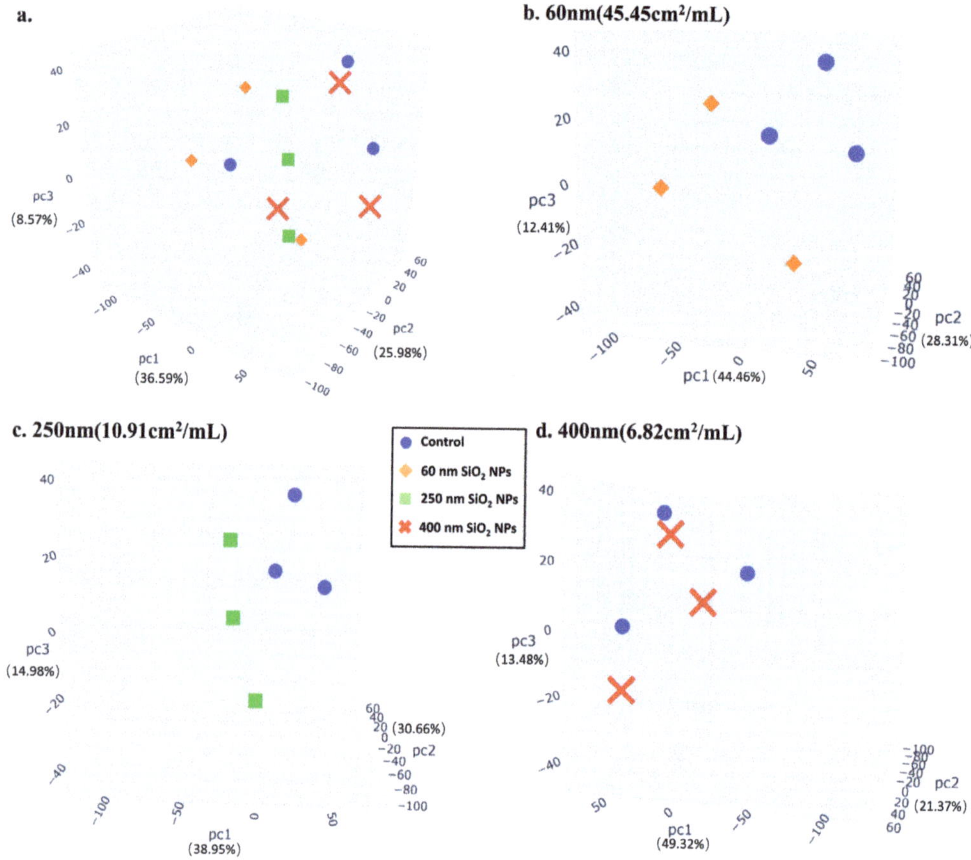


**Figure 3. Multivariate analysis of proteomics in the control group and $SiO_2$ NPs-treated (100 μg/mL) groups.** PCA 3D plots were drawn to compare the difference between the control group and the treatment groups (**a**). Pairwise comparisons between the control group and 60 nm (**b**), 250 nm (**c**), and 400 nm (**d**) treatment groups were also carried out. The control group and the three $SiO_2$ NPs treatment groups were relatively far apart on the score map, revealing significantly separations, especially between the 60 nm or 250 nm $SiO_2$ NPs treatment group and the control group (control-1, control-2, and control-3).

Based on KEGG enrichment pathway analysis (Figure 4d,e and Figure A1c,d), the main pathways that were significantly affected in the 60 nm $SiO_2$ NPs treatment group included cholesterol metabolism, complement and coagulation cascades, alcoholism, etc. Compared with the 250 nm and 400 nm $SiO_2$ NPs, 60 nm $SiO_2$ NPs significantly enhanced pathways such as the Ras signaling pathway and weakened the pathways such as glycosaminoglycan biosynthesis–heparin sulfate/heparin. Therefore, the treatment of $SiO_2$ NPs could induce size-dependent proteomic changes: the smaller the particle size, the greater the impact.

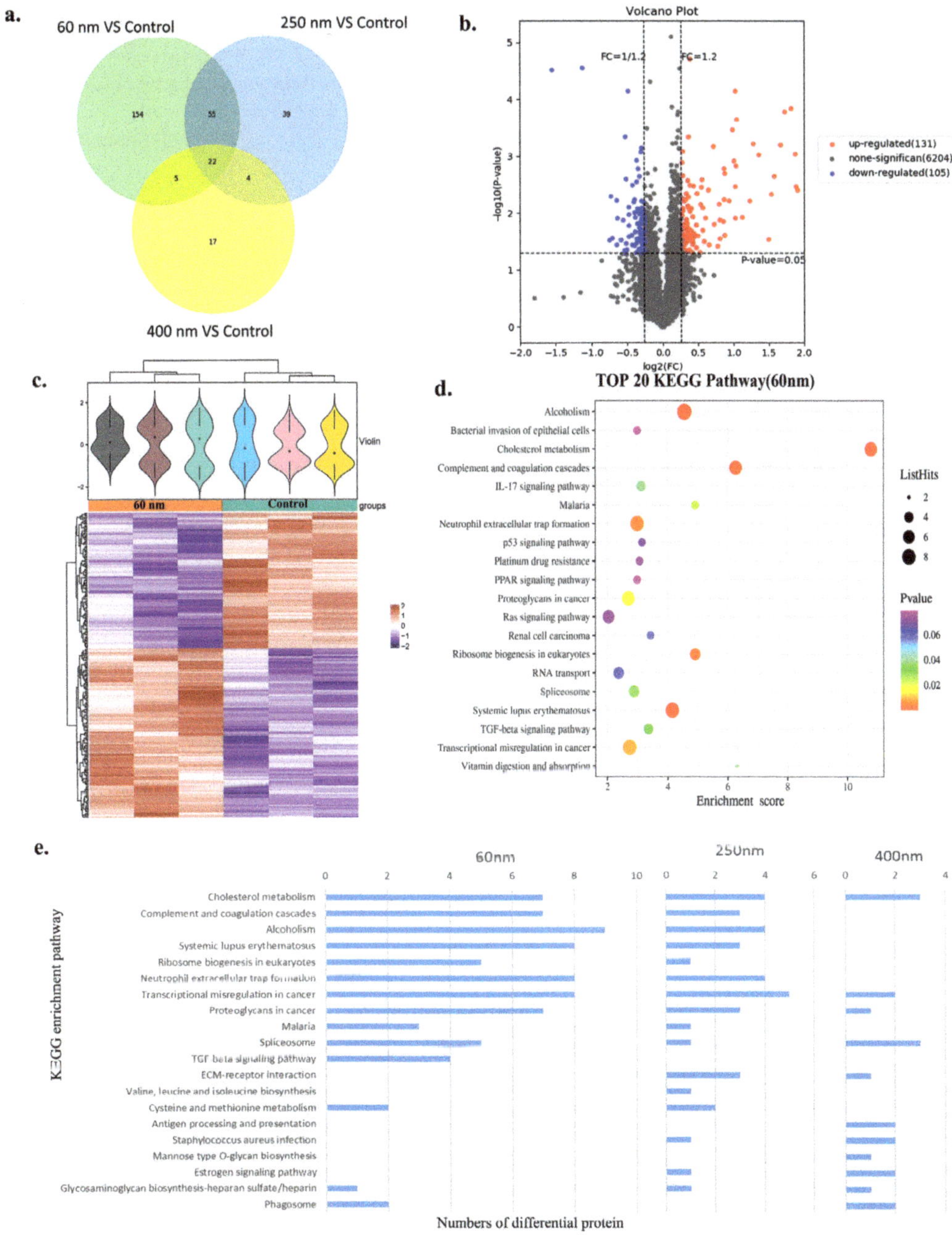


**Figure 4. Proteomics and pathway analysis of $SiO_2$ NPs.** A Venn diagram of the different proteins in three treatment groups compared to the control group showing that the size of $SiO_2$ NPs affected different proteins (**a**). A volcano map of proteins with varying expression levels in the 60 nm treatment group (**b**). A heat map of cluster analysis comparing the 60 nm treatment and control groups revealing a notable difference (**c**). The KEGG enrichment analysis bubble plot, generated in descending order of $-\log10$ *p*-value in the 60 nm $SiO_2$ NPs treatment group (**d**). The bar pattern of different protein numbers in different pathways of KEGG compares the three particle-size treatment groups (**e**).

### 3.4. Metabolomics

After being treated with 100 μg/mL $SiO_2$ NPs for 24 h, HepG2 cells were also digested for untargeted metabolomics in GC-MS. After metabolite identification, 496 metabolites were included in subsequent analysis. As shown in Figure 5, PCA and OPLS-DA plots revealed that the control group and the three $SiO_2$ NPs treatment groups were significantly separated, indicating a difference in metabolic characteristics.

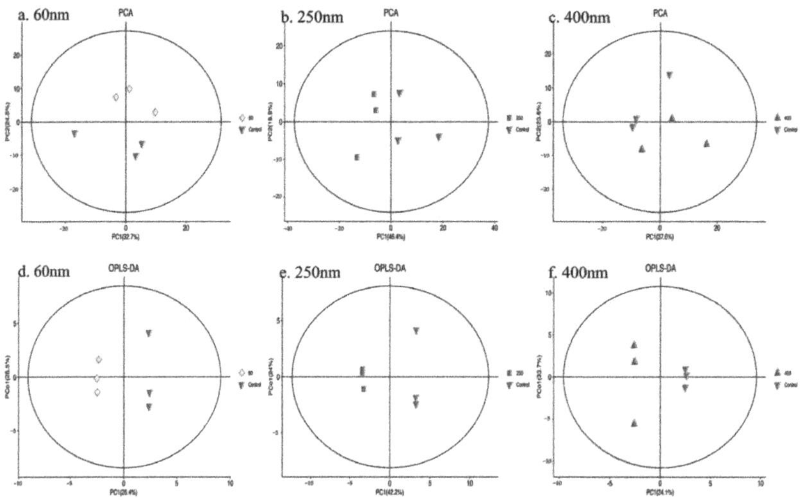


**Figure 5. Multivariate analysis of metabolites in the control group and $SiO_2$ NPs-treated (100 μg/mL) groups.** Pairwise comparisons between the control group and 60 nm (**a**), 250 nm (**b**), and 400 nm (**c**) treatment groups carried out through PCA 2D plots. PCA was performed by the expression of trusted metabolites. The control group and the $SiO_2$ NPs treatment groups of three sizes are significantly separated, indicating the difference in metabolic characteristics. OPLS-DA compares the difference between the control group and the treatment groups of three different sizes, respectively (**d**–**f**).

Then, differentially expressed metabolites between the $SiO_2$ NPs treatment groups and control group were screened. It was found that there were 18, 36, and 24 differential metabolites in the 60 nm, 250 nm, and 400 nm $SiO_2$ NPs treatment groups, respectively (Figure 6a). Among 18 differential metabolites between the 60 nm $SiO_2$ NPs treatment group and control group, which were mainly divided into the category of lipids and lipid-like molecules, 8 proteins were up-regulated, and 10 were down-regulated (Figure 6b). However, most of the differential metabolites (97%) in the 250 nm $SiO_2$ NPs treatment group were down-regulated, while most of the differential metabolites (92%) in the 400 nm $SiO_2$ NPs treatment group were up-regulated. These results also indicate that $SiO_2$ NPs with different particle sizes induced different metabolic changes. The cluster heat maps of the differential metabolites in the 60 nm, 250 nm, and 400 nm $SiO_2$ NPs treatment groups compared with the control group are shown in Figures 6c and A2a,b.

Based on KEGG enrichment pathway analysis (Figure 6d,e and Figure A2c,d), the main metabolic pathways that were significantly affected in the 60 nm $SiO_2$ NPs treatment group included the central carbon metabolism in cancer, arginine biosynthesis, and alanine, aspartate, and glutamate metabolism pathways, among others. Compared with the 250 nm and 400 nm $SiO_2$ NPs, 60 nm $SiO_2$ NPs significantly enhanced pathways such as glyoxylate and dicarboxylate metabolism. Therefore, the treatment of $SiO_2$ NPs could induce metabolic changes, which were shown to vary with the change in particle size.

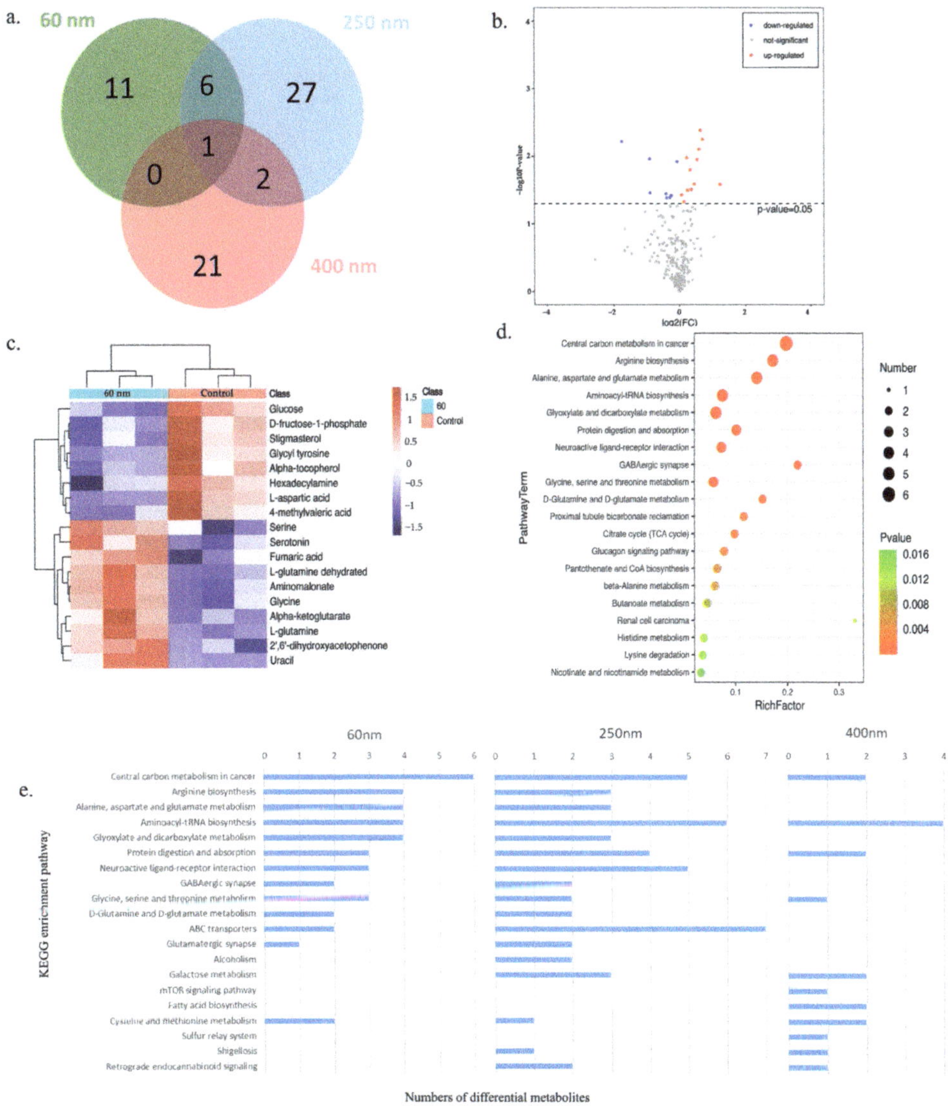


**Figure 6. Metabolomics and pathway analysis of HepG2 cells treated with $SiO_2$ NPs.** A Venn diagram of the different metabolites in treatment groups of three different sizes compared with the control group demonstrates the difference in the size of $SiO_2$ NPs on differential proteins (**a**). Differentially expressed metabolites in the 60 nm treatment group shown on a volcano map (**b**). The characteristic difference between the 60 nm treatment group and control group shown by a cluster analysis heat map (**c**). A KEGG enrichment analysis bubble plot drawn in the descending order of $-\log10$ *p*-value corresponding to each entry in the 60 nm $SiO_2$ NPs treatment group (**d**). The bar graph of different metabolite numbers in different pathways of KEGG comparing the three particle size treatment groups (**e**).

### *3.5. Correlation Analysis of Proteomics and Metabolomics*

We further combined the results of proteomics and metabolomics to find key events at different molecular levels induced by $SiO_2$ NPs. At first, the correlations between differential proteins and differential metabolites were confirmed by Pearson correlation analysis

(Figures 7a and A3). For example, among these differential proteins and metabolites induced by 60 nm $SiO_2$ NPs, more than 86.9% were significantly correlated. According to the results of the correlation analysis between differential proteins and differential metabolites, the correlation network diagram was plotted (Figure 7b). The differential proteins apolipoprotein A-II (APOA2), midkine (MDK), and apolipoprotein E (APOE) and the differential metabolites L-glutamine dehydrated and L-glutamine were found to have the largest numbers of associations, respectively. Moreover, pathways in cancer and central carbon metabolism in cancer were the two pathways that had the largest numbers of associations in the 60 nm $SiO_2$ NPs treatment group (Figure 7c), differing from the other two treatment groups (Figure 7d,e).

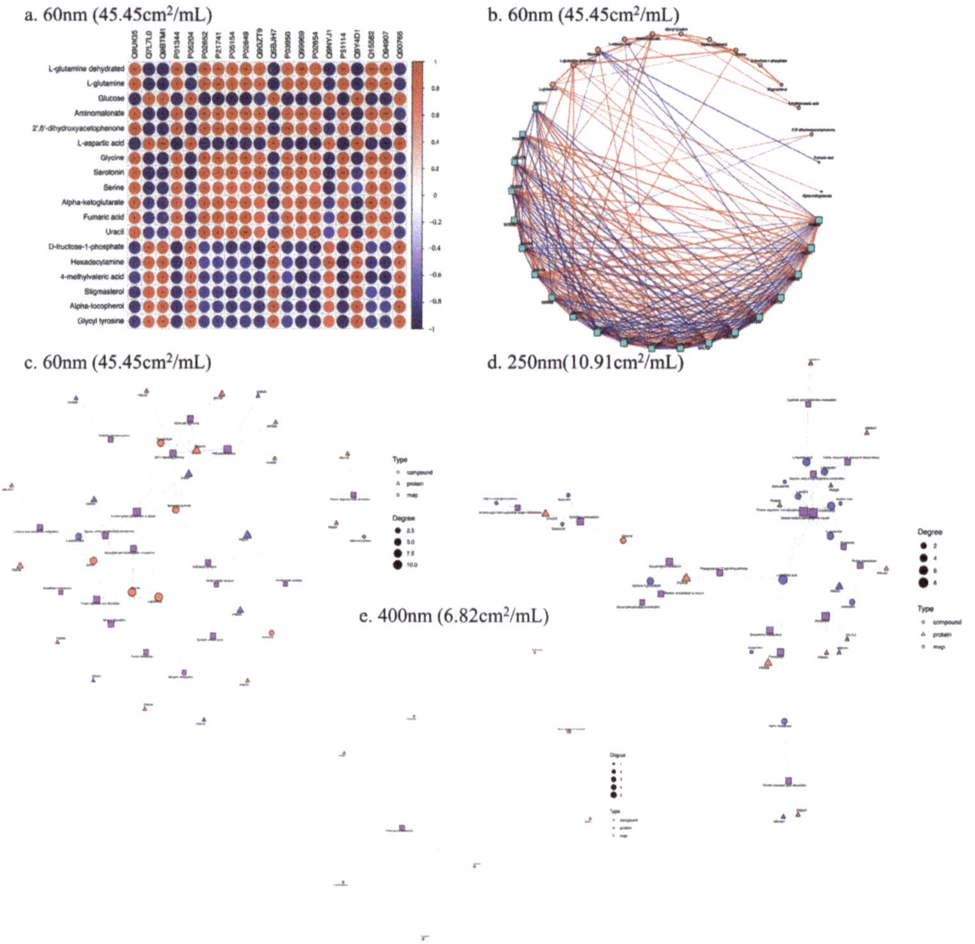


**Figure 7. Correlation analysis of proteomics and metabolomics.** A correlation heat map of differential proteins and differential metabolites treated with 60 nm $SiO_2$ NPs (**a**) (* $p < 0.05$; ** $p < 0.01$, *** $p < 0.001$). The correlation network diagram drawn according to the correlation analysis results of the differential gene and the differential metabolite (**b**). In the figure, the shape size is related to the number of connections, and the thickness of the connection between the shapes represents the degree of correlation. In the KGML network diagrams of differential proteins and metabolites in the 60 nm (**c**), 250 nm (**d**), and 400 nm (**e**) $SiO_2$ NPs treatment groups, the red color indicates up-regulated proteins or metabolites, and the blue color indicates down-regulated proteins or metabolites.

Through the analysis of the combined pathways of protein metabolism, it was found that the significantly enriched pathways were mainly as follows: arginine biosynthesis, complement and coagulation cascades, and cholesterol metabolism in the 60 nm group; galactose metabolism and valine, leucine, and isoleucine biosynthesis in the 250 nm group; and aminoacyl-tRNA biosynthesis in the 400 nm group. The two pathways cholesterol metabolism and central carbon metabolism in cancer were the common pathways between the three size groups. The pathway results of the 250 nm group and the 400 nm group were similar. Moreover, several key metabolic pathways were also screened by KGML analysis, including glyoxylate and dicarboxylate metabolism and amino acid metabolism (glycine, serine, and threonine metabolism). In addition, there were complex interactions between differential proteins (EGLN1 (Egl nine homolog 1) and MET (hepatocyte growth factor receptor)) and metabolites (fumaric acid and alpha-ketoglutarate), which can lead to $SiO_2$ NPs-induced metabolic dysfunction.

## 4. Discussion

Humans experience exposure to $SiO_2$ NPs through various pathways, and many reports are confirming the adverse effects of $SiO_2$ NPs on human health. Therefore, studying the cytotoxic effects and mechanisms of $SiO_2$ NPs is necessary for safety assessment. The liver is the main target organ for $SiO_2$ NPs. The objective of this study was to analyze the effects of $SiO_2$ NPs exposure on cellular metabolism based on proteomics and metabolomics techniques and to explore the mechanism of cytotoxicity. Through the differential proteins and differential metabolites screened after exposure to smaller-sized $SiO_2$ NPs at 100 μg/mL, we found that $SiO_2$ NPs could interfere with cholesterol metabolism, glucose metabolism, and amino acid metabolism, eventually leading to cytotoxicity. This provides clues for the potential mechanism underlying the cytotoxicity induced by $SiO_2$ NPs. This study also helps to deepen our understanding of the potential health risks caused by $SiO_2$ NPs and contributes to the application of combined omics in toxicological assessment. The harmful effects of silica are influenced by the size of the nanoparticles. The 60 nm treatment group in our study exhibited more cytotoxicity than the 250 nm and 400 nm groups. Numerous further in vitro and in vivo investigations have also demonstrated a strong correlation between the size of the particles and the cytotoxicity of $SiO_2$ NPs [41,42]. Yang et al. studied the effects of four different-sized particles (68, 43, 19, and 498 nm) on HepG2 cells and found that smaller silica particles had higher toxic effects for the probable reason that smaller particles on the nanoscale were more easily endocytosed [23]. Demir et al. [43] used *Drosophila melanogaster* to detect the genotoxic activity of different $SiO_2$ NPs with different sizes (6, 15, 30, and 55 nm) and observed significant induction of oxidative DNA damage, which was indirectly related to $SiO_2$ NPs size. In addition, this study found that the omics results of $SiO_2$ NPs are also highly correlated with the size of the particles, consistent with some other findings [44,45]. In proteomics, we found the particle size became smaller, and the number of differential proteins also became smaller (whether the differential proteins were up- or down-regulated). Similarly, Bannuscher et al. [44] treated NR8383 alveolar macrophages with three sizes of $SiO_2$ NPs (7, 15, and 40 nm) and found that the overall clustering structure of the untargeted proteomics results was similar, but the counts of proteins decreased with size. Karkossa et al. [45] found similar results in that the amount of change in protein and metabolomics results was related to the size of the particles. Thus, consistent with previous findings, smaller particles tend to have higher cytotoxicity and bring greater perturbations at the protein or metabolic level than larger ones. At present, nanotoxicology studies are still basically based on mass concentration as the dose unit, and this study is the same. However, the toxicity of nanoparticles is affected by various physicochemical parameters, including size, surface structure, etc., and some studies have found that surface area is more effective as a dose index when studying particles of different size ranges [46,47], which is a follow-up aspect worthy of attention.

Proteomics is essential for understanding complex biochemical processes at the protein level. The results showed that protein synthesis-related pathways were affected by $SiO_2$ NP, including ribosome, translational, and transcriptional pathways. In our study, 60 nm particles disrupted RNA modifications (NOP10, NHP2, and SNU13 down-regulated), splisomes (HNRNPM, RBMX, and SNU13 down-regulated), and ribosome proteins (MRPL11, MRPL14, and MRPL23 down-regulated). In addition, from the proteomics results, we found that $SiO_2$ NP exposure also affected cholesterol metabolism, and the differential proteins related to cholesterol metabolism screened in this study were up-regulated, such as APOB, APOE, APOA1, APOA2, APOC1, ANGPTL8, and LRP2. Some studies have yielded the same or similar results. Duan et al. [48] used an ICR mouse model to find that the level of cholesterol and LDL cholesterol in serum and liver tissue was significantly increased, and the ratio of HDL to LDL cholesterol was significantly reduced A zebrafish biological model was used to find that $SiO_2$ NP could activate lipid metabolism pathways. Chatterjee et al. [49] treated HepG2 with four types of amorphous $SiO_2$ NPs with different surface areas and also found perturbations of steroid-cholesterol biosynthesis. This suggests that repeated exposure to $SiO_2$ NP may be a risk factor for metabolic and cardiovascular diseases such as metabolic syndrome, non-alcoholic fatty liver disease, atherosclerosis, and type II diabetes [50].

$SiO_2$ NPs interfered with several key metabolic pathways, including glyoxylate and dicarboxylate metabolism and glycine, serine, and threonine metabolism, which could exacerbate oxidative stress and lead to liver damage. These results are similar to those of other studies [48,51]. Chatterjee et al. [52] conducted metabolomics with amorphous $SiO_2$ NP-treated HepG2 cells and ICR mouse livers and found that inhibition of glutathione metabolism and oxidative stress were some of the main causes of amorphous $SiO_2$ NPs-mediated hepatotoxicity. Enrichment analysis of differential metabolites showed that arginine biosynthesis and alanine, aspartic acid, and glutamate metabolism were affected by $SiO_2$ NP exposure. The liver is essential for maintaining normal glucose homeostasis, which ensures the energy supply of various tissues in the body through gluconeogenesis, glycogen decomposition, glycogen synthesis, glycolysis, and so on [53]. From the metabolomics results, we found that the differential metabolite (D-fructose-1-phosphate, beta-D-glucose) content associated with glucose metabolism decreased, and the glycolysis/gluconeogenesis pathway was blocked.

Through the joint pathway enrichment analysis of proteomics and metabolomics, it was also found that arginine biosynthesis and cholesterol metabolism were two significantly altered pathways, echoing the results of the above-mentioned single omics results. The correlation analysis showed that amino acid metabolism was also affected by $SiO_2$ NP. In addition to being precursors to numerous metabolic intermediates, amino acids are essential for energy metabolism and protein synthesis. We found the content of α-ketoglutaric acid, fumaric acid, glycine, L-glutamine, and serine increased and the aspartic acid content decreased. Fumarate and α-ketoglutaric acid, the intermediates in the citric acid cycle (TCA), promote the accumulation of fumarate and succinate, respectively [54], diffusing in the cytosol and ultimately promoting a pseudo-hypoxic state that favors tumor development [55]. The three enzymes engaged in the de novo synthesis of purine nucleotides and the two enzymes involved in the de novo synthesis of pyrimidine nucleotides both require glutamine as a substrate [56]. In addition to the fact that a large part of the lactic acid produced in cancer cells comes from glutamine [57], glutamine decomposition and reducing carboxylation can lead to anabolic reactions of fatty acids and cholesterol. The one-carbon route, which involves serine and glycine, is involved in the production of purines and pyrimidines as well as the regulation of cancer cells' epigenetic traits [58,59]. Aspartic acid is the only amino acid that can directly enter gluconeogenesis without entering the TCA cycle [60]; it is a carbon source synthesized by purine and pyrimidine, and the decrease in its expression directly affects the level of purine and pyrimidine [60]. Our results show that $SiO_2$ NPs disrupt energy metabolism in HepG2 cells, similar to the results of previous studies [61].

The advantage of this study is its use of a combination of proteomics and metabolomics analysis, which helped to determine the functional pathways involved in cytotoxicity and elucidate its underlying mechanisms. Systems biology, including proteomics and metabolomics, provides a lot of data that can be used to reveal novel biomarkers and biological pathways involved in the way nanomaterials act. However, the wide range of physicochemical properties of proteins dictates that only a subset of all proteins are detected by current technology, and metabolomics data also show lower sensitivity than commonly used toxicological methods [62]. Therefore, by integrating results from multiple cellular reaction layers from different omics methods, a higher level of confidence can be obtained.

## 5. Conclusions

In summary, the present study focused on cytotoxicity and omics changes in HepG2cells after exposure to $SiO_2$ NPs of different sizes. It was demonstrated that exposure to $SiO_2$ NPs could induce size-dependent cytotoxicity and changes in proteomics and metabolomics, probably mainly by interfering with energy metabolism pathways, including cholesterol metabolism and arginine biosynthesis. Our findings provide scientific insights for the exploration of toxicity mechanisms of $SiO_2$ NPs.

**Author Contributions:** Conceptualization, Z.C. and J.N.; methodology, J.S., H.Z., W.L. and Y.L.; software, J.S., W.L. and Y.L.; writing—original draft preparation, J.S.; data curation, Y.Z., N.Y. and Y.M.; writing—review and editing, J.S., H.Z., Y.Z., N.Y. and Y.M.; visualization, J.S.; supervision, Z.C., J.N. and G.J.; project administration, Z.C., J.N. and G.J.; funding acquisition, Z.C. and G.J. All authors have read and agreed to the published version of the manuscript.

**Funding:** The work was supported by Open Project Fund from Key Laboratory of Coal Environmental Pathogenicity and Prevention (Shanxi Medical University), Ministry of Education, China (No. MEKLCEPP/SXMU-202402), the Open Project Fund from Key Laboratory of Environment & Health (Huazhong University of Science and Technology), Ministry of Education (No. 2024GWKFJJ01), and the Open Fund of Key Laboratory of Chemical Pollution and Health and Safety of Chinese Center for Disease Control and Prevention (2024CDCKL02).

**Institutional Review Board Statement:** Not applicable.

**Informed Consent Statement:** Not applicable.

**Data Availability Statement:** Data are contained within the article and Appendix A.

**Conflicts of Interest:** The authors declare no conflicts of interest. The funders had no role in the design of the study; in the collection, analyses, or interpretation of data; in the writing of the manuscript; or in the decision to publish the results.

## Abbreviations

The following abbreviations are used in this manuscript:

| | |
|---|---|
| $SiO_2$ NPs | Silica nanoparticles |
| HepG2 | Human hepatoma cells |
| WHO | World Health Organization |
| CCK-8 | Cell Counting Kit-8 assay |

| | |
|---|---|
| OD | Optical density |
| HPLC-MS | High-pH reverse-phase separation and mass spectrometry |
| GC-MS | Gas chromatography–mass spectrometry |
| PCA | Principal component analysis |
| OPLS-DA | Orthogonal partial least squares analysis |
| KGML | KEGG markup language |
| SD | Standard deviation |
| TEM | Transmission electron microscopy |
| APOA2 | Apolipoprotein A-II |
| MDK | Midkine |
| APOE | Apolipoprotein E |
| EGLN1 | Egl nine homolog 1 |

## Appendix A

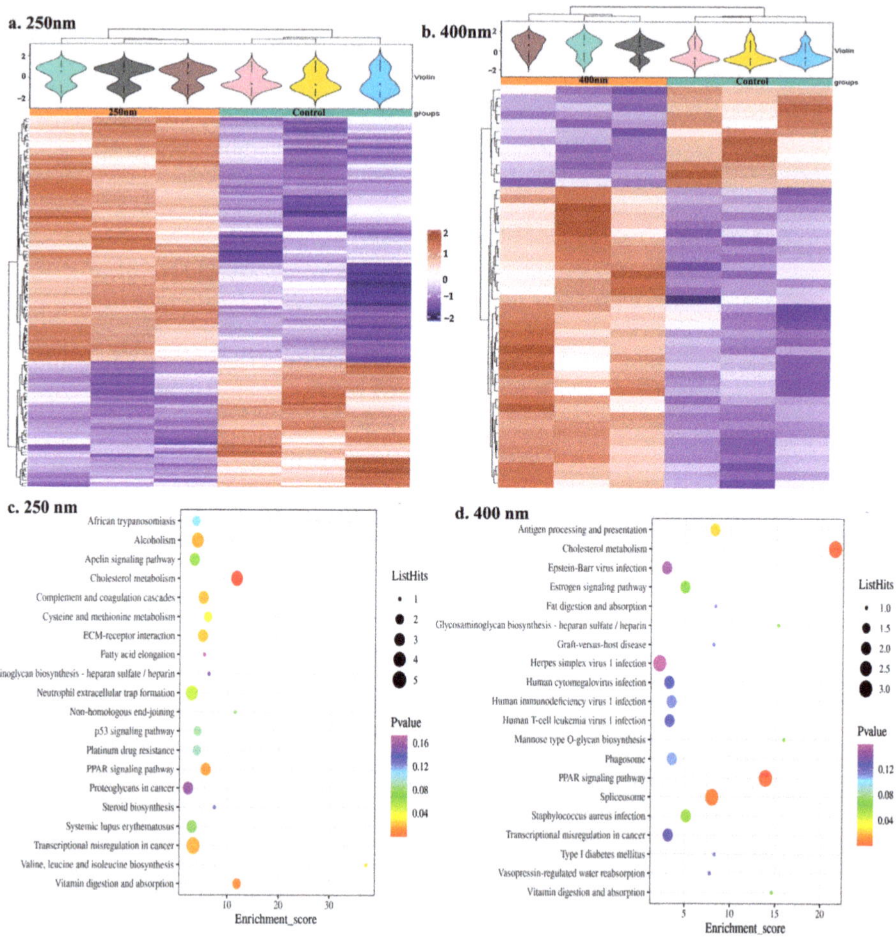


**Figure A1. Proteomics and pathway analysis in 250 nm and 400 nm $SiO_2$ NPs treatment groups.** The heat map of cluster analysis demonstrates the characteristic difference between 250 nm (**a**) or 400 nm (**b**) treatment group and control group. KEGG enrichment analysis bubble plots drawn in the descending order of −log1010 *p*-value corresponding to each entry in 250 nm $SiO_2$ NPs treatment group (**c**) and 400 nm $SiO_2$ NPs treatment group (**d**).

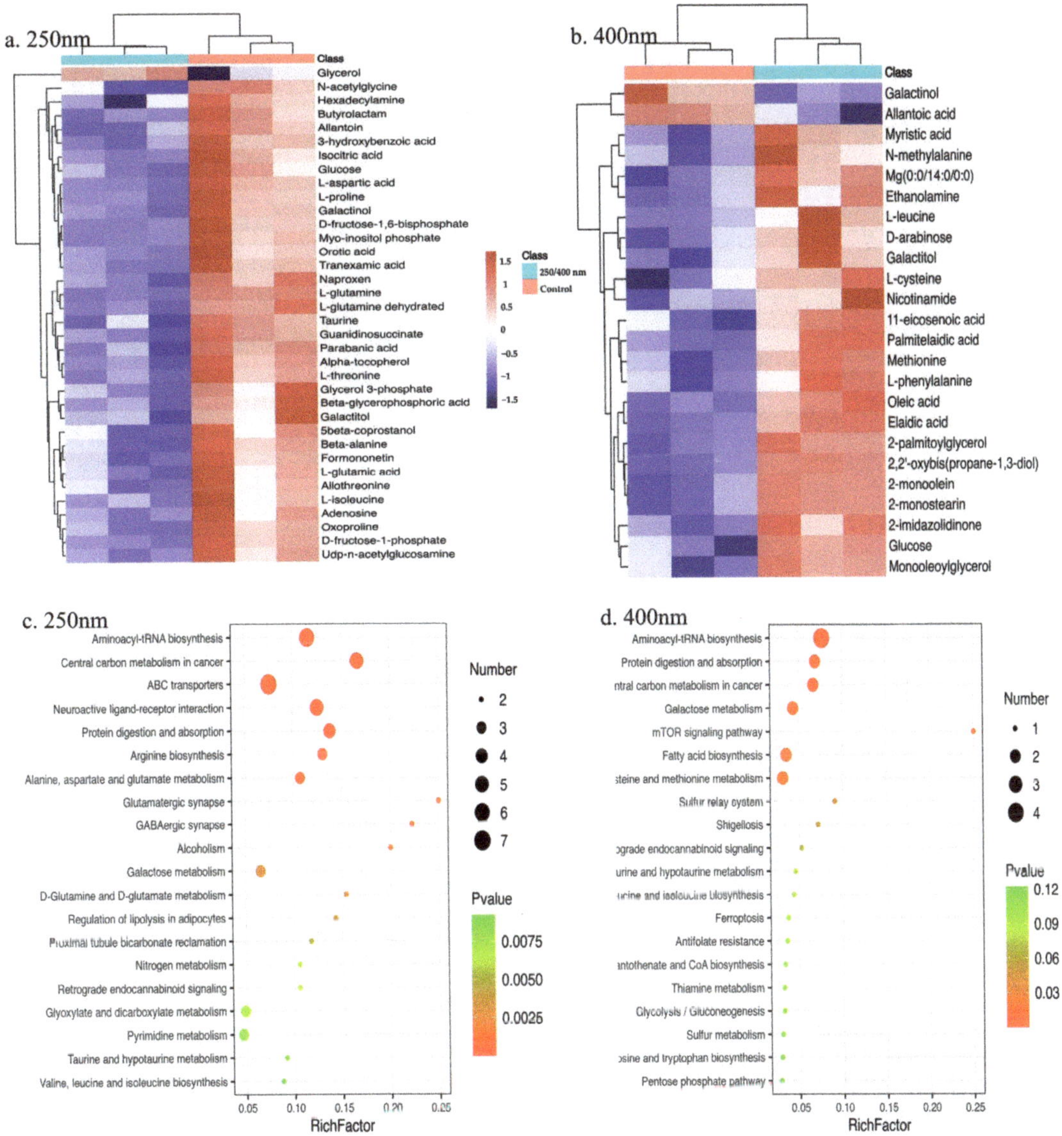


**Figure A2. Metabolomics and pathway analysis in 250 nm and 400 nm $SiO_2$ NPs treatment groups.** The heat map of cluster analysis demonstrates the characteristic difference between 250 nm (**a**) or 400 nm (**b**) treatment group and control group. KEGG enrichment analysis bubble plots drawn in the descending order of −log1010 *p*-value corresponding to each entry in 250 nm (**c**) and 400 nm $SiO_2$ NPs treatment group (**d**).

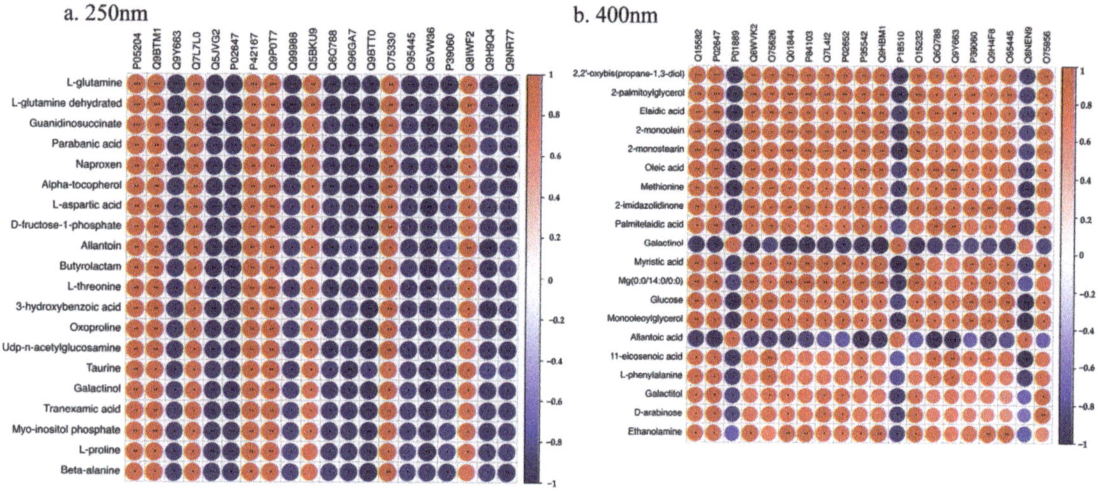


**Figure A3. Correlation heat map of differential proteins and differential metabolites treated with 250 nm (a) or 400 nm (b) $SiO_2$ NPs** (* $p < 0.05$; ** $p < 0.01$; *** $p < 0.001$).

## References


1. Arts, J.H.E.; Muijser, H.; Duistermaat, E.; Junker, K.; Kuper, C.F. Five-day inhalation toxicity study of three types of synthetic amorphous silicas in Wistar rats and post-exposure evaluations for up to 3months. *Food Chem. Toxicol.* **2007**, *45*, 1856–1867. [CrossRef] [PubMed]
2. Vance, M.E.; Kuiken, T.; Vejerano, E.P.; McGinnis, S.P.; Hochella, M.F., Jr.; Rejeski, D.; Hull, M.S. Nanotechnology in the real world: Redeveloping the nanomaterial consumer products inventory. *Beilstein. J. Nanotechnol.* **2015**, *6*, 1769–1780. [CrossRef] [PubMed]
3. Dekkers, S.; Krystek, P.; Peters, R.J.; Lankveld, D.P.; Bokkers, B.G.; van Hoeven-Arentzen, P.H.; Bouwmeester, H.; Oomen, A.G. Presence and risks of nanosilica in food products. *Nanotoxicology* **2011**, *5*, 393–405. [CrossRef]
4. Jain, P.; Hassan, N.; Iqbal, Z.; Dilnawaz, F. Mesoporous Silica Nanoparticles: A Versatile Platform for Biomedical Applications. *Recent. Pat. Drug Deliv. Formul.* **2018**, *12*, 228–237. [CrossRef]
5. Wang, Y.; Zhao, Q.; Han, N.; Bai, L.; Li, J.; Liu, J.; Che, E.; Hu, L.; Zhang, Q.; Jiang, T.; et al. Mesoporous silica nanoparticles in drug delivery and biomedical applications. *Nanomedicine* **2015**, *11*, 313–327. [CrossRef] [PubMed]
6. Martin, C.A.; Lin, Z.; Kumar, A.; Dinneen, S.R.; Osgood, R.M., 3rd; Deravi, L.F. Biomimetic Colorants and Coatings Designed with Cephalopod-Inspired Nanocomposites. *ACS Appl. Bio Mater.* **2021**, *4*, 507–513. [CrossRef]
7. Liu, S.; Han, M.Y. Silica-coated metal nanoparticles. *Chem. Asian J.* **2010**, *5*, 36–45. [CrossRef]
8. SCCS; Hoet, P.H. Opinion of the Scientific Committee on Consumer Safety (SCCS)—Revision of the opinion on the safety of the use of Silica, Hydrated Silica, and Silica Surface Modified with Alkyl Silylates (nano form) in cosmetic products. *Regul. Toxicol. Pharmacol.* **2016**, *74*, 79–80. [CrossRef]
9. Tassinari, R.; Martinelli, A.; Valeri, M.; Maranghi, F. Amorphous silica nanoparticles induced spleen and liver toxicity after acute intravenous exposure in male and female rats. *Toxicol. Ind. Health* **2021**, *37*, 328–335. [CrossRef]
10. Bancos, S.; Stevens, D.L.; Tyner, K.M. Effect of silica and gold nanoparticles on macrophage proliferation, activation markers, cytokine production, and phagocytosis in vitro. *Int. J. Nanomed.* **2015**, *10*, 183–206. [CrossRef]
11. Deng, Y.D.; Zhang, X.D.; Yang, X.S.; Huang, Z.L.; Wei, X.; Yang, X.F.; Liao, W.Z. Subacute toxicity of mesoporous silica nanoparticles to the intestinal tract and the underlying mechanism. *J. Hazard. Mater.* **2021**, *409*, 124502. [CrossRef] [PubMed]
12. Inoue, M.; Sakamoto, K.; Suzuki, A.; Nakai, S.; Ando, A.; Shiraki, Y.; Nakahara, Y.; Omura, M.; Enomoto, A.; Nakase, I.; et al. Size and surface modification of silica nanoparticles affect the severity of lung toxicity by modulating endosomal ROS generation in macrophages. *Part Fibre Toxicol.* **2021**, *18*, 21. [CrossRef]
13. Boey, A.; Ho, H.K. All Roads Lead to the Liver: Metal Nanoparticles and Their Implications for Liver Health. *Small* **2020**, *16*, 2000153. [CrossRef] [PubMed]

14. Waegeneers, N.; Brasseur, A.; Van Doren, E.; Van der Heyden, S.; Serreyn, P.J.; Pussemier, L.; Mast, J.; Schneider, Y.J.; Ruttens, A.; Roels, S. Short-term biodistribution and clearance of intravenously administered silica nanoparticles. *Toxicol. Rep.* **2018**, *5*, 632–638. [CrossRef] [PubMed]
15. Lipka, J.; Semmler-Behnke, M.; Sperling, R.A.; Wenk, A.; Takenaka, S.; Schleh, C.; Kissel, T.; Parak, W.J.; Kreyline, W.G. Biodistribution of PEG-modified gold nanoparticles following intratracheal instillation and intravenous injection. *Biomaterials* **2010**, *31*, 6574–6581. [CrossRef]
16. Azouz, R.A.; Korany, R.M.S. Toxic Impacts of Amorphous Silica Nanoparticles on Liver and Kidney of Male Adult Rats: An In Vivo Study. *Biol. Trace Elem. Res.* **2021**, *199*, 2653–2662. [CrossRef]
17. Javdani, H.; Etemad, L.; Moshiri, M.; Zarban, A.; Hanafi-Bojd, M.Y. Effect of tannic acid-templated mesoporous silica nanoparticles on iron-induced oxidative stress and liver toxicity in rats. *Toxicol. Rep.* **2021**, *8*, 1721–1728. [CrossRef]
18. Smulders, S.; Ketkar-Atre, A.; Luyts, K.; Vriens, H.; Nobre, S.D.; Rivard, C.; Van Landuyt, K.; Baken, S.; Smolders, E.; Golanski, L.; et al. Body distribution of $SiO_2$-$Fe_3O_4$ core-shell nanoparticles after intravenous injection and intratracheal instillation. *Nanotoxicology* **2016**, *10*, 567–574. [CrossRef]
19. Yu, Y.; Duan, J.; Li, Y.; Li, Y.; Jing, L.; Yang, M.; Wang, J.; Sun, Z. Silica nanoparticles induce liver fibrosis via TGF-β(1)/Smad3 pathway in ICR mice. *Int. J. Nanomed.* **2017**, *12*, 6045–6057. [CrossRef]
20. Mahmoud, A.M.; Desouky, E.M.; Hozayen, W.G.; Bin-Jumah, M.; El-Nahass, E.; Soliman, H.A.; Farghali, A.A. Mesoporous Silica Nanoparticles Trigger Liver and Kidney Injury and Fibrosis Via Altering TLR4/NF-kappa B, JAK2/STAT3 and Nrf2/HO-1 Signaling in Rats. *Biomolecules* **2019**, *9*, 528. [CrossRef]
21. Liu, T.L.; Li, L.L.; Fu, C.H.; Liu, H.Y.; Chen, D.; Tang, F.Q. Pathological mechanisms of liver injury caused by continuous intraperitoneal injection of silica nanoparticles. *Biomaterials* **2012**, *33*, 2399–2407. [CrossRef] [PubMed]
22. Isoda, K.; Tetsuka, E.; Shimizu, Y.; Saitoh, K.; Ishida, I.; Tezuka, M. Liver injury induced by thirty- and fifty-nanometer-diameter silica nanoparticles. *Biol. Pharm. Bull.* **2013**, *36*, 370–375. [CrossRef]
23. Li, Y.; Sun, L.; Jin, M.; Du, Z.; Liu, X.; Guo, C.; Li, Y.; Huang, P.; Sun, Z. Size-dependent cytotoxicity of amorphous silica nanoparticles in human hepatoma HepG2 cells. *Toxicol. Vitr.* **2011**, *25*, 1343–1352. [CrossRef]
24. Sun, L.; Li, Y.; Liu, X.; Jin, M.; Zhang, L.; Du, Z.; Guo, C.; Huang, P.; Sun, Z. Cytotoxicity and mitochondrial damage caused by silica nanoparticles. *Toxicol. Vitr.* **2011**, *25*, 1619–1629. [CrossRef]
25. Lu, X.; Qian, J.; Zhou, H.; Gan, Q.; Tang, W.; Lu, J.; Yuan, Y.; Liu, C. In vitro cytotoxicity and induction of apoptosis by silica nanoparticles in human HepG2 hepatoma cells. *Int. J. Nanomed.* **2011**, *6*, 1889–1901. [CrossRef]
26. Yang, H.; Wu, Q.Y.; Lao, C.S.; Li, M.Y.; Gao, Y.; Zheng, Y.; Shi, B. Cytotoxicity and DNA damage in mouse macrophages exposed to silica nanoparticles. *Genet. Mol. Res.* **2016**, *15*, 15039005. [CrossRef]
27. Ahamed, M.; Akhtar, M.J.; Alhadlaq, H.A. Influence of silica nanoparticles on cadmium-induced cytotoxicity, oxidative stress, and apoptosis in human liver HepG2 cells. *Environ. Toxicol.* **2020**, *35*, 599–608. [CrossRef] [PubMed]
28. de Oliveira, A.L.; Miranda, R.G.; Dorta, D.J. Recreational MDMA doses do not elicit hepatotoxicity in HepG2 spheroids under normo- and hyperthermia. *Toxicology* **2024**, *503*, 153761. [CrossRef]
29. He, J.; Liu, H.; Li, Z.; Xu, M.; Zhang, Y.; Jiang, T.; Mo, L. Integrated transcriptomic and metabolomic analysis of the hepatotoxicity of dichloroacetonitrile. *Sci. Total Environ.* **2024**, *927*, 172237. [CrossRef]
30. Lu, J.; Yang, Y.; Zhu, L.; Li, M.; Xu, W.; Zhang, C.; Cheng, J.; Tao, L.; Li, Z.; Zhang, Y. Exposure to environmental concentrations of natural pyrethrins induces hepatotoxicity: Assessment in HepG2 cell lines and zebrafish models. *Chemosphere* **2022**, *288*, 132565. [CrossRef]
31. Lv, H.; Hong, L.; Tian, Y.; Yin, C.; Zhu, C.; Feng, H. Corilagin alleviates acetaminophen-induced hepatotoxicity via enhancing the AMPK/GSK3β-Nrf2 signaling pathway. *Cell Commun. Signal* **2019**, *17*, 2. [CrossRef] [PubMed]
32. Yao, Q.Q.; Li, L.; Xu, M.C.; Hu, H.H.; Zhou, H.; Yu, L.S.; Zeng, S. The metabolism and hepatotoxicity of ginkgolic acid (17:1) in vitro. *Chin. J. Nat. Med.* **2018**, *16*, 829–837. [CrossRef] [PubMed]
33. Johnson, C.H.; Ivanisevic, J.; Siuzdak, G. Metabolomics: Beyond biomarkers and towards mechanisms. *Nat. Rev. Mol. Cell Biol.* **2016**, *17*, 451–459. [CrossRef]
34. Wei, S.; Wei, Y.; Gong, Y.; Chen, Y.; Cui, J.; Li, L.; Yan, H.; Yu, Y.; Lin, X.; Li, G.; et al. Metabolomics as a valid analytical technique in environmental exposure research: Application and progress. *Metabolomics Off. J. Metabolomic Soc.* **2022**, *18*, 35. [CrossRef]
35. Matysiak, M.; Kapka-Skrzypczak, L.; Brzóska, K.; Gutleb, A.C.; Kruszewski, M. Proteomic approach to nanotoxicity. *J. Proteom.* **2016**, *137*, 35–44. [CrossRef]
36. Gallud, A.; Delaval, M.; Kinaret, P.; Marwah, V.S.; Fortino, V.; Ytterberg, J.; Zubarev, R.; Skoog, T.; Kere, J.; Correia, M.; et al. Multiparametric Profiling of Engineered Nanomaterials: Unmasking the Surface Coating Effect. *Adv. Sci.* **2020**, *7*, 2002221. [CrossRef]

37. Gioria, S.; Lobo Vicente, J.; Barboro, P.; La Spina, R.; Tomasi, G.; Urbán, P.; Kinsner-Ovaskainen, A.; François, R.; Chassaigne, H. A combined proteomics and metabolomics approach to assess the effects of gold nanoparticles in vitro. *Nanotoxicology* **2016**, *10*, 736–748. [CrossRef]
38. Cui, L.; Wang, X.; Sun, B.B.; Xia, T.; Hu, S. Predictive Metabolomic Signatures for Safety Assessment of Metal Oxide Nanoparticles. *Acs Nano* **2019**, *13*, 13065–13082. [CrossRef]
39. Vulimiri, S.V.; Sonawane, B.R.; Szabo, D.T. Systems biology application in toxicology. In *Encyclopedia of Toxicology*, 3rd ed.; Wexler, P., Ed.; Academic Press: Oxford, UK, 2014; pp. 454–458. [CrossRef]
40. Fiehn, O. Metabolomics—The link between genotypes and phenotypes. *Plant Mol. Biol.* **2002**, *48*, 155–171.
41. Kim, W.; Kim, W.K.; Lee, K.; Son, M.J.; Kwak, M.; Chang, W.S.; Min, J.K.; Song, N.W.; Lee, J.; Bae, K.H. A reliable approach for assessing size-dependent effects of silica nanoparticles on cellular internalization behavior and cytotoxic mechanisms. *Int. J. Nanomed.* **2019**, *14*, 7375–7387. [CrossRef]
42. Nabeshi, H.; Yoshikawa, T.; Matsuyama, K.; Nakazato, Y.; Arimori, A.; Isobe, M.; Tochigi, S.; Kondoh, S.; Hirai, T.; Akase, T.; et al. Size-dependent cytotoxic effects of amorphous silica nanoparticles on Langerhans cells. *Pharmazie* **2010**, *65*, 199–201. [PubMed]
43. Demir, E.; Aksakal, S.; Turna, F.; Kaya, B.; Marcos, R. In vivo genotoxic effects of four different nano-sizes forms of silica nanoparticles in Drosophila melanogaster. *J. Hazard. Mater.* **2015**, *283*, 260–266. [CrossRef] [PubMed]
44. Bannuscher, A.; Karkossa, I.; Buhs, S.; Nollau, P.; Kettler, K.; Balas, M.; Dinischiotu, A.; Hellack, B.; Wiemann, M.; Luch, A.; et al. A multi-omics approach reveals mechanisms of nanomaterial toxicity and structure-activity relationships in alveolar macrophages. *Nanotoxicology* **2020**, *14*, 181–195. [CrossRef] [PubMed]
45. Karkossa, I.; Bannuscher, A.; Hellack, B.; Bahl, A.; Buhs, S.; Nollau, P.; Luch, A.; Schubert, K.; von Bergen, M.; Haase, A. An in-depth multi-omics analysis in RLE-6TN rat alveolar epithelial cells allows for nanomaterial categorization. *Part. Fibre Toxicol.* **2019**, *16*, 38. [CrossRef]
46. Oberdörster, G.; Oberdörster, E.; Oberdörster, J. Nanotoxicology: An emerging discipline evolving from studies of ultrafine particles. *Environ. Health Perspect.* **2005**, *113*, 823–839. [CrossRef]
47. Waters, K.M.; Masiello, L.M.; Zangar, R.C.; Tarasevich, B.J.; Karin, N.J.; Quesenberry, R.D.; Bandyopadhyay, S.; Teeguarden, J.G.; Pounds, J.G.; Thrall, B.D. Macrophage responses to silica nanoparticles are highly conserved across particle sizes. *Toxicol. Sci. Off. J. Soc. Toxicol.* **2009**, *107*, 553–569. [CrossRef]
48. Duan, J.; Liang, S.; Feng, L.; Yu, Y.; Sun, Z. Silica nanoparticles trigger hepatic lipid-metabolism disorder in vivo and in vitro. *Int. J. Nanomed.* **2018**, *13*, 7303–7318. [CrossRef]
49. Chatterjee, N.; Yang, J.; Atluri, R.; Lee, W.; Hong, J.; Choi, J. Amorphous silica nanoparticle-induced perturbation of cholesterol homeostasis as a function of surface area highlights safe-by-design implementation: An integrated multi-OMICS analysis. *RSC Adv.* **2016**, *6*, 68606–68614. [CrossRef]
50. Willeit, P.; Skroblin, P.; Kiechl, S.; Fernandez-Hernando, C.; Mayr, M. Liver microRNAs: Potential mediators and biomarkers for metabolic and cardiovascular disease? *Eur. Heart J.* **2016**, *37*, 3260–3266. [CrossRef]
51. Sun, M.Q.; Zhang, J.Y.; Liang, S.; Du, Z.; Liu, J.Y.; Sun, Z.W.; Duan, J.C. Metabolomic characteristics of hepatotoxicity in rats induced by silica nanoparticles. *Ecotox Environ. Safe* **2021**, *208*, 111496. [CrossRef]
52. Chatterjee, N.; Jeong, J.; Yoon, D.; Kim, S.; Choi, J. Global metabolomics approach in in vitro and in vivo models reveals hepatic glutathione depletion induced by amorphous silica nanoparticles. *Chem.-Biol. Interact.* **2018**, *293*, 100–106. [CrossRef]
53. Petersen, M.C.; Vatner, D.F.; Shulman, G.I. Regulation of hepatic glucose metabolism in health and disease. *Nat. Rev. Endocrinol.* **2017**, *13*, 572–587. [CrossRef] [PubMed]
54. Bonora, M.; Patergnani, S.; Rimessi, A.; De Marchi, E.; Suski, J.M.; Bononi, A.; Giorgi, C.; Marchi, S.; Missiroli, S.; Poletti, F.; et al. ATP synthesis and storage. *Purinergic Signal* **2012**, *8*, 343–357. [CrossRef]
55. King, A.; Selak, M.A.; Gottlieb, E. Succinate dehydrogenase and fumarate hydratase: Linking mitochondrial dysfunction and cancer. *Oncogene* **2006**, *25*, 4675–4682. [CrossRef] [PubMed]
56. Moffatt, B.A.; Ashihara, H. Purine and pyrimidine nucleotide synthesis and metabolism. *Arab. Book* **2002**, *1*, e0018. [CrossRef]
57. DeBerardinis, R.J.; Mancuso, A.; Daikhin, E.; Nissim, I.; Yudkoff, M.; Wehrli, S.; Thompson, C.B. Beyond aerobic glycolysis: Transformed cells can engage in glutamine metabolism that exceeds the requirement for protein and nucleotide synthesis. *Proc. Natl. Acad. Sci. USA* **2007**, *104*, 19345–19350. [CrossRef] [PubMed]
58. Ducker, G.S.; Rabinowitz, J.D. One-Carbon Metabolism in Health and Disease. *Cell Metab.* **2017**, *25*, 27–42. [CrossRef]
59. Meiser, J.; Vazquez, A. Give it or take it: The flux of one-carbon in cancer cells. *FEBS J.* **2016**, *283*, 3695–3704. [CrossRef]
60. Varahan, S.; Sinha, V.; Walvekar, A.; Krishna, S.; Laxman, S. Resource plasticity-driven carbon-nitrogen budgeting enables specialization and division of labor in a clonal community. *eLife* **2020**, *9*, e57609. [CrossRef]

61. Zhu, Y.; Zhang, Y.; Li, Y.; Guo, C.; Fan, Z.; Li, Y.; Yang, M.; Zhou, X.; Sun, Z.; Wang, J. Integrative proteomics and metabolomics approach to elucidate metabolic dysfunction induced by silica nanoparticles in hepatocytes. *J. Hazard. Mater.* **2022**, *434*, 128820. [CrossRef]
62. van Ravenzwaay, B.; Montoya, G.A.; Fabian, E.; Herold, M.; Krennrich, G.; Looser, R.; Mellert, W.; Peter, E.; Strauss, V.; Walk, T.; et al. The sensitivity of metabolomics versus classical regulatory toxicology from a NOAEL perspective. *Toxicol. Lett.* **2014**, *227*, 20–28. [CrossRef] [PubMed]

toxics

MDPI

Article

# ZnO Nanoparticles-Induced MRI Alterations to the Rat Olfactory Epithelium and Olfactory Bulb after Intranasal Instillation

**Lifeng Gao [1], Yuguang Meng [2], Xiaowen Luo [1], Jiangyuan Chen [1] and Xuxia Wang [2,*]**

[1] Department of Medical Imaging, School of Medicine, Jianghan University, Wuhan 430056, China; gao_lifeng@jhun.edu.cn (L.G.); aquariuswind@jhun.edu.cn (X.L.); chenjiangyuan@jhun.edu.cn (J.C.)

[2] State Key Laboratory of Magnetic Resonance and Atomic and Molecular Physics, National Center for Magnetic Resonance in Wuhan, Key Laboratory of Magnetic Resonance in Biological Systems, Innovation Academy for Precision Measurement Science and Technology, Chinese Academy of Sciences, Wuhan 430071, China; mengyg@gmail.com

* Correspondence: wangxuxia@apm.ac.cn

**Abstract:** Since zinc oxide (ZnO) nanoparticles (NPs) have been widely applied, the nano community and the general public have paid great attention to the toxicity of ZnO NPs. We detected 20-nm ZnO NPs biotoxicity following nasal exposure utilizing the non-invasive and real-time magnetic resonance imaging (MRI) technique. MR images were scanned in the rat olfactory epithelium (OE) and olfactory bulb (OB) on a 4.7 T scanner following the treatment (as early as 1 day and up to 21 days after), and the histological changes were evaluated. The influence of the size of the ZnO NPs and chemical components was also investigated. Our study revealed that 20-nm ZnO NPs induced obvious structural disruption and inflammation in the OE and OB at the acute stage. The results suggest that the real-time and non-invasive advantages of MRI allow it to observe and assess, directly and dynamically, the potential toxicity of long-term exposure to ZnO NPs in the olfactory system. These findings indicate the size-dependent toxicity of ZnO NPs with respect to the olfactory bulb. Further study is needed to reveal the mechanism behind ZnO NPs' toxicity.

**Keywords:** zinc oxide; nanoparticles; toxicity; olfactory system; magnetic resonance imaging

## 1. Introduction

Zinc oxide (ZnO) nanoparticles (NPs) have been employed in a wide range of rubber, cosmetic, foods, medical, and biological fields [1,2]. The potential health risks of mass-produced nanomaterials have received great public and academic attention. ZnO NPs' aerosol exposure can originate from welding fumes and manufacturing processing [3,4], which has been proven to cause pulmonary impairment [5,6] and metal fume fever [7].

Studies have shown the translocation of nanosized particles from the nose to the central nervous system (CNS), an important mechanism by which these particles enter the brain. An early study demonstrated the anterograde axonal transport of 50-nm silver-coated gold colloids along the olfactory nerve to the olfactory bulb in the squirrel monkey after intranasal instillation [8]. Oberdörster, G. et. al. investigated the migration of inhaled ultrafine $^{13}C$ particles (36 nm) in the rat brain and found that after 6 h of inhalation exposure, there was a significant and sustained increase in $^{13}C$ concentration in the olfactory bulb, from which they inferred that the migration of $^{13}C$ particles from the nasal cavity to the CNS was mainly accomplished via olfactory sensory neurons [9]. Likewise, metal oxide NPs such as manganese oxide (MnO) and iron oxide have been found to translocate into the brain via the olfactory route [10–12]. Therefore, we hypothesized that environmental and occupational exposures to ZnO NPs by the respiratory system, by virtue of their extremely small size, may enter the nasal cavity and affect the CNS via the olfactory pathway.

Nano-sized particles may exhibit distinct biological responses in contrast to bulk-sized particles of the same chemical composition [13]. Some cellular studies have reported the high cytotoxicity of ZnO NPs compared with larger-sized ZnO particles [14,15]. NPs were found to cause more immune function, inflammation, and transcriptomic responses than larger particles of the same material within the in vivo studies focused on nasal olfactory epithelium (OE), the respiratory tract, and oral exposure [16–18]. Tin-Tin-Win-Shwe et. al. demonstrated the size-dependent immune function of ultrafine carbon black in mice's olfactory bulb (OB) following intranasal instillation [16]. After oral administration, ZnO NPs showed more transcriptomic responses than bulk-sized ZnO in rat liver [18]. Studies addressing the possibility of the effects of ZnO NPs versus larger-sized particles on the OB are very limited.

ZnO NPs have been manufactured in bulk and widely applied. The potential health risks of the mass-produced nanomaterials prompted us to pay attention to the NP's safety application. ZnO NPs belong to highly soluble metal oxide. The results from cellular experiments demonstrate that ZnO NPs are more toxic than other metal oxide NPs [19–21]. Our understanding of how the ZnO NPs may disturb the olfactory pathway is poor. Cellular studies co-incubating human nasal mucosa cells with ZnO NPs illustrated cytotoxic, pro-inflammatory, and apoptosis responses in these cells [22,23]. Short-term inhalation exposure to ZnO NPs caused nasal necrosis in rats [24]. In the previous study, we proved that 30-nm ZnO NPs instilled in the nasal cavities of rats caused cellular injury and inflammation to the OE [25].

In this study, to further identify the influence of particle scale on the olfactory system (OE and OB), we applied magnetic resonance imaging (MRI) and histochemical methods to investigate the size effect of the intranasal exposure of nano-sized and submicron-sized ZnO particles (20 and 500 nm) on rats. Moreover, the influence of the chemical properties of the ZnO NPs and the zinc ions dissolved before the instillation was also considered.

The novelty of this article is that our study identifies the ZnO NPs-induced adverse effect on the olfactory bulb. As far as we know, olfactory bulb damage caused by ZnO NPs has never been reported before. The olfactory impairment caused by NPs could be screened by MRI. This work will facilitate the study of the link between ZnO NPs exposure and neurodegenerative disease.

## 2. Materials and Methods

### 2.1. Chemicals

ZnO NPs with a diameter of 20 nm and $Fe_2O_3$ NPs with a diameter of 30 nm were purchased from Haitai Nano Material Co., Ltd., Nanjing, China, and ZnO NPs with a diameter of 500 nm were purchased from National Pharmaceutical Chemical Reagent Co., Ltd., Beijing, China. We used sodium carboxymethyl cellulose (CMC) as an agent to suspend the NPs, which was manufactured by Sinopharm Chemical Reagent Co., Ltd., Shanghai, China. CMC is a water-soluble polymer that increases the viscosity of a solution, thereby helping to disperse nanoparticles and prevent aggregation. By forming a viscous solution, CMC effectively reduces the settling rate of the particles and therefore provides a good suspension aid.

### 2.2. Characterization of NPs

For the particle size characterization, the ZnO and $Fe_2O_3$ NPs were measured using JEM-200CX transmission electron microscopy (JEOL, Japan). The purity of the NPs was evaluated via an X-ray fluorescence spectrometer (Bruker, Germany). For the crystalline phase characterization, the NPs were analyzed via D/MAX 2000 X-ray diffraction (Rigaku, Japan). The specific surface area of the NPs was measured using an ASAP2010 Brunauer–Emmett–Teller technique. ZnO NP-CMC suspension was prepared by dispersing the ZnO NPs within 1 wt% CMC saline solution. The $Fe_2O_3$ NPs were also dispersed within the same solution to prepare $Fe_2O_3$ NP-CMC suspension. The concentration of $Zn^{2+}$ in the supernatant of ZnO NP-CMC suspension was determined using complexometric titration: ammonia–ammonium chloride buffer solution (pH 10.0) was added to the suspension, followed by the addition of Chromium Black T indicator, and titration was carried out with a standard solution of 9.92 mM $Na_2EDTA$. The endpoint of the titration was reached when the color of the mixture changed from sky blue to purplish red. The concentration of $Zn^{2+}$ in the 20-nm and 500-nm ZnO NP-CMC suspensions was to be about 0.065 mg·mL$^{-1}$ in both cases. The ZnO NP-CMC suspensions were centrifuged at 12,000× g rpm and/or 16,099× g for 10 min; then, the supernatants were extracted.

### 2.3. Animals

All experimental animals were handled in accordance with the National Committee for the Ethics and Use of Laboratory Animals. Male Sprague-Dawley rats (140–200 g in weight) were bought from the Animal Laboratory of Zhongnan Hospital of Wuhan University. The rats were group-housed in clean polypropylene cages in the SPF-level laboratory animal room. They are maintained within a light-cycle-controlled and temperature-controlled environment. Relative humidity was kept at 50 ± 5%. Rats are free to commercial rodent food and water. The animals were subjected to experimental studies following at least 5 days of laboratory domestication.

### 2.4. Experimental Preparation

Animals without obvious nasal structural abnormalities were chosen for intranasal exposure. Exposure doses were designed in the same way as our previous study [25]. Animals were randomly separated into five groups to receive unilateral intranasal drops of one of the following 40 μL of solution/suspension (given with a 20 μL pipette tip):

(1) 1 wt% saline solution of CMC, n = 8;
(2) Supernatant of 40 mg ZnO $mL^{-1}$ 20-nm ZnO NP-CMC suspension (S-ZnO20), n = 5;
(3) 40 mg $Fe_2O_3$ $mL^{-1}$ $Fe_2O_3$ NP-CMC suspension ($Fe_2O_3$), n = 8;
(4) 40 mg ZnO $mL^{-1}$ 20-nm ZnO NP-CMC suspension (ZnO20), n = 8;
(5) 40 mg ZnO $mL^{-1}$ 500-nm ZnO NP-CMC suspension (ZnO500), n = 8.

Before the intranasal exposure, all suspensions were sonicated for 10 min.

### 2.5. MRI Study

A Bruker Biospec 4.7 T/30 cm small animal scanner was utilized to perform all MRI scans. A 12 cm diameter Helmholtz volume coil was used for radiofrequency (RF) pulse transmission, and a 2.5 cm diameter single loop surface coil was used for signal reception, both of which were decoupled. The nasal structures of the animals were scanned via the spin-echo $T_1$-weighted MRI sequence to avoid including unsuitable animals in the trials. At 0 days (before) and 1 day (1 d), 4 days (4 d), and 7 days (7 d) after intranasal instillation, $T_2$-weighted image acquisition screening for OE defects and quantitative measurement of $T_1$ values were performed on the OE of all rats under chloral hydrate anesthesia (5 wt% solution, 7 mL $kg^{-1}$ dosage), respectively, to monitor changes in the OE dynamically in the following five groups: CMC (n = 6), S-ZnO20 (n = 5), $Fe_2O_3$ (n = 6), ZnO20 (n = 6), and ZnO500 (n = 6). At the same time points, $T_2$-weighted images were acquired to monitor OB alterations in five groups (n = 3 in each group). At 21 days (21 d), the damage to the olfactory bulbs of the ZnO20 (n = 3) and ZnO500 (n = 3) groups were scanned with $T_2$-weighted and $T_1$ inversion recovery images. The spin-echo $T_1$-weighted image parameters were as follows: repetition time: 400 ms; echo time: 15 ms; field of view: 1.5 cm × 1.5 cm; matrix size: 128 × 128; slice thickness: 0.8 mm; and number of averages: 2. The $T_2$-weighted image parameters were as follows: a repetition time of 3000 ms; 6 echoes, with echo times ranging from 25 to 175 ms; and an echo interval of 25 ms. $T_1$ values of the OE were measured by the fast Look–Locker $T_1$ imaging measurement sequence (LL $T_1$) with a repetition time of 5000 ms. The $T_1$ values were fitted by 24 small-angle gradient echo signals acquired with an excitation interval of 150 ms. The imaging parameters for the $T_1$ inversion recovery sequence were as follows: repetition time: 5000 ms; echo time: 15 ms; inversion recovery time: 450 ms. In the other MRI scans, the field of view parameters, matrix size, slice thickness, and number of averages are the same as those in the spin-echo $T_1$-weighted image.

### 2.6. Histologic Examination

At 1 and 22 days after treatment, except for the S-ZnO20 group, two typical rats in every group were executed for pathohistological evaluation of the OE and OB. For hematoxylin–

eosin staining, animals were perfused with 0.9 wt% NaCl and 4 wt% paraformaldehyde solutions through the left ventricular aorta. The OE and OB of each animal were then dissected, sampled, and fixed in 4 wt% paraformaldehyde solutions for one night. For the next 7 days, the fixed OE samples were decalcified within 15% EDTA. After that, the OE and OB specimens were embedded in paraffin and sliced to a thickness of 4 μm. The sections were deparaffinized, rehydrated, and stained with hematoxylin and eosin. At last, the sections were dehydrated, cleared, and covered with a neutral balsam.

### 2.7. Statistical Analysis

The region of interest (ROI) on the LL $T_1$ image was selected in ectoturbinate 2 (susceptible region) of the instilled side of the OE in the CMC group, and the $T_1$ value of ROI was fitted using a house-made MATLAB program. The data were expressed as mean ± standard deviation and statistically analyzed using the SPSS19.0 software package. Two-way analysis of variance (ANOVA) was used to analyze $T_1$ value data. Two-tailed Student's *t*-tests were used to evaluate the statistical significance of inter- and intro-group differences. The significance level was set at $p < 0.05$ with Bonferroni correction for multiple comparisons.

## 3. Results

### 3.1. Characterization Results of NPs

In Table 1, the range of the diameter of the ZnO NPs (20 nm) was between 15 and 30 nm, and the length range was between 20 and 40 nm. The purity was 99.9 wt%. The specific surface area was 31.5 $m^2 \cdot g^{-1}$. The crystalline structure was a zincite phase crystal. Figure 1B shows representative transmission electron microscopy images of 20-nm ZnO NPs. The characterization results of the $Fe_2O_3$ NPs and the ZnO NPs (500 nm) are shown in Table 1 and Figure 1.

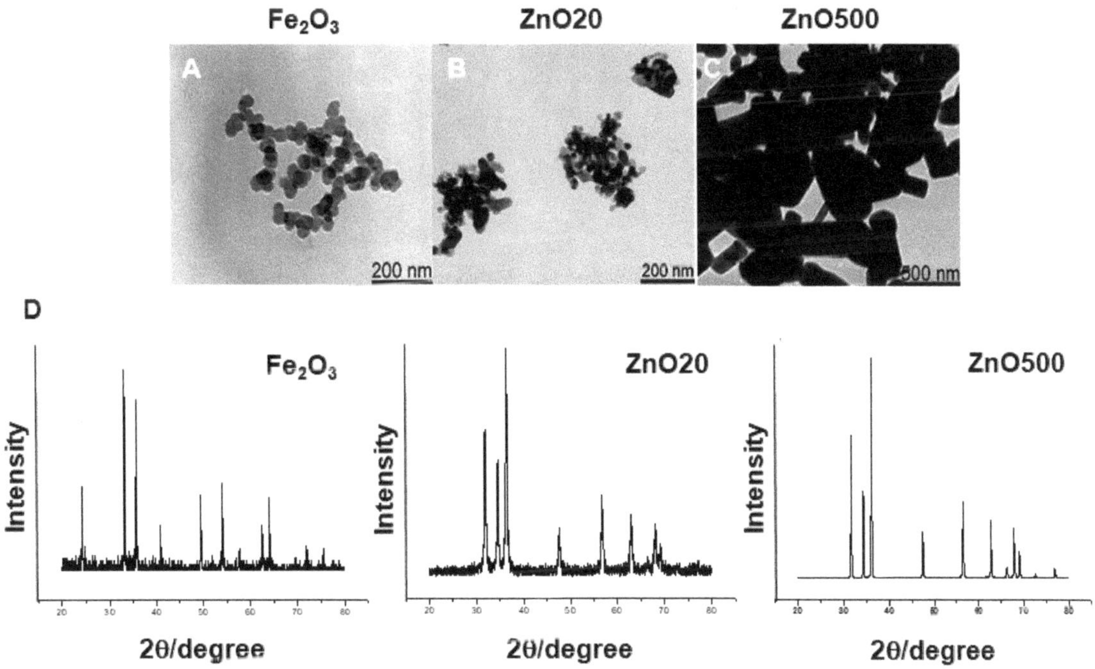


**Figure 1.** Representative transmission electron microscopy images and X-ray diffraction spectra of $Fe_2O_3$ nanoparticles (NPs), 20-nm zinc oxide (ZnO) NPs, and 500-nm ZnO NPs. (**A–C**) transmission

electron microscopy images; (**D**) X-ray diffraction spectra. A and B: bar 200 nm; C: bar 500 nm. The TEM images and X-ray diffraction spectra of $Fe_2O_3$ NPs and 500-nm ZnO NPs are from the literature [25].

**Table 1.** The characterization results of $Fe_2O_3$ NPs, 20-nm and 500-nm ZnO NPs (the data of $Fe_2O_3$ and 500-nm ZnO NPs are from the literature [25]).

| Samples | Purity (%) | Diameter (nm) | Specific Surface Area ($m^2 \cdot g^{-1}$) | Crystalline Structure |
|---|---|---|---|---|
| $Fe_2O_3$ | 97.9 | 25–40 | 10.0 | Maghemite |
| ZnO20 | 99.9 | Width = 15–30<br>Length = 20–40 | 31.5 | Zincite |
| ZnO500 | >99.9 | Width = 240–440<br>Length = 360–660 | 51.1 | Zincite |

### 3.2. *Toxic Effects of 20-nm ZnO NPs*

$T_2$-weighted images of the OE are shown in Figure 2. At 1 d, 4 d, and 7 d after intranasal exposure, the rats instilled with CMC, S-ZnO20, and $Fe_2O_3$ exhibited no evident abnormities in the OE compared to before the treatment (0 d). At 1 d, the rats treated with ZnO20 occasionally exhibited hyperintensity in areas of the OE in the bilateral turbinates, which can be explained by the septal window connecting two sides of the nasal cavity. The regions with hyperintensity were visible at 4 d and 7 d after the exposure to ZnO20. At 1 d, compared with the rats instilled with ZnO20, those treated with ZnO500 exhibited less-pronounced edema in OE. Edema was less apparent on $T_2$-weighted images at 4 d and 7 d after the exposure to ZnO500.

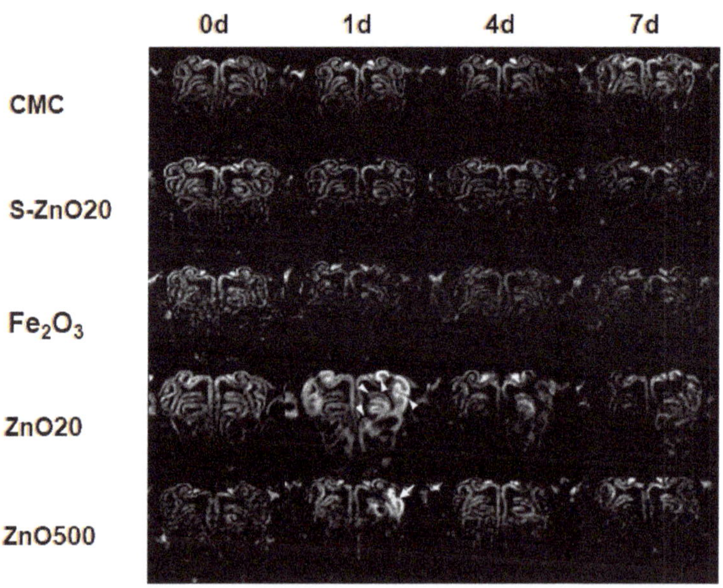


**Figure 2.** $T_2$-weighted images of the OE before (0 d) and at 1, 4, and 7 days after exposure to CMC, S-ZnO20, $Fe_2O_3$, ZnO20, and ZnO500. The white arrow indicates the bright signal in the turbinate at 1 d in the ZnO20 group, while the white arrowhead marks the bright signal in the turbinate at 1 d in the ZnO500 group, suggesting different extents of edema.

Figure 3 shows the $T_1$ relaxation time ($T_1$ value) changes in the ectoturbinate 2 of the instilled side of the OE in the CMC, S-ZnO20, $Fe_2O_3$, ZnO20, and ZnO500 group rats over time.

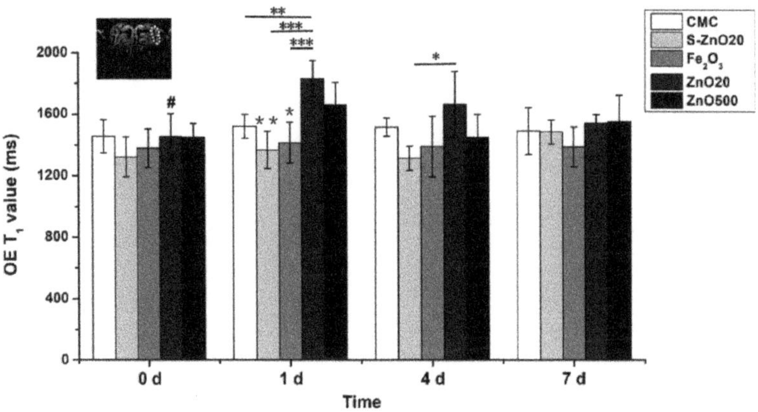


**Figure 3.** Histogram graph showing the $T_1$ relaxation time ($T_1$ value) of the region of interest (ROI) in the olfactory epithelium (OE) before (0 d) and after intranasal instillation in each group of rats. The white dashed line indicates the ROI in the ectoturbinate 2 of the OE in the CMC group. At 1 d, in the ZnO20 group, the $T_1$ value of the ROI significantly increases compared with its baseline at 0 d (#, $p = 0.003$), which is significantly higher than that of the CMC, S-ZnO20, and $Fe_2O_3$ groups, respectively (**, $p < 0.005$, ***, $p < 0.001$). At 1 d, the $T_1$ value in the ROI of the ZnO500 group is significantly higher than that of the $Fe_2O_3$ and S-ZnO groups, respectively (*, $p < 0.05$; **, $p < 0.01$). At 4 d, the $T_1$ value of the ZnO20 group is significantly higher than that of the S-ZnO20 group (*, $p < 0.05$).

Two-way ANOVA revealed that the main effects of time, group, and time × group interaction were statistically significant for $T_1$ value. At 1 d, the $T_1$ value of the ZnO20 group significantly increased compared to its baseline (0 day) (1830.3 ± 118.5 ms vs. 1453.8 ± 148.6 ms, $p = 0.003$). It also significantly increased compared to the CMC group (vs. 1521.67 ± 78.2 ms, $p < 0.005$), S-ZnO20 group (vs. 1368.6 ± 121.3 ms, $p < 0.001$), and $Fe_2O_3$ group (vs. 1415.7 ± 132.4 ms, $p < 0.001$) at 1 d, respectively. There was a trend of a rise in the OE's $T_1$ value in the ZnO20 group relative to that in the ZnO500 group. After that, the $T_1$ value of the ZnO20 group gradually decreased to 1664.3 ± 213.5 ms at 4 d and 1543.7 ± 54.7 ms at 7 d, respectively. At 4 d, the $T_1$ value of the ZnO20 group was higher than that of the S-ZnO20 group (1664.3 ± 213.5 ms vs. 1314.8 ± 78.0 ms, $p < 0.05$). In the ZnO500 group at 1 d, a significant $T_1$ value increase was seen compared to the $Fe_2O_3$ group (1661.2 ± 145.8 ms vs. 1415.7 ± 132.4 ms, $p < 0.05$) and S-ZnO20 (vs. 1368.6 ± 121.3 ms, $p < 0.01$), respectively. An upward trend was shown compared to its baseline (0 day) (vs. 1450.7 ± 88.2 ms). Then, the $T_1$ value of the ZnO500 group returned to the normal level.

Figure 4 shows the $T_2$-weighted images of the OB in one representative rat from the CMC, S-ZnO20, $Fe_2O_3$, ZnO20, and ZnO500 groups at each time point before and after intranasal instillation. At 4 d, bright signal intensity was shown in the ZnO20 group along part of the lateral and dorsal borders of the treated OB, which became more pronounced at 21 d. Transient bright signal intensity on the lateral border in the ZnO500 group was shown at 4 d. However, it returned to a normal level at 21 d. At 21 d, the treated OB size in the ZnO20 group showed a significant decrease compared with left untreated OB, while no apparent shrinkage was observed in the ZnO500 group. The treated OB in CMC, S-ZnO20, and $Fe_2O_3$ groups had not shown any changes in $T_2$ signal intensity until 7 d.

Figure 5 shows the inversion recovery $T_1$-weighted images of the rat OB at 1, 4, 7, and 21 days after intranasal instillation of ZnO20. At 7 d, there was an apparent region of low signal intensity along the lateral border of the instilled side of the OB, indicating tissue edema and inflammation. At 21 d, the instilled side of the OB significantly shrunk compared with the control side, probably due to the thinning of the olfactory nerve layer (ONL) to some extent.

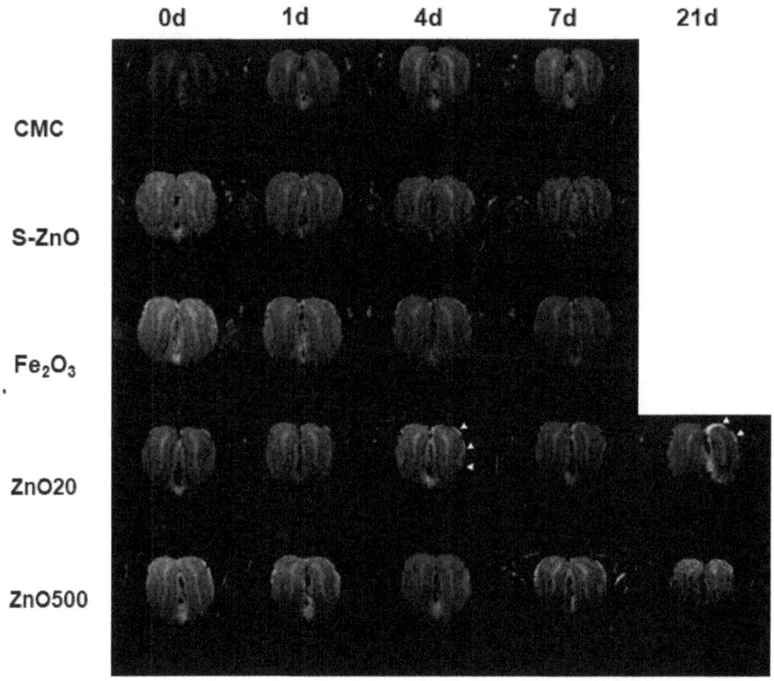


**Figure 4.** The $T_2$-weighted image of the olfactory bulb (OB) before and after exposure to CMC, S-ZnO20, $Fe_2O_3$, ZnO20, and ZnO500. At 4 d and 21 d, the white arrow indicates the region of high signal intensity along the lateral and dorsal border of the right treated OB in the ZnO20 group, suggesting edema.

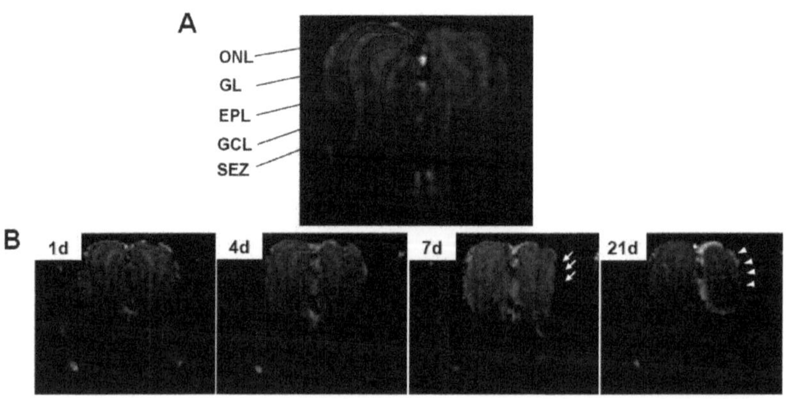


**Figure 5.** The inversion recovery $T_1$-weighted images of the rat olfactory bulb (OB). In panel (**A**), the black dashed line outlines the distinct layer structure of the control side of the OB in the CMC group, from the outer layer to the inner layer, including the ONL (olfactory nerve layer), GL (glomerular layer), EPL (external plexiform layer), GCL (granule cell layer), and SEZ (subependymal zone). In panel (**B**), the inversion recovery $T_1$-weighted images of the OB in the ZnO20 group at 1 d, 4 d, 7 d, and 21 d are shown. The arrow indicates the region of low signal intensity in the inversion recovery $T_1$-weighted image on the instilled side, and the arrowhead reveals the thinning of the ONL.

*3.3. Structural Changes of the OE and OB*

In Figure 6, cellular damage and inflammation in OE, as well as olfactory nerve fiber losses in OB, are induced by 20-nm ZnO NPs. The normal structure of the OE in the CMC-treated rat is presented in Figure 6A, which is composed of epithelial cells (E), lamina propria (LP), and turbinate (TB). The olfactory axons penetrate and terminate in the olfactory glomeruli after traveling across the surface of the OB, which constitute the ONL (Figure 6F). The ZnO20 group showed an acute inflammatory cell infiltration in the OE at 1 d, with disorganized epithelial cells, accompanied by the disappearance or reduction of olfactory axons. At 22 d, it was likely an epithelial cell reproduction originating from the LP, indicating a recovery state of the injured OE. A vacuole was apparent in the ONL on the lateral OB as early as 1 day after the treatment. By 22 days after the treatment, the olfactory axons no longer formed an intact layer, and the thickness of the ONL was thinner than before. The blood vessels in the OE and OB of the ZnO20-treated rats were significantly dilated, suggesting increased vascular permeability due to inflammatory reactions. At 22 d, the hematoxylin–eosin staining results of the OE and OB in both the $Fe_2O_3$ and ZnO500 groups illustrated well-organized columnar epithelial cells and the compact structure of the ONL.

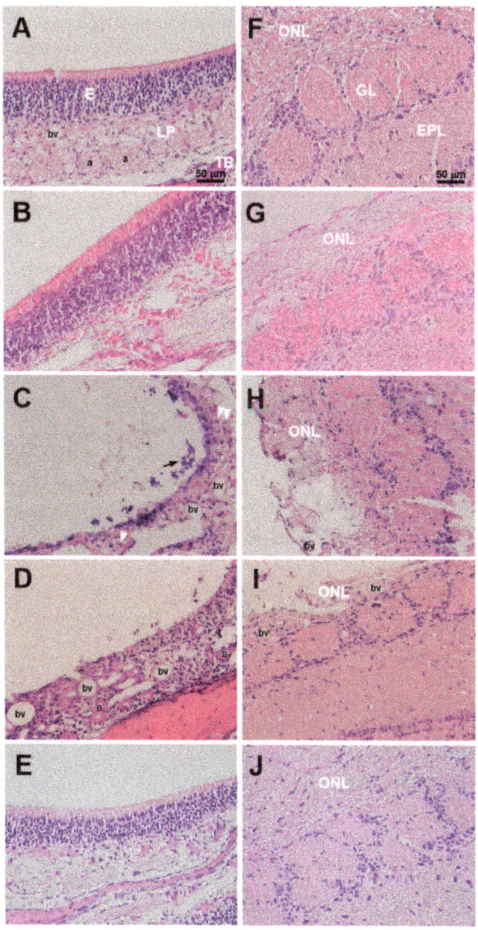


**Figure 6.** The hematoxylin–eosin staining images of rat olfactory epithelium (OE) and olfactory bulb (OB) after exposure to CMC, $Fe_2O_3$, ZnO20, and ZnO500. (**A–E**) represent the stainings of the OE at 1 d

after exposure to CMC, at 22 d after exposure to $Fe_2O_3$, at 1 d and 22 d after exposure to ZnO20, and at 22 d after exposure to ZnO500, respectively. (**F–J**) represent the correspondent stainings of OB. The white arrowheads mark infiltrated phagocyte cells, and the black arrow points out the cellular debris in (**C**). TB: turbinate; LP: lamina propria; E: epithelial cells; a: bundles of olfactory axons; bv: blood vessel; ONL: olfactory nerve layer; GL: glomerular layer; EPL: external plexiform layer (bar: 50 μm).

## 4. Discussion

The main findings of this study are that the qualitative and quantitative analysis on the OE and OB in rats using MRI and combined with histopathological examination confirm that intranasally instilled 20-nm ZnO NPs acutely results in cellular damage and inflammation in the OE, accompanied with edema and atrophy in the OB.

Our experimental results are consistent with the viewpoint of particle size as a major factor influencing the toxic effects of nanomaterials. The size of the NPs makes their movement in the body across cell membranes and normal diffusion barriers possible. We found that 20-nm ZnO NPs caused the most severe damage to the rat OE and OB. Quantitative $T_1$ value measurement illustrated that at 1 d, the $T_1$ value of the OE in the ZnO20 group increased compared to those in all of the other groups at the same time point, which was consistent with the $T_2$-weighted imaging results, suggesting most severe edema [26] in the OE of the ZnO20 group. An obvious low signal intensity was observed in the inversion recovery $T_1$-weighted image on the lateral side of the OB of the ZnO20 group at 7 d, which may mark tissue edema, followed by atrophy at 21 d. The MRI findings were identified via the histological results. Typical pathological features of the OE in the ZnO20 group were structural disorganization of the epithelial cell layer, disappearance or shrinkage of the olfactory axons, and infiltration of inflammatory cells; the OB was characterized by the thinning of the ONL. Changes in vascular permeability induced by inflammatory responses were present in both the OE and OB. For the 500-nm ZnO NPs, the instilled side of the OE and OB did not appear to be very obviously damaged, either from the MRI findings (only a transient olfactory epithelial edema highlight signal was visible on the $T_2$ weighted image) or from the hematoxylin–eosin pathology findings. These results suggest that 20-nm ZnO NPs exert more toxicity responses to the OE and OB than those induced by 500-nm ZnO NPs. The olfactory nerve axon diameter is <200 nm [27], which may be the "threshold" limiting the uptake of particulate matter into the olfactory nerve terminals. Elder et al. [10] found that inhaled 30-nm MnO NPs could enter the OB via the olfactory nerve. Then, there were increases in Mn concentrations in the OB, striatum, frontal cortex, and cerebellum. Tumor necrosis factor-α protein, macrophage inflammatory protein-2, and glial fibrillary acidic protein were also increased in the OB. Bermudez et al. [28,29] found that 20-nm $TiO_2$ NPs induced inflammatory responses and cytotoxicity in rats at a rate 5–10 times higher than 300-nm $TiO_2$ NPs. Our results also found that the smaller the particle size, the more likely they were to cause injury to the OE and OB. Wang et al. [11] reported the TEM results of neurodendron degeneration, membranous structure disruption, and the lysosome increase in the OB after long-term and low-dose intranasal exposure to nano-sized $Fe_2O_3$ (21 nm). However, in our study, the MRI results at each time point did not show any signal abnormality in the OE and OB after $Fe_2O_3$ NPs exposure, and the hematoxylin–eosin pathology results did not show any significant damage (except for vasodilatation). Therefore, we conclude that $Fe_2O_3$ NPs did not cause obvious damage to the olfactory system of the rats in the present experiment. $Fe_2O_3$ NP was designed as a negative control in our study because it is classified as insoluble metal oxide. The element-dependent nanotoxicity of metal oxide NPs implies that the Zn element might be the toxicant form. $Zn^{2+}$ could inhibit cellular energy production by blocking mitochondrial respiration and could even induce neuronal death. Given that ZnO NP is a kind of highly soluble metal oxide, we infer that the releases of zinc ions will rise as the particle size decreases. We suggest that the dissolution should be regarded as a crucial step in producing the toxicity of ZnO NPs.

There are some arguments about the induction of the adverse effects of ZnO NPs. Due to the high solubility of ZnO NPs, some in vitro studies have suggested that ZnO-NP cytotoxicity stems mainly from the release of $Zn^{2+}$ ions [24,30,31]. However, several studies suggest that particle dependence is another important toxicity mechanism for ZnO NPs [32–35]. A review discussed that ZnO NP-induced genotoxicity could originate from the release of $Zn^{2+}$ ions and particle form [36]. Given that the smaller the particles of substances with the same chemical properties are, the greater solubility they have, the $[Zn^{2+}]$ in both the supernatants of the 20-nm and 500-nm ZnO NP-CMC suspensions was measured in our study. Exceeding our expectations, the $[Zn^{2+}]$ is equal in both suspensions. Furthermore, the $[Zn^{2+}]$ in the supernatant of the 20-nm ZnO NP-CMC suspension did not induce significant defects to the OE and OB. We show that the dissolved fraction of the ZnO NPs in suspension does not account for the toxicity of the ZnO NP-CMC suspensions to the rat olfactory system, which is consistent with the results of our previous research [25] and the toxicity of the ZnO NP suspensions to Daphnia magna [33].

ZnO NPs are among the more soluble metal oxide nanomaterials. Therefore, it is more likely to be transformed into soluble zinc ions after in vivo treatment. Except for the particle size factor, dissolved $Zn^{2+}$, as the other negligible aspect, may play a major role in the ZnO NPs' toxicity to nasal mucosal cells [22]. Previous studies have found that intranasal instilled $ZnSO_4$ can destroy OE, leading to peripheral afferent nerve deafferentation [37]. Persson et al. reported that $Zn^{2+}$ (as $ZnCl_2$) could be translocated along the olfactory nerves of the rat into the olfactory bulb and even the anterior portion of the olfactory cortex, and that zinc ions have been found to accumulate in the olfactory glomerulus axon terminals of primary olfactory neurons [38]. We speculate that the slightly acidic environment (pH 5.5–6.5) of the nasal mucosa [39] and the low pH within cytoplasmic vesicles (e.g., lysosomes, pH 5.2) facilitate the dissolution of ZnO NPs [40]. In line with this opinion, surface coatings on the ZnO nanoparticles mitigated cellular responses such as cell stress, inflammatory, and apoptosis [23]. Interestingly, accumulated Zn in the form of ZnO in rat liver has recently been revealed, demonstrating some overlaps and considerable specificity in metabolism profiles related to the antioxidant systems and energy metabolism pathways versus $ZnSO_4$ exposure [35]. ZnO in particulate form in the OB synaptosomes and brain has been found following nasal exposure of rats to airborne ZnO NPs (12–14 nm particle size), demonstrating an OB–brain translocation pathway for ZnO NPs [41]. However, the brain-region-specific distribution of exogenous ZnO NPs was not further clarified in that study. In a sense, our study located the ZnO NPs-induced adverse effect in OB.

In clinics, olfactory impairment and deficits have been reported in neurodegenerative disorders such as Parkinson's disease (PD) and Alzheimer's disease (AD) [42,43]. Damage to the olfactory pathway may be an early sign of AD and PD [44,45]. Epidemiologic investigations have shown a link between excessive zinc exposure and demyelinating diseases [46]. Zinc dysregulation will lead to an increase in extracellular $Zn^{2+}$ concentration, which may precipitate β amylase and play a role in Alzheimer's disease [47]. Van Denderen et al. [48] suggested that a decrease in the metabolic activity in the olfactory brain would result in a drop of the nerve fiber density in the anterior cerebral artery after $ZnSO_4$-induced loss of olfaction. A decrease in nerve fiber density in the precommunicating part of the anterior cerebral artery was also found in patients with Alzheimer's disease [49]. Moreover, ZnO NPs have been reported to be involved in the pathogenesis of neuronal diseases [50] and cause neural stem cell apoptosis [51]. For occupational workers chronically exposed to zinc-containing powders, fumes from zinc-plating factories, and welding environments, ZnO NPs might deposit in the nasal mucosa and subsequently undergo cellular uptake of primary olfactory sensory neurons, enter the olfactory bulb via axonal transport, and arrive at the olfactory cortex or even deeper brain regions via the axonal transmission of secondary olfactory neurons, resulting in excessive Zn element overload in the brain. Suppose that inhalation of ZnO NPs adversely affects the olfactory system and induces or aggravates the development of neurodegenerative disorders; in this case, the health of the occupationally exposed population should be given more attention.

As a well-established technique in medical and biological applications, the value of MRI has been greatly underestimated for nanotoxicology studies. The results of this study indicate that MRI could be used as a bio-screening tool to assess the reverse consequences of nasal exposure to ZnO NPs. It is important to ensure the safe application of nanomaterials [52] by elucidating the biological effects of nanomaterials and then exploring ways to eliminate and avoid their nanotoxicity.

## 5. Conclusions

The global rise in nanomaterials production has prompted people to pay attention to the safe application of NPs. We found acute toxicity effects on the rat olfactory system using MRI technology via nasally instilled 20-nm ZnO NPs. Our study revealed that 20-nm ZnO NPs caused obvious structural disruption and inflammation to the OE and OB at the acute stage. The results of our study support the viewpoint of the size-dependent toxic effect of NPs. The $T_1$ value of the OE in the ZnO20 group increased at 1 d, consistent with the $T_2$-weighted imaging results, suggesting severe edema. OB edema and atrophy were illustrated in the inversion recovery $T_1$-weighted images following cellular damage and inflammation in the OE. The MRI findings were identified via the histological results. Structural disorganization of the epithelial cell layer, shrinkage of the olfactory axons, and infiltration of inflammatory cells are typical pathological features in the OE; the OB was characterized by the thinning of the ONL. Changes in vascular permeability were present in both the OE and OB. To the best of our knowledge, OB damage caused by ZnO NPs has never been reported before. The results suggest that the real-time and non-invasive advantages of MRI allow it to directly and dynamically observe and assess the potential toxicity of long-term exposure to ZnO NPs in the olfactory system. More studies are required to pinpoint the mechanism behind the ZnO NPs' toxicity.

In the future, our research will focus on the biosafety assessment of manufactured nanoparticles, including, but not limited to, the nanoparticle toxicity of long-term nasal exposure and the transport mechanism of nanoparticles in neurodegenerative disease.

**Author Contributions:** Conceptualization, X.W. and L.G.; methodology, L.G.; software, Y.M.; validation, X.L.; formal analysis, X.L.; investigation, J.C.; resources, Y.M.; data curation, X.W.; writing—original draft preparation, L.G.; writing—review and editing, X.W.; visualization, X.L.; supervision, J.C.; project administration, J.C.; funding acquisition, L.G. and X.W. All authors have read and agreed to the published version of the manuscript.

**Funding:** This research was funded by the Natural Science Foundation of China (No. 81601204), the Research Fund of Jianghan University (No. 2022SXZX26), and the Project in the Field of Laboratory Animal Research in Hubei Province (No. 2023CFA002).

**Institutional Review Board Statement:** The animal study protocol was approved by the Ethics Committee of the Department of Medicine, Jianghan University (No: JHDXLL2022-069).

**Data Availability Statement:** The data are contained within the article.

**Conflicts of Interest:** The authors declare no conflicts of interest.

## References

1. Sabir, S.; Arshad, M.; Chaudhari, S.K. Zinc oxide nanoparticles for revolutionizing agriculture: Synthesis and applications. *Sci. World J.* **2014**, *2014*, 925494. [CrossRef] [PubMed]
2. Raha, S.; Ahmaruzzaman, M. ZnO nanostructured materials and their potential applications: Progress, challenges and perspectives. *Nanoscale Adv.* **2022**, *4*, 1868–1925. [CrossRef]
3. Fine, J.M.; Gordon, T.; Chen, L.C.; Kinney, P.; Falcone, G.; Sparer, J.; Beckett, W.S. Characterization of clinical tolerance to inhaled zinc oxide in naive subjects and sheet metal workers. *J. Occup. Environ. Med.* **2000**, *42*, 1085–1091. [CrossRef] [PubMed]
4. Osmond, M.J.; Mccall, M.J. Zinc oxide nanoparticles in modern sunscreens: An analysis of potential exposure and hazard. *Nanotoxicology* **2010**, *4*, 15–41. [CrossRef] [PubMed]
5. Kuschner, W.G.; D'Alessandro, A.; Wong, H.; Blanc, P.D. Early pulmonary cytokine responses to zinc oxide fume inhalation. *Environ. Res.* **1997**, *75*, 7–11. [CrossRef]

6. Lam, H.F.; Conner, M.W.; Rogers, A.E.; Fitzgerald, S.; Amdur, M.O. Functional and morphologic changes in the lungs of guinea pigs exposed to freshly generated ultrafine zinc oxide. *Toxicol. Appl. Pharmacol.* **1985**, *78*, 29–38. [CrossRef]
7. Beckett, W.S.; Chalupa, D.F.; Pauly-Brown, A.; Speers, D.M.; Stewart, J.C.; Frampton, M.W.; Utell, M.J.; Huang, L.S.; Cox, C.; Zareba, W.; et al. Comparing inhaled ultrafine versus fine zinc oxide particles in healthy adults: A human inhalation study. *Am. J. Resp. Crit. Care* **2005**, *171*, 1129–1135. [CrossRef]
8. De Lorenzo, A.J.D. The olfactory neuron and the blood-brain barrier. In *Ciba Foundation Symposium—Internal Secretions of the Pancreas (Colloquia on Endocrinology)*; John Wiley & Sons, Ltd.: London, UK, 1970.
9. Oberdörster, G.; Sharp, Z.; Atudorei, V.; Elder, A.; Gelein, R.; Kreyling, W.; Cox, C. Translocation of inhaled ultrafine particles to the brain. *Inhal. Toxicol.* **2004**, *16*, 437–445. [CrossRef]
10. Elder, A.; Gelein, R.; Silva, V.; Feikert, T.; Opanashuk, L.; Carter, J.; Potter, R.; Maynard, A.; Finkelstein, J.; Oberdörster, G. Translocation of inhaled ultrafine manganese oxide particles to the central nervous system. *Environ. Health Perspect.* **2006**, *114*, 1172–1178. [CrossRef]
11. Wang, B.; Feng, W.Y.; Zhu, M.T.; Wang, Y.; Wang, M.; Gu, Y.Q.; Ouyang, H.; Wang, H.J.; Li, M.; Zhao, Y.L.; et al. Neurotoxicity of low-dose repeatedly intranasal instillation of nano- and submicron-sized ferric oxide particles in mice. *J. Nanopart. Res.* **2009**, *11*, 41–53. [CrossRef]
12. Wu, J.; Ding, T.T.; Sun, J. Neurotoxic potential of iron oxide nanoparticles in the rat brain striatum and hippocampus. *Neurotoxicology* **2013**, *34*, 243–253. [CrossRef] [PubMed]
13. Aillon, K.L.; Xie, Y.M.; El-Gendy, N.; Berkland, C.J.; Forrest, M.L. Effects of nanomaterial physicochemical properties on toxicity. *Adv. Drug Deliv. Rev.* **2009**, *61*, 457–466. [CrossRef] [PubMed]
14. Hsiao, I.L.; Huang, Y.J. Effects of serum on cytotoxicity of nano- and micro-sized ZnO particles. *J. Nanopart. Res.* **2013**, *15*, 1829. [CrossRef]
15. Sahu, D.; Kannan, G.M.; Vijayaraghavan, R. Size-Dependent Effect of Zinc Oxide on Toxicity and Inflammatory Potential of Human Monocytes. *J. Toxicol. Environ. Health A* **2014**, *77*, 177–191. [CrossRef] [PubMed]
16. Tin-Tin-Win-Shwe; Yamamoto, S.; Ahmed, S.; Kakeyama, M.; Kobayashi, T.; Fujimaki, H. Brain cytokine and chemokine mRNA expression in mice induced by intranasal instillation with ultrafine carbon black. *Toxicol. Lett.* **2006**, *163*, 153–160. [CrossRef] [PubMed]
17. Donaldson, K.; Duffin, R.; Langrish, J.P.; Miller, M.R.; Mills, N.L.; Poland, C.A.; Raftis, J.; Shah, A.; Shaw, C.A.; Newby, D.E. Nanoparticles and the cardiovascular system: A critical review. *Nanomedicine* **2013**, *8*, 403–423. [CrossRef] [PubMed]
18. Yu, J.; Choi, S.J. Particle size and biological fate of ZnO do not cause acute toxicity, but affect toxicokinetics and gene expression profiles in the rat livers after oral administration. *Int. J. Mol. Sci.* **2021**, *22*, 1698. [CrossRef]
19. Gojova, A.; Guo, B.; Kota, R.S.; Rutledge, J.C.; Kennedy, I.M.; Barakat, A.I. Induction of inflammation in vascular endothelial cells by metal oxide nanoparticles: Effect of particle composition. *Environ. Health Perspect.* **2007**, *115*, 403–409. [CrossRef]
20. Jeng, H.A.; Swanson, J. Toxicity of metal oxide nanoparticles in mammalian cells. *J. Environ. Sci. Health Part A Toxic Hazard. Subst. Environ. Eng.* **2006**, *41*, 2699–2711. [CrossRef]
21. Kahru, A.; Dubourguier, H.C. From ecotoxicology to nanoecotoxicology. *Toxicology* **2010**, *269*, 105–119. [CrossRef]
22. Hackenberg, S.; Scherzed, A.; Technau, A.; Kessler, M.; Froelich, K.; Ginzkey, C.; Koehler, C.; Burghartz, M.; Hagen, R.; Kleinsasser, N. Cytotoxic, genotoxic and pro-inflammatory effects of zinc oxide nanoparticles in human nasal mucosa cells. *Toxicol. Vitr.* **2011**, *25*, 657–663. [CrossRef] [PubMed]
23. Osmond-McLeod, M.J.; Osmond, R.I.W.; Oytam, Y.; McCall, M.J.; Feltis, B.; Mackay Sim, A.; Wood, S.A.; Cook, A.L. Surface coatings of ZnO nanoparticles mitigate differentially a host of transcriptional, protein and signalling responses in primary human olfactory cells. *Part Fibre Toxicol.* **2013**, *10*, 54. [CrossRef] [PubMed]
24. Landsiedel, R.; Ma-Hock, L.; Kroll, A.; Hahn, D.; Schnekenburger, J.; Wiench, K.; Wohlleben, W. Testing Metal-Oxide Nanomaterials for Human Safety. *Adv. Mater.* **2010**, *22*, 2601–2627. [CrossRef] [PubMed]
25. Gao, L.F.; Yang, S.T.; Li, S.R.; Meng, Y.G.; Wang, H.F.; Lei, H. Acute toxicity of zinc oxide nanoparticles to the rat olfactory system after intranasal instillation. *J. Appl. Toxicol.* **2013**, *33*, 1079–1088. [CrossRef]
26. Loubinoux, I.; Volk, A.; Borredon, J.; Guirimand, S.; Tiffon, B.; Seylaz, J.; Méric, P. Spreading of vasogenic edema and cytotoxic edema assessed by quantitative diffusion and $T_2$ magnetic resonance imaging. *Stroke* **1997**, *28*, 419–427. [CrossRef]
27. Griff, E.R.; Greer, C.A.; Margolis, F.; Ennis, M.; Shipley, M.T. Ultrastructural characteristics and conduction velocity of olfactory receptor neuron axons in the olfactory marker protein-null mouse. *Brain Res.* **2000**, *866*, 227–236. [CrossRef]
28. Bermudez, E.; Mangum, J.B.; Asgharian, B.; Wong, B.A.; Reverdy, E.E.; Janszen, D.B.; Hext, P.M.; Warheit, D.B.; Everitt, J.I. Long-term pulmonary responses of three laboratory rodent species to subchronic inhalation of pigmentary titanium dioxide particles. *Toxicol. Sci.* **2002**, *70*, 86–97. [CrossRef]
29. Bermudez, E.; Mangum, J.B.; Wong, B.A.; Asgharian, B.; Hext, P.M.; Warheit, D.B.; Everitt, J.I. Pulmonary responses of mice, rats, and hamsters to subchronic inhalation of ultrafine titanium dioxide particles. *Toxicol. Sci.* **2004**, *77*, 347–357. [CrossRef]
30. Brunner, T.J.; Wick, P.; Manser, P.; Spohn, P.; Grass, R.N.; Limbach, L.K.; Bruinink, A.; Stark, W.J. In vitro cytotoxicity of oxide nanoparticles: Comparison to asbestos, silica, and the effect of particle solubility. *Environ. Sci. Technol.* **2006**, *40*, 4374–4381. [CrossRef]
31. De Berardis, B.; Civitelli, G.; Condello, M.; Lista, P.; Pozzi, R.; Arancia, G.; Meschini, S. Exposure to ZnO nanoparticles induces oxidative stress and cytotoxicity in human colon carcinoma cells. *Toxicol. Appl. Pharmacol.* **2010**, *246*, 116–127. [CrossRef]

32. Poynton, H.C.; Lazorchak, J.M.; Impellitteri, C.A.; Smith, M.E.; Rogers, K.; Patra, M.; Hammer, K.A.; Allen, H.J.; Vulpe, C.D. Differential gene expression in Daphnia magna suggests distinct modes of action and bioavailability for ZnO nanoparticles and Zn ions. *Environ. Sci. Technol.* **2011**, *45*, 762–768. [CrossRef] [PubMed]
33. Hua, J.; Vijver, M.G.; Richardson, M.K.; Ahmad, F.; Peijnenburg, W.J.G.M. Particle-specific toxic effects of differently shaped zinc oxide nanoparticles to zebrafish embryos (Danio rerio). *Environ. Toxicol. Chem.* **2014**, *33*, 2859–2868. [CrossRef] [PubMed]
34. Khare, P.; Sonane, M.; Nagar, Y.; Moin, N.; Ali, S.; Gupta, K.C.; Satish, A. Size dependent toxicity of zinc oxide nano-particles in soil nematode Caenorhabditis elegans. *Nanotoxicology* **2015**, *9*, 423–432. [CrossRef] [PubMed]
35. Guo, Z.L.; Luo, Y.L.; Zhang, P.; Chetwynd, A.J.; Xie, H.D.Q.H.; Monikh, F.A.; Tao, W.Q.; Xie, C.J.; Liu, Y.Y.; Xu, L.; et al. Deciphering the particle specific effects on metabolism in rat liver and plasma from ZnO nanoparticles versus ionic Zn exposure. *Environ. Int.* **2020**, *136*, 105437. [CrossRef] [PubMed]
36. Scherzad, A.; Meyer, T.; Kleinsasser, N.; Hackenberg, S. Molecular mechanisms of zinc oxide nanoparticle-induced genotoxicity short running title: Genotoxicity of ZnO NPs. *Materials* **2017**, *10*, 1427. [CrossRef] [PubMed]
37. Burd, G.D. Morphological study of the effects of intranasal zinc sulfate irrigation on the mouse olfactory epithelium and olfactory bulb. *Microsc. Res. Tech.* **1993**, *24*, 195–213. [CrossRef]
38. Persson, E.; Henriksson, J.; Tallkvist, J.; Rouleau, C.; Tjälve, H. Transport and subcellular distribution of intranasally administered zinc in the olfactory system of rats and pikes. *Toxicology* **2003**, *191*, 97–108. [CrossRef]
39. Mei, D.; Mao, S.R.; Sun, W.; Wang, Y.J.; Kissel, T. Effect of chitosan structure properties and molecular weight on the intranasal absorption of tetramethylpyrazine phosphate in rats. *Eur. J. Pharm. Biopharm.* **2008**, *70*, 874–881. [CrossRef]
40. Xia, T.; Kovochich, M.; Liong, M.; Mädler, L.; Gilbert, B.; Shi, H.B.; Yeh, J.I.; Zink, J.I.; Nel, A.E. Comparison of the mechanism of toxicity of zinc oxide and cerium oxide nanoparticles based on dissolution and oxidative stress properties. *ACS Nano* **2008**, *2*, 2121–2134. [CrossRef]
41. Kao, Y.Y.; Cheng, T.J.; Yang, D.M.; Wang, C.T.; Chiung, Y.M.; Liu, P.S. Demonstration of an olfactory bulb-brain translocation pathway for ZnO nanoparticles in rodent cells in vitro and in vivo. *J. Mol. Neurosci.* **2012**, *48*, 464–471. [CrossRef]
42. Duda, J.E.; Moberg, P.J.; Balderston, C.; Roalf, D.R.; Doty, R.L.; Stern, M.B. Meta-analysis of olfactory dysfunction in Alzheimer's, Parkinson's and Huntington's Diseases. *Neurobiol. Aging* **2004**, *25*, S95. [CrossRef]
43. Ibarretxe-Bilbao, N.; Junque, C.; Marti, M.J.; Valldeoriola, F.; Vendrell, P.; Bargallo, N.; Zarei, M.; Tolosa, E. Olfactory impairment in Parkinson's disease and white matter abnormalities in central olfactory areas: A voxel-based diffusion tensor imaging study. *Mov. Disord.* **2010**, *25*, 1888–1894. [CrossRef] [PubMed]
44. Roberts, E.; Junque, C.; Marti, M.J.; Valldeoriola, F.; Vendrell, P.; Bargallo, N.; Zarei, M.; Tolosa, E. Alzheimer's disease may begin in the nose and may be caused by aluminosilicates. *Neurobiol. Aging* **1986**, *7*, 561–567. [CrossRef] [PubMed]
45. Doty, R.L.; Bromley, S.M.; Stern, M.B. Olfactory testing as an aid in the diagnosis of Parkinson's disease: Development of optimal discrimination criteria. *Neurodegeneration* **1995**, *4*, 93–97. [CrossRef] [PubMed]
46. Prodan, C.I.; Holland, N.R. CNS demyelination from zinc toxicity? *Neurology* **2000**, *54*, 1705–1706. [CrossRef] [PubMed]
47. Frederickson, C.J.; Bush, A.I. Synaptically released zinc: Physiological functions and pathological effects. *Biometals* **2001**, *14*, 353–366. [CrossRef]
48. van Denderen, J.C.M.; van Wieringen, G.W.; Hillen, B.; Bleys, R.L.A.W. Zinc sulphate-induced anosmia decreases the nerve fibre density in the anterior cerebral artery of the rat. *Auton. Neurosci.* **2001**, *94*, 102–108. [CrossRef]
49. Bleys, R.L.; Cowen, T.; Groen, G.J.; Hillen, B. Perivascular nerves of the human basal cerebral arteries: II. Changes in aging and Alzheimer's disease. *J. Cereb. Blood Flow Metab.* **1996**, *16*, 1048–1057. [CrossRef]
50. Frederickson, C.J.; Koh, J.Y.; Bush, A.I. The neurobiology of zinc in health and disease. *Nat. Rev. Neurosci.* **2005**, *6*, 449–462. [CrossRef]
51. Deng, X.Y.; Luan, Q.X.; Chen, W.T.; Wang, Y.L.; Wu, M.H.; Zhang, H.J.; Jiao, Z. Nanosized zinc oxide particles induce neural stem cell apoptosis. *Nanotechnology* **2009**, *20*, 115101. [CrossRef]
52. Gandhi, S.; Shastri, D.H.; Shah, J.G.; Nair, A.B.; Jacob, S. Nasal Delivery to the Brain: Harnessing Nanoparticles for Effective Drug Transport. *Pharmaceutics* **2024**, *16*, 481. [CrossRef] [PubMed]

*toxics*

MDPI

*Article*

# The Impact of Ambient Air Pollution on Allergic Rhinitis Symptoms: A Prospective Follow-Up Study

**Wen Sun [1], Chan Ding [1], Zhuoying Jiang [1], Xinliang Zheng [1], Jinlan Jiang [2,*] and Huadong Xu [1,*]**

1 School of Public Health, Hangzhou Medical College, 182 Tianmushan Road, Xihu District, Hangzhou 310013, China; 881012022125@hmc.edu.cn (W.S.); 130232023252@hmc.edu.cn (C.D.); jiangzhuoying0304@163.com (Z.J.); zxl2695291160@163.com (X.Z.)

2 The Second School of Clinical Medicine, Zhejiang Chinese Medical University, 548 Binwen Road, Binjiang District, Hangzhou 310053, China

* Correspondence: 502536834@ucas.ac.cn (J.J.); xuhuadong@hmc.edu.cn (H.X.)

**Abstract:** Air pollution has become a serious public health problem and there is evidence that air pollution affects the incidence of allergic rhinitis. To further investigate the effect of ambient air pollutants on the severity of allergic rhinitis symptoms, a prospective follow-up study in patients with allergic rhinitis was conducted. A total of 167 allergic rhinitis patients with a mean age of 35.4 years, who were visiting the hospital, were enrolled. The daily symptom severity of allergic rhinitis and the concentrations of six air pollutants, including $PM_{2.5}$, $PM_{10}$, $SO_2$, CO, $O_3$ and $NO_2$, were collected through follow-up investigations. The impact of ambient air pollutants on symptom severity was assessed via multi-pollutant models. Among several typical ambient air pollutants, we observed correlations of allergic rhinitis symptoms with $PM_{2.5}$, $PM_{10}$, CO, $SO_2$ and $NO_2$, whereas $O_3$ showed no such correlation. Specifically, $PM_{2.5}$ and $PM_{10}$ were significantly associated with sneezing and nasal blockage. $NO_2$ was significantly correlated with symptoms of rhinorrhea, itchy nose and itchy eyes. CO was significantly linked to sneezing and nasal blockage symptoms. These air pollutants not only had a direct impact on allergic rhinitis symptoms but also exhibited a lagging effect. This study indicates that short-term exposure to air pollutants is associated with exacerbation of nasal symptoms in patients with allergic rhinitis, leading to a decline in their quality of life.

**Keywords:** allergic rhinitis; ambient air pollution; prospective study; nasal symptoms

## 1. Introduction

Since the onset of global industrialization, the pollution problem has become increasingly serious. To date, air pollution remains a major public health problem. In fact, according to a report released by the World Health Organization (WHO) in 2022, 99% of the global population lived in places that failed to meet the air quality guidelines of the WHO [1]. It was further estimated that outdoor ambient air pollution contributed to 4.2 million premature deaths globally in 2019 [2]. Research on air pollution and respiratory health has been extensive, driven by the direct impact of air pollutants on the human respiratory system. Numerous studies have demonstrated associations between air pollution and health issues such as acute lower respiratory infections, chronic obstructive pulmonary disease (COPD), asthma, lung cancer and allergic rhinitis [3]. These studies also highlight that there is no identified threshold below which exposure to air pollution can be deemed safe [4,5].

Allergic rhinitis, one of the most prevalent chronic diseases globally, is typically characterized by sneezing, nasal itching, nasal blockage and runny nose. It affects an estimated 10–40% of the global population, annually contributing to approximately USD 17.5 billion in health-related economic losses [6]. For those afflicted, allergic rhinitis can cause sleep disturbances, fatigue, mood depression, reduced sense of smell and cognitive impairment, thereby profoundly impacting their quality of life and productivity in both learning and work settings [7,8]. Furthermore, allergic rhinitis stands as a notable risk factor for asthma, otitis media and allergic conjunctivitis. Prolonged exposure to allergic rhinitis can exacerbate or precipitate lower respiratory tract disorders, particularly asthma [9]. Allergic rhinitis is a multifactorial disease determined by a combination of genetics and the environment. In recent decades, the prevalence of allergic rhinitis among populations has risen steadily, with atmospheric pollution increasingly recognized as a pivotal environmental risk factor [10]. Epidemiological investigations have revealed that exposure to airborne fine particulate matter ($PM_{2.5}$) was associated with heightened rates of clinic visits for allergic rhinitis [11]. Animal studies demonstrated that $PM_{2.5}$ exposure exacerbated nasal allergy symptoms in an ovalbumin (OVA) sensitized murine model of allergic rhinitis [12].

The role of $PM_{2.5}$ in allergic rhinitis has been extensively studied, revealing its capacity to induce cellular oxidative stress and inflammatory responses, particularly in inflamed nasal mucosal epithelial cells [11,13]. $PM_{2.5}$-induced oxidative stress is postulated as a mechanism exacerbating allergic rhinitis symptoms [14]. An allergic rhinitis mouse model study demonstrated that *N*-acetylcysteine, as an antioxidant agent, alleviated $PM_{2.5}$-induced symptoms, underscoring involvement of $PM_{2.5}$ in oxidative stress and inflammation [14]. With advancing research, the epigenetic impacts of $PM_{2.5}$ have been gaining attention in the last decade. Exposure to $PM_{2.5}$ in the nasal mucosa of allergic rhinitis rats induced oxidative stress, which triggered autophagy through the damage of DNA, RNA and proteins. This process potentially exacerbated the condition by intensifying autophagy activity. Furthermore, they discovered that miR-338-3p effectively suppressed the autophagy induced by $PM_{2.5}$ [15]. In an allergic rhinitis mouse model, it was shown that $PM_{2.5}$ exposure led to the elevated DNA methylation of the IFN-$\gamma$ gene promoter in $CD4^+$ T cells, mediated by the ERK-DNMT pathway. This resulted in a reduction in Th1 cell numbers, a perpetuation of the Th1/Th2 imbalance and the exacerbation of allergic rhinitis [16].

Unlike the case with $PM_{2.5}$, epidemiological inquiries into the relationship between sulfur dioxide ($SO_2$) and allergic rhinitis have produced a heterogenous set of results: whereas certain studies have discerned a connection between $SO_2$ exposure and the onset of allergic rhinitis [17], others fail to corroborate this association [18], thereby highlighting an inconclusive landscape. Besides variations in research methodologies, factors such as geographical differences, distinct time frames and the diversity of study populations have also contributed to the complexity of understanding how $SO_2$ impacts allergic rhinitis. In an experiment utilizing an HDM-induced allergic rhinitis mouse model, brief exposure to $SO_2$ not only augmented nasal symptom severity but also elevated serum Immunoglobulin E (IgE) levels and increased the infiltration of eosinophils in allergic rhinitis mice, alongside up-regulated expression of Th1/Th2/Th17 cytokines in the nasal mucosa. Strikingly, they found that prolonged $SO_2$ exposure had the opposing effect of reducing serum IgE levels in these mice [19]. While numerous studies attest to the influence of ozone ($O_3$), nitrogen dioxide ($NO_2$), carbon monoxide (CO) and $SO_2$ on the progression of allergic rhinitis, there is still a relative dearth of dedicated research in this area.

In the realm of epidemiological explorations of allergic rhinitis in relation to air pollution, numerous researchers have employed retrospective studies [20–22] as well as cohort study designs [23,24] to explore the relationships between ambient pollutant concentrations and outpatient-visit frequencies. Existing epidemiological and experimental research has illuminated the link between air pollution and allergic rhinitis, but many questions remain undetermined. One such question pertains to whether a discernible time-delay exists between pollutant exposure and allergic rhinitis symptoms. More attention has been paid to the effects of air pollutants on the incidence and prevalence of allergic rhinitis [25,26], whereas less environmental epidemiological research has been conducted on the effects of ambient air pollutants on the severity of allergic rhinitis symptoms—essentially, on the progression and exacerbation of the condition. These knowledge gaps limit our comprehensive understanding of disease mechanisms and hinder the development of precise prevention and treatment strategies.

In view of the above background, this study aimed to investigate in depth the dynamic relationship between ambient air pollution levels and allergic rhinitis symptoms through a prospective study, with a special focus on the effect on symptoms of fluctuations in pollutants. By integrating data from multiple sources, including air quality monitoring records and the medical records of allergic rhinitis patients, this study could provide new evidence to elucidate the impact of air pollution on allergic rhinitis.

## 2. Materials and Methods

### 2.1. Study Design and Participants

This panel study, conducted from May 2023 to January 2024, recruited patients with allergic rhinitis who visited the same hospital and had lived continuously in Hangzhou city, China, for at least one year. Ultimately, 167 participants agreed to and completed the research study, all of whom lived within 5 km of the hospital. The age range of the participants was around 35 years. Baseline investigations were conducted to gather the demographic details, the medical histories, the family histories and the lifestyle habits of the subjects, which were considered as control variables in the analysis. All included subjects were diagnosed with allergic rhinitis by professional physicians according to the guidelines for the Diagnosis and Treatment of Allergic Rhinitis in China [9]; these guidelines encompass recurrent symptoms such as sneezing, rhinorrhea, nasal blockage and nasal itching, alongside serological confirmation of specific IgE antibodies to allergens. Individuals with severe cardiopulmonary conditions, immune system disorders, those undergoing immunosuppressive therapies, pregnant or breastfeeding individuals and those with non-allergic rhinitis, nasal polyps, or chronic sinusitis were excluded from this study. During the entire study period, the allergic rhinitis symptoms were tracked daily through questionnaires (Table S1). All patients completed the survey and had complete symptom data. Ethical clearance for this research was obtained from the Ethics Committee of Hangzhou Medical College and written informed consent was secured from all participants prior to their enrollment in this study.

### 2.2. Measurement of Ambient Air Pollution Data

Atmospheric quality monitoring data were collected from the China National Environmental Monitoring Center (CNEMC, http://www.cnemc.cn/ (accessed on 24 April 2024)), as announced by the local environmental protection monitoring center. The data were obtained from the average daily air monitoring report in Hangzhou City, where the daily average concentration of ambient air pollutants is calculated as the arithmetic mean of the hourly concentrations over a 24 h period ($O_3$ concentration value is the arithmetic mean of the ozone concentration over the largest consecutive 8 h period of the day). This study focused on the main air pollutants monitored in daily life, including $PM_{10}$, $PM_{2.5}$, $O_3$, $SO_2$, $NO_2$ and CO. This study employed the daily average concentrations of these pollutants as reported by the monitoring center.

### 2.3. Health Effect Measurements

Throughout the follow-up period of this study, information on the allergic rhinitis symptoms of the study subjects was collected. In accordance with the Chinese Guideline for Allergic Rhinitis [9], symptoms included sneezing (the number of episodes of paroxysmal sneezing in a day), rhinorrhea (the number of episodes of nose blowing in a day), nasal blockage and nasal itching, as well as eye itching. The symptom scoring system ranged from a minimum of 0 to a maximum of 3. Details of the specific allergic rhinitis symptom scoring system are presented in Table S1.

### 2.4. Statistical Analysis

All data were expressed as mean ± standard deviation (SD) for the continuous variables or as percentages for the categorical variables. Spearman correlation analysis was used to investigate the correlation between the pollutants. Based on the previous literature [27], generalized linear mixed models (GLMMs) were employed to analyze the nasal symptom changes according to air pollutants among patients, incorporating each unique identifier of the study subject (as a random intercept model) to account for the repeated measurements of symptoms. Guided by the Akaike Information Criterion (AIC), this study exhaustively examined various pollutants and ultimately constructed models encompassing the six atmospheric pollutants, with stratification based on the included pollutants. Given the interdependence among levels of air pollutants, we compared each optimal multi-pollutant model based on the number of pollutants included. The formula for the GLMM is as follows:

$$Y_{it} = b_0 + u_i + A_1X_1 + \ldots + A_nX_n + \beta \text{ Pollutants} + \varepsilon_{it}$$

where $Y_{it}$ is the allergic rhinitis symptom score in the i-th subject at time t, $b_0$ means the total intercept, $u_i$ means the random intercept for the subject i, $X_1$–$X_n$ mean covariates, $A_1$–$A_n$ are regression coefficients for $X_1$–$X_n$, $\beta$ means the regression coefficient for air pollutant and $\varepsilon_{it}$ is the error for the i-th subject at time t.

The corresponding symptoms were represented by $\beta$-values, which can be positive or negative: positive values indicate an increase in the health effect with an increase in pollutant concentration, while negative values indicate a decrease in the health effect. When the 95% confidence intervals of the $\beta$-values include zero, there is no significant correlation between the level of exposure to the pollutant and the health outcome. All statistical analyses were conducted using R software version 4.4.1 (R Foundation for Statistical Computing) and a two-tailed $p$-value < 0.05 was deemed statistically significant.

## 3. Results

### 3.1. Participants

The baseline characteristics of the participants and their symptom scores at enrollment are presented in Table 1. A total of 167 participants were enrolled in this study, with a mean age of 35.4 years. In total, 60 of the participants (35.9%) were male and 107 (64.1%) were female. The mean body mass index (BMI) was 23.9 ± 3.9 kg/m$^2$ for males and 21.1 ± 2.5 kg/m$^2$ for females. The mean serum IgE level among participants was 376.5 IU/mL. Among the participants, 13 (7.8%) were smokers, while 154 (92.2%) were non-smokers. Additionally, 24 (14.4%) participants were alcohol consumers and 143 (85.6%) were non-drinkers. At the time of enrollment, the study participants exhibited symptom scores for allergic rhinitis as follows: sneezing scored 1.4 ± 0.8, nasal blockage scored 2.3 ± 0.8, rhinorrhea scored 1.7 ± 0.7, an itchy nose scored 1.5 ± 0.8 and itchy eyes scored 1.4 ± 0.9. These scores indicate that allergic rhinitis was indeed affecting the daily lives of the study subjects.

**Table 1.** Baseline characteristics of the study population (*N* = 167).

| Variable | Mean ± SD or *N* (%) |
|---|---|
| Age (years) | 35.4 ± 12.1 |
| Gender | |
| Male | 60 (35.9%) |
| Female | 107 (64.1%) |
| High (cm) | |
| Male | 175 ± 5.2 |
| Female | 160.9 ± 5.6 |
| Weight (kg) | |
| Male | 73.4 ± 12.7 |
| Female | 55 ± 7.3 |

**Table 1.** *Cont.*

| Variable | Mean ± SD or *N* (%) |
|---|---|
| BMI (kg/m$^2$) | |
| Male | 23.9 ± 3.9 |
| Female | 21.1 ± 2.5 |
| IgE (IU/mL) | 376.5 ± 398 |
| Smoking status | |
| Smoker | 13 (7.8%) |
| Never smoker | 154 (92.2%) |
| Drinking status | |
| Drinker | 24 (14.4%) |
| Never drinker | 143 (85.6%) |
| Sneezing [a] | 1.4 ± 0.8 |
| Nasal blockage [a] | 2.3 ± 0.8 |
| Rhinorrhea [a] | 1.7 ± 0.7 |
| Itchy nose [a] | 1.5 + 0.8 |
| Itchy eyes [a] | 1.4 ± 0.9 |

[a] The symptom scores at enrollment.

### 3.2. *Ambient Air Pollution*

Table 2 illustrates the daily average concentrations of ambient air pollutants on a monthly basis during the follow-up study period. Notably, $PM_{2.5}$, $PM_{10}$, $SO_2$ and $NO_2$ exhibited evident variations over the progression of months. Specifically, concentrations in the atmosphere demonstrated a gradual decline from May through July, followed by an upward trend from July until January of the following year. Figure 1 depicts the correlations among these air pollutants. These included significant correlations between $PM_{2.5}$ and $PM_{10}$ ($r$ = 0.96), $PM_{2.5}$ and $SO_2$ ($r$ = 0.69), $PM_{2.5}$ and $NO_2$ ($r$ = 0.82), $PM_{2.5}$ and CO ($r$ = 0.66), $PM_{10}$ and $SO_2$ ($r$ = 0.74), $PM_{10}$ and $NO_2$ ($r$ = 0.82), $PM_{10}$ and CO ($r$ = 0.55), $SO_2$ and $NO_2$ ($r$ = 0.73), $SO_2$ and CO ($r$ = 0.32), $NO_2$ and CO ($r$ = 0.55), $NO_2$ and $O_3$ ($r$ = −0.20) and CO and $O_3$ ($r$ = −0.17).

**Table 2.** The means of the ambient air pollutants by month during the follow-up study period.

| | May | June | July | August | September | October | November | December | January |
|---|---|---|---|---|---|---|---|---|---|
| $PM_{2.5}$ (μg/m$^3$) [a] | 27.6 ± 9.8 | 23.2 ± 9.4 | 14.4 ± 5.4 | 19.1 ± 7.7 | 22.1 ± 9.3 | 29.7 ± 15.3 | 34.5 ± 13.6 | 53.4 ± 37.1 | 66.8 ± 32 |
| $PM_{10}$ (μg/m$^3$) [a] | 49.6 ± 18.1 | 39.2 ± 15.4 | 25.8 ± 7.9 | 31.8 ± 10.9 | 34 ± 12.9 | 47.3 ± 19.7 | 63.1 ± 22.1 | 81.1 ± 50.8 | 93 ± 42.4 |
| $SO_2$ (μg/m$^3$) [a] | 6.2 ± 0.8 | 5.9 ± 0.8 | 5.6 ± 0.5 | 5.7 ± 0.4 | 5.9 ± 0.6 | 7.1 ± 0.6 | 7.3 ± 1 | 7.5 ± 1.2 | 7.6 ± 1.3 |
| $NO_2$ (μg/m$^3$) [a] | 26 ± 6.3 | 22.2 ± 4.4 | 16 ± 3.7 | 16.6 ± 3.3 | 19.5 ± 3.2 | 32.4 ± 11.2 | 41.3 ± 12.2 | 49.2 ± 21.2 | 47.3 ± 14.7 |
| CO (mg/m$^3$) [a] | 0.6 ± 0.1 | 0.6 ± 0.1 | 0.6 ± 0.1 | 0.6 ± 0.1 | 0.7 ± 0.1 | 0.6 ± 0.1 | 0.7 ± 0.1 | 0.8 ± 0.2 | 0.9 ± 0.2 |
| $O_3$ (μg/m$^3$) [b] | 128.7 ± 37.5 | 131.9 ± 57.6 | 96.1 ± 33.5 | 130.5 ± 45.7 | 123.9 ± 43.8 | 126.5 ± 29.7 | 77.6 ± 27.9 | 51 ± 22.8 | 57.5 ± 21.4 |

[a] The arithmetic means of the daily average concentrations. [b] The arithmetic means of the daily maximum continuous 8 h concentrations.

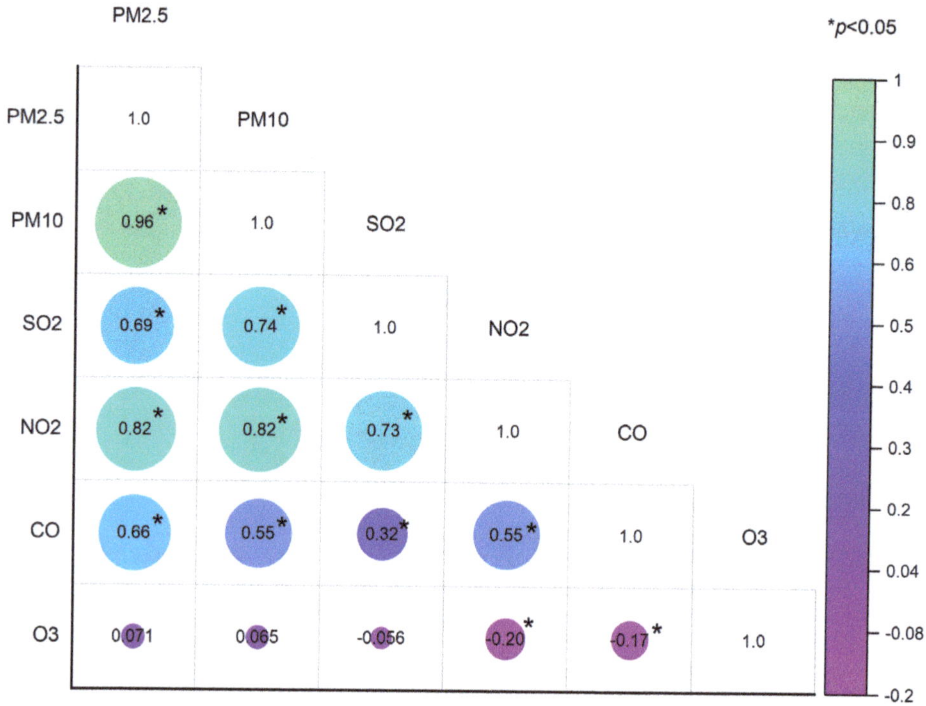


**Figure 1.** The correlation between the air pollutants on lag 0. The numbers of the figure are spearman correlation coefficients. $PM_{2.5}$, particulate matter with diameter < 2.5 μm; $PM_{10}$, particulate matter with diameter < 10 μm; $SO_2$, sulfur dioxide; $NO_2$, nitrogen dioxide; $O_3$, ozone; CO, carbon monoxide.

### 3.3. Lagged Effects of Ambient Air Pollutants on Allergic Rhinitis Symptoms

The lagged effects of the ambient air pollutants on allergic rhinitis symptoms are shown in Figures 2 and S1 and in Table S2. The symptom scores indicate the severity of the symptoms, with higher scores indicating greater severity (Table S1). The $\beta$-values represent the change in symptom scores for each unit increase in pollutant concentration. $PM_{2.5}$ emerged as a prominent influencer, showing statistically significant links with both sneezing ($\beta$ ranging from 0.072 to 0.141, with $p$-values between <0.001 and 0.041) and nasal blockage ($\beta$ ranging from 0.068 to 0.123, $p$-values from 0.006 to 0.034) across lags 0 to 4, peaking in impact at lag 3 for sneezing ($\beta = 0.141, p = 0.019$) and nasal blockage ($\beta = 0.123$, $p = 0.006$). $PM_{10}$ also demonstrated a significant association with sneezing across lags 0 to 3 ($\beta$ ranging from 0.052 to 0.082, $p$-values from 0.009 to 0.045) and with nasal blockage from lags 0 to 2 ($\beta$ ranging from 0.071 to 0.081, $p$-values from 0.002 to 0.024). $NO_2$ exhibited significant correlations with rhinorrhea over lags 0 to 1 ($\beta$ ranging from 0.006 to 0.008, $p$-values from 0.030 to 0.048). CO showed significant correlations with sneezing from lags 0 to 2 ($\beta$ ranging from 0.122 to 0.283, $p$-values from 0.001 to 0.021), with the highest impact observed at lag 2 ($\beta = 0.283, p = 0.001$) and it was correlated with nasal blockage from lag 1 to lag 3 ($\beta$ ranging from 0.101 to 0.236, $p$-values from 0.008 to 0.032), reaching its maximum effect on nasal blockage at lag 2 ($\beta = 0.236, p = 0.008$). $SO_2$ was significantly correlated with sneezing specifically at lag 4 ($\beta = 0.093, p = 0.025$).

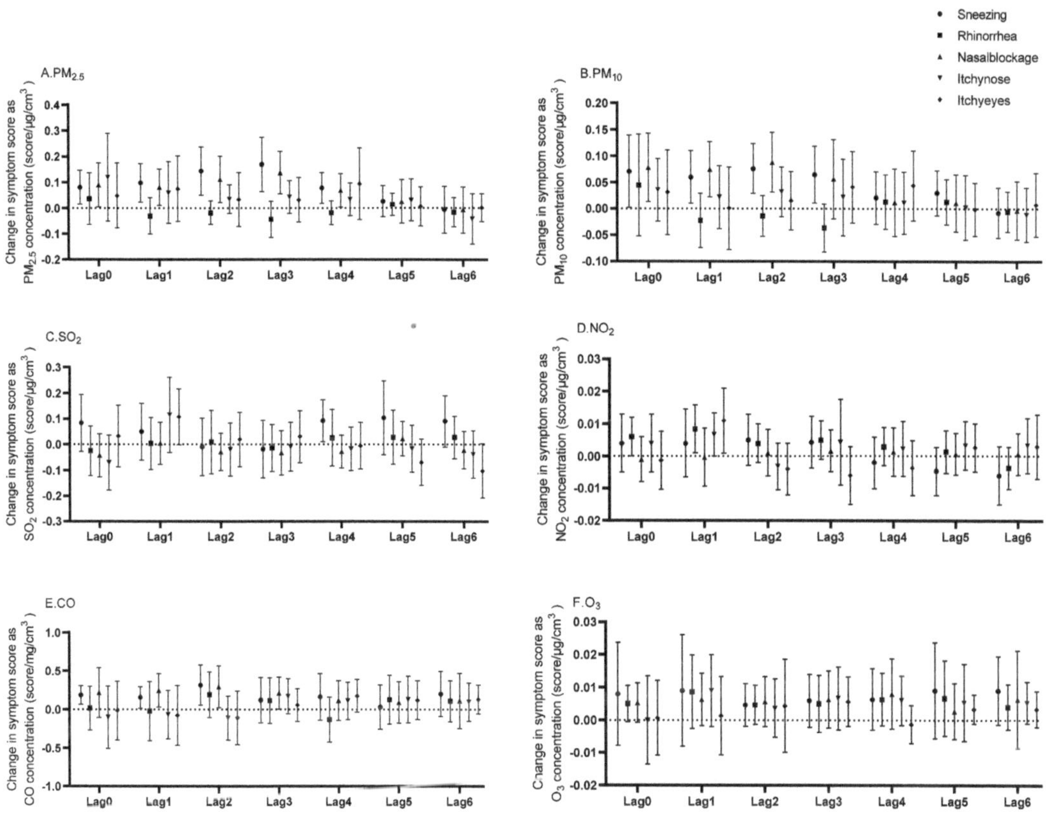


**Figure 2.** Lagged effects of air pollutants on allergic rhinitis symptom scores in patients with allergic rhinitis. Lagged effects of $PM_{2.5}$ (**A**), $PM_{10}$ (**B**), $SO_2$ (**C**), $NO_2$ (**D**), CO (**E**), and $O_3$ (**F**) on allergic rhinitis symptoms are presented. $PM_{2.5}$, particulate matter with diameter < 2.5 μm; $PM_{10}$, particulate matter with diameter < 10 μm; $SO_2$, sulfur dioxide; $NO_2$, nitrogen dioxide; $O_3$, ozone; CO, carbon monoxide.

## 4. Discussion

This study investigated the association between allergic rhinitis symptoms and the levels of ambient air pollutants by tracking changes in the severity of rhinitis symptoms among 167 patients based on the panel design, concurrently monitoring fluctuations in pollutant concentrations during this timeframe. Our findings suggest that certain ambient air pollutants are not only correlated with allergic rhinitis symptoms, but they also show delayed or lagged effects.

In the WHO Global Air Quality Guidelines issued in December 2021 [1], the air quality guideline levels of $PM_{2.5}$, $PM_{10}$, $O_3$, $NO_2$, $SO_2$ and CO were 15 $\mu g/m^3$, 45 $\mu g/m^3$, 100 $\mu g/m^3$, 25 $\mu g/m^3$, 40 $\mu g/m^3$ and 4 $\mu g/m^3$, respectively. During the study period, the concentrations of $PM_{2.5}$, $PM_{10}$ and $NO_2$ were slightly below the guideline levels on some days, generally remaining at the same level. The levels of $SO_2$ and CO were lower than the guideline levels throughout the study period. Therefore, our study has a certain degree of generalizability. Vehicle exhaust emissions, kerosene combustion, industrial emissions and biomass combustion are common sources of ambient air pollutants. Whereas NOx and CO are the main precursors of surface $O_3$ [28], NOx and $SO_2$ are important precursors of $PM_{2.5}$ and their oxidized product $NO_3$ may be the main driver of $PM_{2.5}$ [29,30]. The correlation of PM with CO, $SO_2$ and $NO_2$ was also found in our study, which makes it difficult to isolate the effect of a single pollutant on allergic rhinitis symptoms. This intricate interplay among pollutants explains why the results of related epidemiological studies frequently show inconsistencies and have yet to be fully reconciled.

Considering the complex interactions and potential synergistic effects between pollutants, we used multi-pollutant modeling and found that $PM_{2.5}$, $PM_{10}$, $NO_2$ and CO were each associated with allergic rhinitis symptoms. Specifically, our findings indicate that $PM_{2.5}$, $PM_{10}$ and CO cumulatively affect sneezing and nasal blockage, while $NO_2$ shows a cumulative effect on rhinorrhea, itchy nose and itchy eyes. Consistent with our results, Tang et al. reported that short-term exposures to ambient air pollutants, including $PM_{2.5}$, $PM_{10}$ and CO, were linked to a heightened frequency of outpatient visits for allergic rhinitis [31]. Moreover, elevated outdoor concentrations of $NO_2$ and $PM_{10}$ were correlated with a higher likelihood of airway allergies and allergic rhinitis in children [32]. Luo and colleagues utilized Cox proportional hazard models to evaluate the relationship between long-term air pollutant exposure and allergic rhinitis risk, concluding that prolonged exposure to $PM_{2.5}$, $PM_{10}$ and $NO_2$ elevated the likelihood of developing allergic rhinitis [33]. In alignment with our findings, a cohort investigation revealed a dose–response relationship between chronic air pollution exposure and rhinitis severity in adults. Furthermore, heightened levels of exposure to $PM_{2.5}$, $PM_{10}$ and $NO_2$ were directly linked to intensified rhinitis symptoms [34]. Regarding $SO_2$ and $O_3$, a population-based study found a positive correlation between ambient $SO_2$ levels and allergic rhinitis risk in primary school children [17]. Meanwhile, a strong association between prolonged environmental $O_3$ exposure and an augmented allergic rhinitis symptom risk was reported in children [35]. Conversely, a time-series study reported that exposure to $PM_{10}$, $NO_2$ and $O_3$ significantly elevated the hospitalization risk due to allergic rhinitis, whereas $SO_2$ did not emerge as a significant risk factor for allergic rhinitis-related hospital admissions [18]. Intriguingly, despite $SO_2$ and CO concentrations being well below air quality guideline levels during the study period, we still found a weak correlation between these pollutants and allergic rhinitis symptoms. The association between $O_3$ and increased allergic rhinitis symptoms, however, was not significant. Differences in the results of similar studies might be attributed to variations in the study population, geographic location and timing. These factors can influence the levels and proportions of ambient air pollutants, as well as the age demographics of the study populations. Additionally, regional climate differences may also contribute to these discrepancies.

Regarding the lagged effects of air pollutants on allergic rhinitis, discrepancies in results across different regions, time periods and research methodologies have been observed. In this study, we found that $PM_{2.5}$ was significantly associated with sneezing and nasal blockage symptoms from lag 0 to lag 4. A previous study reported that $PM_{2.5}$ concentrations were associated with an increased risk of allergic rhinitis, occurring at lags 1 and 2, partly aligning with our findings [36]. In a study conducted in Lanzhou, China, short-term exposure to air pollutants was linked to a rise in allergic rhinitis visits, specifically with $O_3$ influencing visits at a lag of 0–6 days and CO at 0–7 days [37]. Another study identified significant associations between CO and $O_3$ exposure and respiratory outpatient visits across lags 0 to 4, but found no significant link between $SO_2$ exposure and such visits. In addition, $NO_2$ was relevant to respiratory outpatient visits only at lag 1 [38]. In this study, $NO_2$ showed a significant correlation with rhinorrhea symptoms at lags 0 to 1, indicating an escalating trend. It also correlated with itchy nose and eye symptoms at lag 1. CO was significantly correlated with nasal symptoms from lag 0 to lag 2, while $SO_2$ was found to have a significant correlation with sneezing symptoms at lag 4. In addition to aligning with previous research findings, the significance of our study lies in its extension beyond the scope of earlier works, which primarily focused on the incidence of allergic rhinitis and hospital visits. Our research narrows the gap by delving into a less-explored realm of nasal allergy symptoms.

In this study, we innovatively employed a panel research methodology to investigate the impact of ambient air pollutants on symptoms of allergic rhinitis, thereby enhancing the credibility of our results and refining our understanding of how individual pollutants affect several typical symptoms of the disease. Nonetheless, it is important to acknowledge its limitations. Our sample solely comprised patients from a single hospital, numbering only 167 individuals, which may limit the generalizability. Additionally, unlike clinical trials, ecological studies cannot directly measure individual exposure levels to ambient air pollutants. For descriptive studies on air pollutants, we used data from atmospheric monitoring stations and applied GLMMs to assess relationships between exposure levels and symptoms. This approach might lead to less accurate study results due to the indirect estimation of exposure. Allergens may have a correlation with pollutants that can also have an effect on allergic rhinitis symptoms. There is no way for this study to assess daily, individual-specific allergen exposure levels. Although allergens may act as a confounding factor, potentially affecting the results, this is a common limitation of ecological research. Similarly, the fact that our survey did not explore the effects of temperature and humidity on the study subjects makes it impossible to determine the effects of temperature and humidity on the results, which is also a limitation of this paper. We plan to recruit more patients to further investigate the impact of air pollution on different types of allergic rhinitis.

## 5. Conclusions

This study employed a prospective follow-up design to investigate the association between a mixture of various ambient air pollutants and the symptoms of allergic rhinitis in patients. This study found that ambient air pollutants were correlated with the severity of allergic rhinitis symptoms, with air pollutants exhibiting delayed effects in the multi-pollutant model. This finding thereby added to the evidence regarding the associations between short-term concurrent exposure to air pollutants and allergic rhinitis symptoms.

**Supplementary Materials:** The following supporting information can be downloaded at https://www.mdpi.com/article/10.3390/toxics12090663/s1. Table S1: Score for allergic rhinitis symptoms; Figure S1: Symptom-by-symptom plot of association between air pollutants and allergic rhinitis symptom scores in patients with allergic rhinitis; and Table S2: Lagged effects of air pollutants on allergic rhinitis symptom scores.

**Author Contributions:** Conceptualization, W.S., J.J. and H.X.; methodology, W.S., J.J. and H.X.; formal analysis, W.S. and C.D.; investigation, W.S., C.D., Z.J. and X.Z.; data curation, W.S. and H.X.; writing—original draft preparation, W.S.; writing—review and editing, W.S., C.D., Z.J. and H.X.; visualization, W.S.; supervision, H.X.; project administration, H.X.; funding acquisition, H.X. All authors have read and agreed to the published version of the manuscript.

**Funding:** This research was funded by the Zhejiang Provincial Natural Science Foundation of China (LQ23H260007), the Scientific Research Fund of Zhejiang Provincial Education Department (Y202249200), the Basic Scientific Research Funds of Department of Education of Zhejiang Province (KYYB202202) and the Key Discipline of Zhejiang Province in Public Health and Preventive Medicine (First Class, Category A).

**Institutional Review Board Statement:** This study was approved by the Ethics Committee of Hangzhou Medical College (No.LL2023-04) and followed the principles of the Helsinki Declaration.

**Informed Consent Statement:** Written informed consent has been obtained from the patients to publish this paper.

**Data Availability Statement:** The data of this study are available upon reasonable request to the corresponding authors.

**Acknowledgments:** All authors sincerely thank all the participants from the hospitals.

**Conflicts of Interest:** The authors declare that they have no competing interests.

## References

1. World Health Organization. Ambient (Outdoor) Air Pollution. Available online: https://www.who.int/news-room/fact-sheets/detail/ambient-(outdoor)-air-quality-and-health (accessed on 24 April 2024).
2. Adamkiewicz, G.; Liddie, J.; Gaffin, J.M. The Respiratory Risks of Ambient/Outdoor Air Pollution. *Clin. Chest Med.* **2020**, *41*, 809–824. [CrossRef] [PubMed]

3. Tran, H.M.; Tsai, F.; Lee, Y.; Chang, J.; Chang, L.; Chang, T.; Chung, K.F.; Kuo, H.; Lee, K.; Chuang, K.; et al. The impact of air pollution on respiratory diseases in an era of climate change: A review of the current evidence. *Sci. Total Environ.* **2023**, *898*, 166340. [CrossRef] [PubMed]
4. Eguiluz-Gracia, I.; Mathioudakis, A.; Bartel, S.; Vijverberg, S.; Fuertes, E.; Comberiati, P.; Cai, Y.; Tomazic, P.; Diamant, Z.; Vestbo, J.; et al. The need for clean air: The way air pollution and climate change affect allergic rhinitis and asthma. *Allergy* **2020**, *75*, 2170–2184. [CrossRef] [PubMed]
5. Maio, S.; Sarno, G.; Tagliaferro, S.; Pirona, F.; Stanisci, I.; Baldacci, S.; Viegi, G. Outdoor air pollution and respiratory health. *Int. J. Tuberc. Lung Dise.* **2023**, *27*, 7–12. [CrossRef] [PubMed]
6. Blaiss, M.S.; Hammerby, E.; Robinson, S.; Kennedy-Martin, T.; Buchs, S. The burden of allergic rhinitis and allergic rhinoconjunctivitis on adolescents: A literature review. *Ann. Allergy Asthma Immunol.* **2018**, *121*, 43–52.e3. [CrossRef] [PubMed]
7. Meltzer, E.O. Allergic Rhinitis: Burden of Illness, Quality of Life, Comorbidities, and Control. *Immunol. Allergy Clin.* **2016**, *36*, 235–248.
8. Zhang, Y.; Zhang, L. Increasing Prevalence of Allergic Rhinitis in China. *Allergy Asthma Immunol. Res.* **2019**, *11*, 156–169. [CrossRef]
9. Cheng, L.; Chen, J.; Fu, Q.; He, S.; Li, H.; Liu, Z.; Tan, G.; Tao, Z.; Wang, D.; Wen, W.; et al. Chinese Society of Allergy Guidelines for Diagnosis and Treatment of Allergic Rhinitis. *Allergy Asthma Immunol. Res.* **2018**, *10*, 300–353. [CrossRef]
10. Nur Husna, S.M.; Tan, H.T.; Md Shukri, N.; Mohd Ashari, N.S.; Wong, K.K. Allergic Rhinitis: A Clinical and Pathophysiological Overview. *Front. Med.-Lausanne* **2022**, *9*, 874114. [CrossRef]
11. Lin, L.; Li, T.; Sun, M.; Liang, Q.; Ma, Y.; Wang, F.; Duan, J.; Sun, Z. Effect of particulate matter exposure on the prevalence of allergic rhinitis in children: A systematic review and meta-analysis. *Chemosphere* **2021**, *268*, 128841. [CrossRef]
12. Piao, C.H.; Fan, Y.; Nguyen, T.V.; Shin, H.S.; Kim, H.T.; Song, C.H.; Chai, O.H. PM(2.5) Exacerbates Oxidative Stress and Inflammatory Response through the Nrf2/NF-κB Signaling Pathway in OVA-Induced Allergic Rhinitis Mouse Model. *Int. J. Mol. Sci.* **2021**, *22*, 8173. [CrossRef] [PubMed]
13. Li, S.; Wu, W.; Wang, G.; Zhang, X.; Guo, Q.; Wang, B.; Cao, S.; Yan, M.; Pan, X.; Xue, T.; et al. Association between exposure to air pollution and risk of allergic rhinitis: A systematic review and meta-analysis. *Environ. Res.* **2022**, *205*, 112472. [CrossRef] [PubMed]
14. Wang, J.; Guo, Z.; Zhang, R.; Han, Z.; Huang, Y.; Deng, C.; Dong, W.; Zhuang, G. Effects of N-acetylcysteine on oxidative stress and inflammation reactions in a rat model of allergic rhinitis after $PM_{2.5}$ exposure. *Biochem. Biophys. Res. Commun.* **2020**, *533*, 275–281. [CrossRef] [PubMed]
15. Wang, J.; Huang, Y.; Zhang, R.; Han, Z.; Zhou, L.; Sun, N.; Dong, W.; Zhuang, G. miR-338-3p inhibits autophagy in a rat model of allergic rhinitis after $PM_{2.5}$ exposure through AKT/mTOR signaling by targeting UBE2Q1. *Biochem. Biophys. Res. Commun.* **2021**, *554*, 1–6. [CrossRef]
16. Li, Y.; Zhou, J.; Rui, X.; Zhou, L.; Mo, X. $PM_{2.5}$ exposure exacerbates allergic rhinitis in mice by increasing DNA methylation in the IFN-γ gene promoter in CD4+T cells via the ERK-DNMT pathway. *Toxicol. Lett.* **2019**, *301*, 98–107. [CrossRef]
17. Kim, S.H.; Lee, J.; Oh, I.; Oh, Y.; Sim, C.; Bang, J.; Park, J.; Kim, Y. Allergic rhinitis is associated with atmospheric SO2: Follow-up study of children from elementary schools in Ulsan, Korea. *PLoS ONE* **2021**, *16*, e0248624. [CrossRef]
18. Dąbrowiecki, P.; Chciałowski, A.; Dąbrowiecka, A.; Piórkowska, A.; Badyda, A. Exposure to ambient air pollutants and short-term risk for exacerbations of allergic rhinitis: A time-stratified, case-crossover study in the three largest urban agglomerations in Poland. *Respir. Physiol. Neurobiol.* **2023**, *315*, 104095. [CrossRef]
19. Ye, M.; Liu, H.; Li, H.; Liu, Q.; Zhou, Z.; Wang, T.; Tan, G. Long-Term Exposure to Sulfur Dioxide Before Sensitization Decreased the Production of Specific IgE in HDM-Sensitized Allergic Rhinitis Mice. *J. Inflamm. Res.* **2022**, *15*, 2477–2490. [CrossRef]
20. Wang, J.; Lu, M.; An, Z.; Jiang, J.; Li, J.; Wang, Y.; Du, S.; Zhang, X.; Zhou, H.; Cui, J.; et al. Associations between air pollution and outpatient visits for allergic rhinitis in Xinxiang, China. *Environ. Sci. Pollut. Res. Int.* **2020**, *27*, 23565–23574. [CrossRef]
21. Wang, M.; Wang, S.; Wang, X.; Tian, Y.; Wu, Y.; Cao, Y.; Song, J.; Wu, T.; Hu, Y. The association between PM(2.5) exposure and daily outpatient visits for allergic rhinitis: Evidence from a seriously air-polluted environment. *Int. J. Biometeorol.* **2020**, *64*, 139–144. [CrossRef]
22. Wu, R.; Guo, Q.; Fan, J.; Guo, C.; Wang, G.; Wu, W.; Xu, J. Association between air pollution and outpatient visits for allergic rhinitis: Effect modification by ambient temperature and relative humidity. *Sci. Total Environ.* **2022**, *821*, 152960. [CrossRef] [PubMed]
23. Chen, J.; Zeng, Y.; Lau, A.K.; Guo, C.; Wei, X.; Lin, C.; Huang, B.; Lao, X.Q. Chronic exposure to ambient $PM_{2.5}/NO_2$ and respiratory health in school children: A prospective cohort study in Hong Kong. *Ecotoxicol. Environ. Saf.* **2023**, *252*, 114558. [CrossRef] [PubMed]
24. Lu, C.; Wang, F.; Liu, Z.; Li, B.; Yang, W.; Liao, H. Intrauterine and early postnatal exposure to air pollution associated with childhood allergic rhinitis. *Chemosphere* **2023**, *336*, 139296. [CrossRef] [PubMed]
25. Rosario, C.S.; Urrutia-Pereira, M.; Murrieta-Aguttes, M.; D'Amato, G.; Chong-Silva, D.C.; Godoi, R.H.M.; Rosario Filho, N.A. Air pollution and rhinitis. *Front. Allergy* **2024**, *5*, 1387525. [CrossRef]
26. Zhang, S.; Fu, Q.; Wang, S.; Jin, X.; Tan, J.; Ding, K.; Zhang, Q.; Li, X. Association between air pollution and the prevalence of allergic rhinitis in Chinese children: A systematic review and meta-analysis. *Allergy Asthma Proc.* **2022**, *43*, e47–e57. [CrossRef] [PubMed]

27. Lee, H.Y.; Kim, H.; Kim, H.J.; Na, G.; Jang, Y.; Kim, S.H.; Kim, N.H.; Kim, H.C.; Park, Y.; Kim, H.C.; et al. The impact of ambient air pollution on lung function and respiratory symptoms in elite athletes. *Sci. Total Environ.* **2023**, *855*, 158862. [CrossRef]
28. Sharma, A.; Mandal, T.K.; Sharma, S.; Shukla, D.; Singh, S.N. Relationships of surface ozone with its precursors, particulate matter and meteorology over Delhi. *J. Atmos. Chem.* **2017**, *74*, 451–474. [CrossRef]
29. Kelly, J.T.; Reff, A.; Gantt, B. A method to predict $PM_{2.5}$ resulting from compliance with national ambient air quality standards. *Atmos. Environ.* **2017**, *162*, 1–10. [CrossRef]
30. Su, T.; Li, J.; Tian, C.; Zong, Z.; Chen, D.; Zhang, G. Source and formation of fine particulate nitrate in South China: Constrained by isotopic modeling and online trace gas analysis. *Atmos. Environ.* **2020**, *231*, 117563. [CrossRef]
31. Tang, W.; Sun, L.; Wang, J.; Li, K.; Liu, S.; Wang, M.; Cheng, Y.; Dai, L. Exploring Associations Between Short-Term Air Pollution and Daily Outpatient Visits for Allergic Rhinitis. *Risk Manag. Healthc. Policy* **2023**, *16*, 1455–1465. [CrossRef]
32. Liu, W.; Cai, J.; Fu, Q.; Zou, Z.; Sun, C.; Zhang, J.; Huang, C. Associations of ambient air pollutants with airway and allergic symptoms in 13,335 preschoolers in Shanghai, China. *Chemosphere* **2020**, *252*, 126600. [CrossRef] [PubMed]
33. Luo, P.; Ying, J.; Li, J.; Yang, Z.; Sun, X.; Ye, D.; Liu, C.; Wang, J.; Mao, Y. Air Pollution and Allergic Rhinitis: Findings from a Prospective Cohort Study. *Environ. Sci. Technol.* **2023**, *57*, 15835–15845. [CrossRef] [PubMed]
34. Burte, E.; Leynaert, B.; Marcon, A.; Bousquet, J.; Benmerad, M.; Bono, R.; Carsin, A.; de Hoogh, K.; Forsberg, B.; Gormand, F.; et al. Long-term air pollution exposure is associated with increased severity of rhinitis in 2 European cohorts. *J. Allergy Clin. Immunol.* **2020**, *145*, 834–842.e6. [CrossRef] [PubMed]
35. Zhou, P.; Qian, Z.; McMillin, S.; Vaughn, M.; Xie, Z.; Xu, Y.; Lin, L.; Hu, L.; Yang, B.; Zeng, X.; et al. Relationships between Long-Term Ozone Exposure and Allergic Rhinitis and Bronchitic Symptoms in Chinese Children. *Toxics* **2021**, *9*, 221. [CrossRef]
36. Chai, G.; He, H.; Sha, Y.; Zhai, G.; Zong, S. Effect of PM(2.5) on daily outpatient visits for respiratory diseases in Lanzhou, China. *Sci. Total Environ.* **2019**, *649*, 1563–1572. [CrossRef] [PubMed]
37. Ji, J.; Chen, K.; Dong, J.; Yu, H.; Zhang, Y. Associations between air pollution and outpatient visits for allergic rhinitis in Lanzhou, China. *Environ. Sci. Pollut. Res. Int.* **2023**, *30*, 91453–91465. [CrossRef]
38. Liu, C.; Liu, Y.; Zhou, Y.; Feng, A.; Wang, C.; Shi, T. Short-term effect of relatively low level air pollution on outpatient visit in Shennongjia, China. *Environ. Pollut.* **2019**, *245*, 419–426. [CrossRef]

*toxics*

MDPI

*Article*

# Lentinan Alleviated PM2.5 Exposure-Induced Epithelial–Mesenchymal Transition in Pulmonary Epithelial Cells by Inhibiting the GARP/TGF-β/Smad Pathway

**Zhi Wang [1], Shiqing Xu [1], Bohao Bian [2], Zhida Hu [3], Feiyang Wu [1], Siqi Zhao [1], Xiaohui Wang [1], Li Wang [1,*] and Teng Ma [1,*]**

[1] School of Public Health, Baotou Medical College, Inner Mongolia University of Science & Technology, Baotou 014040, China; 2022200104@stu.btmc.edu.cn (Z.W.); 2022200097@stu.btmc.edu.cn (S.X.); 17302256519@163.com (F.W.); sqtjzy@163.com (S.Z.); 102018909@btmc.edu.cn (X.W.)

[2] Hulunbuir Center for Disease Control and Prevention, Hulun Buir 021000, China; 13604749342@163.com

[3] Cangzhou People's Hospital, Department of Hospital Infection Management, Cangzhou 061000, China; 2021400116@stu.btmc.edu.cn

* Correspondence: 101995002@btmc.edu.cn (L.W.); 102018924@btmc.edu.cn (T.M.)

**Abstract:** PM2.5 (fine particulate matter) is an air pollutant widely present in urban and industrial areas, which has emerged as a significant threat to human health. Specifically, long-term exposure to PM2.5 could lead to various lung diseases, including pulmonary fibrosis and Chronic Obstructive Pulmonary Disease (COPD). The Glycoprotein A Repetitions Predominant (GARP) protein, a key receptor and regulator for TGF-β1, has recently emerged as a vital cytokine in PM2.5-induced pulmonary pathological changes. As a membrane glycoprotein, GARP binds to TGF-β, keeping it in an active state. Herein, PM2.5 treatment upregulated GARP and promoted Epithelial–Mesenchymal Transition (EMT) via TGF-β/SMAD signaling pathway activation. Conversely, lentinan (a shiitake mushroom-derived polysaccharide) effectively reversed the PM2.5-induced GARP upregulation, alleviating EMT. This study elucidates the role of GARP in PM2.5-induced EMT through the TGF-β/SMAD pathway in pulmonary epithelial cells and discusses the therapeutic potential of lentinan.

**Keywords:** COPD; PM2.5; lentinan; GARP; EMT

## 1. Introduction

Lung diseases account for a substantial proportion of morbidities and mortalities worldwide, posing significant health risks [1]. Air pollution—especially by fine particulate matter (PM2.5)—is among the many factors that contribute to the development of respiratory illnesses [2]. Owing to the fact that they are small enough to penetrate deep into the lungs and enter the bloodstream, PM2.5 particles have been linked to various respiratory conditions, ranging from chronic bronchitis to more severe complications such as emphysema and lung fibrosis [3–5]. According to the research, long-term exposure to PM2.5 could exacerbate inflammation in the airways [6], triggering symptoms such as coughing [7], wheezing [8], and shortness of breath [9]. Moreover, prolonged PM2.5 exposure could increase the risk of developing more severe lung conditions, with its impact also extending to the cardiovascular system, further complicating overall health [10]. Therefore, given the ubiquity of PM2.5 in urban and industrial areas, addressing air pollution could be crucial to reducing the burden of lung diseases and improving public health.

The specific mechanism of PM2.5 exposure in lung diseases involves the exacerbation of airway inflammation and remodeling, which activates Epithelial–Mesenchymal Transition (EMT) processes in lung epithelial cells [11]. The cellular alterations that follow promote airway obstruction and pulmonary fibrosis, which are hallmarks of Chronic Obstructive Pulmonary Disease (COPD) [12]. According to research, EMT contributes to the loss of epithelial integrity, elevating the risk of respiratory infections and causing a further decline in lung function [13]. Therefore, understanding the mechanisms through which PM2.5 mediates EMT could provide crucial insights into the treatment of lung diseases. Regarding tumorigenesis, PM2.5 could also induce chronic inflammation and Oxidative Stress (OS), which are crucial factors that promote EMT in various cancer types [14]. Furthermore, PM2.5 exposure could trigger signaling pathways such as TGF-β and NF-κB [15], a transition that enhances cancer cell migratory and invasive capabilities, contributing to metastasis and a poor prognosis [16,17].

Lentinan, a polysaccharide derived from the cell wall of shiitake mushrooms, could strengthen the host immune system, helping in preventing various illnesses. Lentinan has been shown to exert anti-inflammatory effects via immune response modulation [18]. Specifically, it could inhibit the secretion of pro-inflammatory cytokines such as TNF-α, IL-6, and IL-1β, thus reducing inflammation. Lentinan achieves this effect through the regulation of key signaling pathways, including the NF-κB and MAPK pathways, which are crucially involved in inflammatory responses [19]. Research has reported lentinan's potential in alleviating chronic inflammatory illnesses, such as Rheumatoid Arthritis (RA) and Inflammatory Bowel Disease (IBD), highlighting its potential utility as an adjunctive therapy to conventional anti-inflammatory treatments [20]. The anti-inflammatory properties of lentinan could also help reduce airway hyper-responsiveness and tissue damage in asthma and COPD patients. Additionally, lentinan could play an anti-tumor role by alleviating inflammatory response and reducing the production of EMT [21]. Nonetheless, research on the role of lentinan in alleviating air pollutant-induced EMT is relatively scarce.

The Glycoprotein A Repetitions Predominant (GARP) protein is a transmembrane protein that regulates TGF-β on the cell surface by binding to it, thus activating the TGF-β signaling pathway [22]. In cancer, GARP enhances TGF-β activation, thus promoting EMT, which, in turn, leads to increased tumor cell migration and invasion, ultimately promoting tumor progression and metastasis [23]. Moreover, GARP upregulation has been associated with immune evasion in various malignancies, further supporting tumor growth [24,25]. In respiratory diseases, particularly COPD and asthma, GARP upregulation might contribute to airway remodeling and fibrosis via TGF-β-mediated EMT, resulting in airway obstruction and reduced lung function [26]. Furthermore, GARP could influence inflammatory responses within the airways, exacerbating symptoms of pertinent conditions [27]. However, the role of GARP in PM2.5-induced lung diseases remains unclear. Although the role of GARP in immune modulation and cancer has been extensively studied, its involvement in particulate matter-induced EMT, particularly in respiratory diseases, remains largely unexplored. This study is the first to identify GARP as a key regulator of PM2.5-induced EMT and to investigate the therapeutic potential of lentinan, in mitigating this process. The results offer new perspectives on PM2.5's pathological effects on lungs, suggesting GARP's promise in treating airway illnesses.

## 2. Materials and Methods

### 2.1. Cell Culture and PM2.5 Sampling and Preparation

Beas-2B human bronchial epithelial cells were obtained from Pricella Life Science and Technology Co., Ltd. (Wuhan, China). The cell culture was maintained in Dulbecco's Modified Eagle Medium (DMEM) (Gibco, Gaithersburg, MD, USA). To create the complete medium, we supplemented the DMEM with 10% Fetal Bovine Serum (FBS) (Gibco, Gaithersburg, MD, USA) and a 1% antibiotic solution [containing 100 IU/mL penicillin and 100 μg/mL streptomycin (Beyotime, Shanghai, China)]. The cells were grown in a humidified incubator (Thermo Scientific, Waltham, MA, USA), maintaining a temperature of 37 °C and a 5% $CO_2$ atmosphere. Upon reaching 80–90% confluency, the Beas-2B cells were trypsinized to detach them, then replated uniformly in well plates or culture dishes. Subsequently, these cells were exposed to varying concentrations of PM2.5 culture solution for a 24 h period before being harvested for further experimentation.

Herein, PM2.5 was sampled 1.5 m above the ground on the roof of Baotou Medical College's laboratory building using an air sampler KB-6210 with a flow rate of 100 L/min. The sampling lasted 21 h (from 9:00 to 6:00 the next day), and the sampling temperature, air pressure, and site conditions were recorded. The collected samples were folded in half twice using tweezers, placed in tinfoil, and balanced in a dryer for 24 h. We previously conducted a chemical analysis of the composition of PM2.5. Research showed that rare earth elements exhibit a strong positive correlation with inorganic elements, indicating a consistent source or shared anthropogenic influences, primarily from coal and oil combustion as well as industrial pollution. The high enrichment factors of Se, Cd, Ag, Pb, and As in PM2.5 suggest that their origins are largely attributed to anthropogenic pollution, with minimal influence from crustal sources [28]. After removing the filter membrane, the samples were weighed with the same electronic balance as before sampling, and stored in a refrigerator at 20 °C, awaiting further tests. Subsequently, the particles were dissolved in DMEM at a concentration of 1000 μg/mL and stored at 4 °C in the laboratory, awaiting further study. Finally, the cells were treated with different concentrations of PM2.5 (0, 6.25, 12.5, and 25 μg/mL) for 24 h.

### 2.2. Cell Proliferation Assay

Cell viability was evaluated utilizing the Cell Counting Kit-8 (CCK-8) assay (Biosharp, Hefei, China). In summary, BEAS-2B cells were plated at a density of 5000 cells per well in 96-well plates and exposed to different concentrations of PM2.5 for 24 h. For the experimental group, the culture medium was continuously refreshed with a new solution containing lentinan. After the incubation period, the old medium was discarded and substituted with an equal volume of fresh medium enriched with 10% CCK-8 reagent. The cells were then further incubated for 2 h at 37 °C. Ultimately, the absorbance was recorded at 450 nm using a microplate reader (Multiskan MK3, Thermo Fisher Scientific, Waltham, MA, USA).

### 2.3. Wound Healing Assay (WHA)

First, Beas-2B cells from each group were inoculated into 6-well plates. At 70–80% growth, a straight line was evenly drawn in the pores with a 200 μL gun tip. After cleaning the cell fragments with PBS, a serum-free medium was added. The images of cells were observed at 0 and 24 h and photographed using a microscope. The scratch area was quantified using ImageJ version 1.50 software.

### 2.4. Transwell Assay (TWA)

Cellular invasion was evaluated using a Transwell chamber setup. Initially, Matrigel was mixed with DMEM at a dilution of 1:8. This blend was then placed into cold Transwell chambers (8 μm pore size, Corning, New York, NY, USA) and left to incubate at 37 °C for 2 h to facilitate gel solidification. Subsequently, a cell suspension at a concentration of $1 \times 10^5$/mL was prepared, and 100 μL of this suspension was introduced into the upper chamber containing serum-free medium. Meanwhile, the lower chamber was filled with 700 μL of DMEM enriched with 10% FBS. After a 48 h incubation period, cells that migrated to the lower side of the membrane were counted using an inverted microscope and stained with crystal violet. To fix the cells, a 4% Paraformaldehyde (PFA) solution was applied for 15 min.

### 2.5. Real-Time Polymerase Chain Reaction (RT-PCR)

Herein, RT-PCR was performed using the Applied Biosystems GeneAmp 9700 PCR system (Applied Biosystems), with human GAPDH employed as an internal control. All real-time data were analyzed using the comparative Ct method and normalized to GAPDH. The primers for the amplification of GARP cDNA were as follows: forward (5′–3′): GCATAGCAACGTGCTGATGGAC; reverse (5′–3′): GATGCTGTTGCAGCTCAGGTCT. The primers for the amplification of TGF-β1 cDNA were as follows: forward (5′–3′): TACCTGAACCCGTGTTGCTCTC; reverse (5′–3′): GTTGCTGAGGTATCGCCAGGAA. The primers used to amplify GAPDH were as follows: forward (5′–3′): ACAACTTTGGTATCGTGGAAGG; reverse (5′–3′): GCCATCACGCCACAGTTTC.

### 2.6. Western Blot (WB) Assay

Cells were collected, and protein levels were quantified via the BCA assay kit (Beyotime, Beijing, China). Following this, proteins underwent separation using SDS-PAGE, which were subsequently transferred onto PVDF membranes (Millipore, Burlington, NJ, USA). The membranes were then blocked with 5% non-fat milk for a duration of 2 h before being incubated overnight at 4 °C with primary antibodies targeting Vimentin (1:1000; Affinity, Cincinnati, OH, USA), E-Cadherin (1:1000; Affinity, Cincinnati, OH, USA), N-Cadherin (1:1000; Affinity, Cincinnati, OH, USA), GARP (1:1000; Proteintech, Wuhan, China), TGF-β1 (1:800; Abcam, Cambridge, UK), p-SMAD2/3 (1:1000; Abcam, Cambridge, UK), and β-Actin (1:10,000; Affinity, Cincinnati, OH, USA). After this incubation, the membranes were treated with HRP-conjugated secondary antibodies (1:5000; Affinity, Cincinnati, OH, USA) at room temperature for an hour. Lastly, the membranes were visualized using ECL reagent (APPLYGEN, Beijing, China).

### 2.7. RNA Interference

GARP inhibitor (si-GARP) and si-GARP Negative Control (si-NC) were sourced from IGEBio (Guangzhou, China). Liposome 2000 reagent (Invitrogen) was used to complete the transfection. Briefly, the cells were first inoculated onto a six-well plate. Afterward, a MEM solution infused with either si-GARP or si-NC was combined with another MEM solution containing Liposome 2000 reagent. This concoction was then employed to transfect the cells over a 6 h period. Once the transfection was complete, the cells were subjected to PM2.5 exposure for 24 h, after which they were harvested and stored, ready for subsequent experimental procedures.

### 2.8. Statistical Analysis

Each experiment was conducted three separate times. We used GraphPad Prism 9.0 for all statistical analyses. When comparing the two groups, we ran a Student's $t$-test. For comparisons involving more than two groups, we used a one-way ANOVA followed by Tukey's post hoc test. We considered results with * $p < 0.05$ to be statistically significant, and those with ** $p < 0.01$ to be highly significant.PM2.5

## 3. Results

### *3.1. Lentinan Reversed the PM2.5-Induced Decrease in Cell Activity*

Following exposure to varying levels of PM2.5 and lentinan, cell viability was evaluated using the CCK-8 assay. The findings revealed that, when compared to the control group, cells treated with a PM2.5 concentration of 12.5 μg/mL showed a notable decline in proliferation activity ($p < 0.01$) (Figure 1A). For subsequent experiments, PM2.5 doses of 6.25, 12.5, and 25 μg/mL were chosen as the focus groups. In contrast, while treatment with 50/100 μg/mL lentinan failed to counteract the diminished cell viability caused by PM2.5 exposure, a significant improvement was observed at a lentinan concentration of 200 μg/mL ($p < 0.05$) (Figure 1B). As a result, 200 μg/mL lentinan was selected for further experimental treatments.

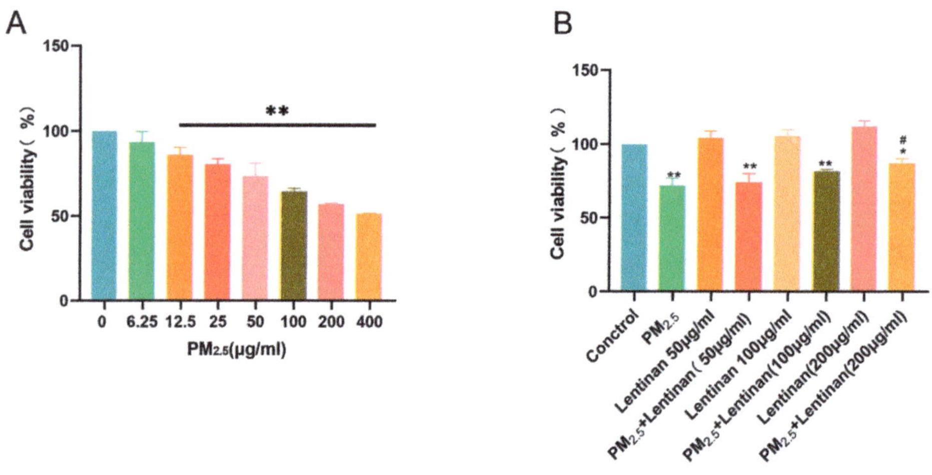


**Figure 1.** Lentinan reversed the PM2.5-induced decreased cell activity: (**A**) CCK-8-detected effect of different concentrations of PM2.5 on Beas-2B cell viability after 24 h of treatment; and (**B**) CCK-8-assessed protective effect of lentinan onPM2.5-induced cell damage. Compared to the control group, *: $p < 0.05$, **: $p < 0.01$. Compared to the PM2.5 group, #: $p < 0.05$. n = 3.

### *3.2. PM2.5 Promoted Invasive, Migratory, and EMT Induction Abilities in Beas-2B Cells*

After treatment with different concentrations of PM2.5 (0, 6.25, 12.5, and 25 μg/mL) for 24 h, Beas-2B cells were assessed for their migratory, invasive, and EMT induction abilities using WHA, TWA, and WB. Compared to the control group, Beas-2B cells exposed to PM2.5 exhibited higher migratory and invasive abilities (Figure 2A,B). Furthermore, PM2.5 significantly upregulated N-Cadherin and Vimentin, and downregulated E-Cadherin, in a dose-dependent manner, suggesting that it induced the EMT process in Beas-2B cells (Figure 2C).

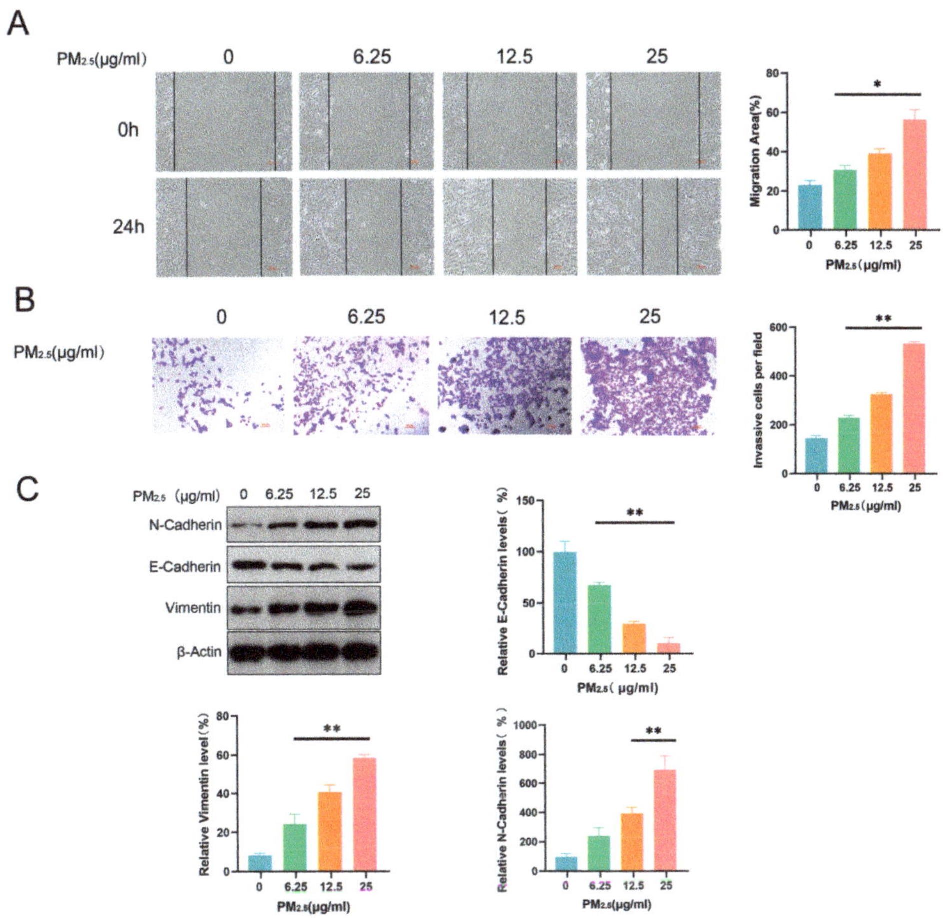


**Figure 2.** PM2.5 enhanced the invasive, migratory, and EMT induction abilities of Beas-2B cells. (**A**) WHA-detected migratory ability of Beas-2B cells; (**B**) TWA-detected invasive ability of Beas-2B cells; and (**C**) WB-detected expression of EMT-related proteins N-Cadherin, E-Cadherin, and Vimentin. *: $p < 0.05$, **: $p < 0.01$.

### *3.3. PM2.5 Activated the GARP/TGF-β/Smad Pathway*

Herein, network-based predictions were performed using Genemania databases to investigate the potential interaction between GARP and TGF-β. We found that GARP (LRRC32) could interact with TGF-β, implying the former's direct or indirect involvement in the regulation of the TGF-β/SMAD pathway under PM2.5 exposure (Figure 3A). To establish whether PM2.5 impacted the GARP/TGF-β/Smad pathway, proteins related to this pathway were detected through WB after exposure to PM2.5 for 24 h. According to the results, the GARP, TGF-β1, and p-Smad2/3 proteins in the cells were significantly upregulated after exposure to PM2.5 (Figure 3B). Subsequently, the mRNA contents of GARP and TGF-β1 were detected using PCR, revealing that the mRNA expression levels of GARP and TGF-β1 increased with the PM2.5 exposure dose (Figure 3C,D). These findings suggest that PM2.5 can activate the GARP/TGF-β/Smad pathway.

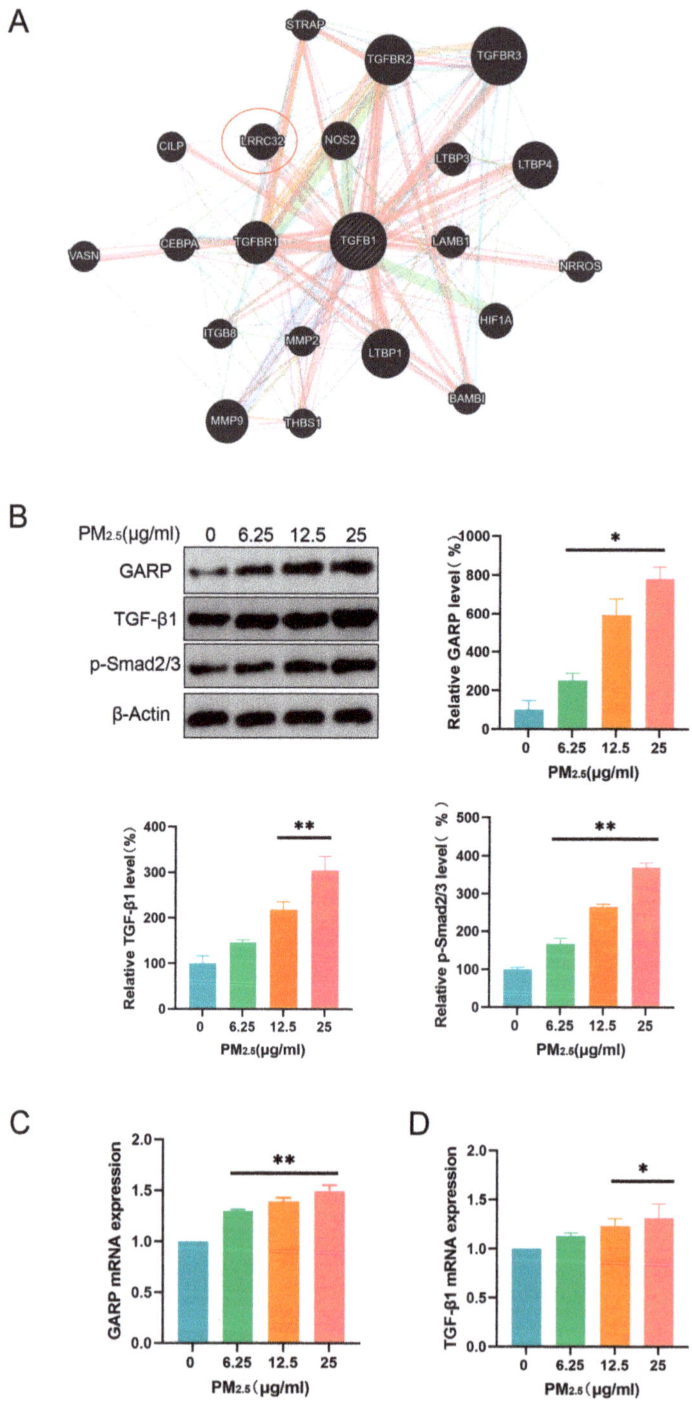


**Figure 3.** PM2.5 activated the GARP/TGF-β/Smad pathway: (**A**) Protein binding was predicted using Genemania databases; (**B**) WB analysis of GARP/TGF-β/Smad pathway-associated proteins; (**C**) PCR-detected relative GARP mRNA expression; and (**D**) PCR-detected relative TGF-β1 mRNA expression. *: $p < 0.05$, **: $p < 0.01$.

### *3.4. GARP Knockdown Reversed the Effects of PM2.5 on Beas-2B Cell Migratory, Invasive, and EMT Induction Abilities*

To establish whether the GARP/TGF-β/Smad axis correlated with the effect of PM2.5 on Beas-2B cells, we successfully constructed a GARP knockdown cell model (Figure 4A). According to the results, GARP downregulation inhibited the migratory and invasive abilities of PM2.5-exposed cells (Figure 4B,C). Furthermore, N-Cadherin and Vimentin were significantly downregulated, while E-Cadherin was upregulated, suggesting that inhibiting the GARP/TGF-β/Smad pathway could reverse the PM2.5-induced EMT process in Beas-2B cells (Figure 4D).

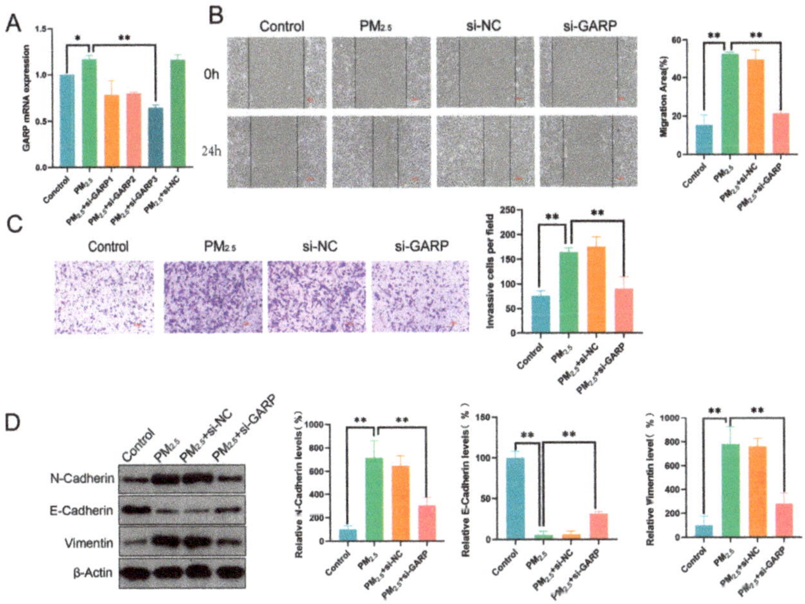

**Figure 4.** GARP knockdown reversed the effects of PM2.5 on Beas-2B cell migratory, invasive, and EMT induction abilities: (**A**) PCR-detected GARP expression; (**B**) WHA-detected migratory ability of Beas-2B cells; (**C**) TWA-detected invasive ability of Beas-2B cells; and (**D**) WB-detected expression of EMT-related proteins N-Cadherin, E-Cadherin, and Vimentin. *: $p < 0.05$, **: $p < 0.01$.

### *3.5. Lentinan Mitigated the Impact of PM2.5 on Beas-2B Cells*

Herein, Beas-2B cells were exposed to PM2.5 for 24 h and then treated with lentinan for an additional 24 h to establish whether the latter treatment could mitigate the effect of PM2.5 on the cells. Subsequently, the migratory, invasive, and EMT induction abilities of the cells were detected using WHA, TWA, and WB. According to the results, lentinan effectively suppressed the migratory and invasive properties of cells exposed to PM2.5 (Figure 5A,B). Additionally, in comparison to the PM2.5 group, treatment with lentinan led to a marked decrease in the expression of N-Cadherin and Vimentin, while simultaneously increasing the expression of E-Cadherin. This suggests that lentinan has the potential to reverse the EMT process induced by PM2.5 in Beas-2B cells (Figure 5C).

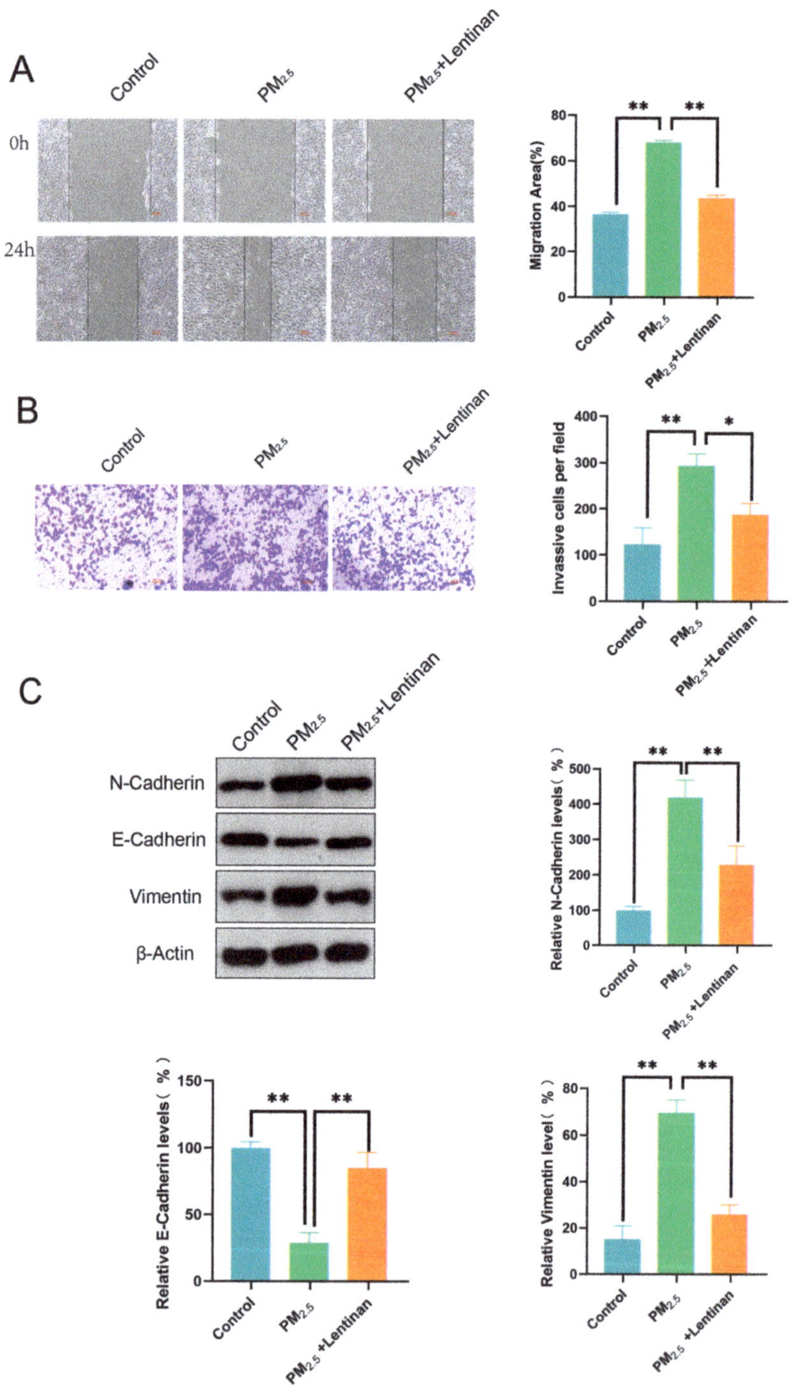


**Figure 5.** Lentinan inhibited the PM2.5-induced migratory, invasive, and EMT induction abilities of Beas-2B cells: (**A**) WHA-detected migratory ability of Beas-2B cells; (**B**) TWA-detected invasive ability of Beas-2B cells; and (**C**) WB-detected expression of EMT-related proteins N-Cadherin, E-Cadherin, and Vimentin. *: $p < 0.05$, **: $p < 0.01$.

### 3.6. Lentinan Inhibited the PM2.5-Induced GARP/TGF-β/Smad Pathway Activation

To establish whether lentinan treatment could impact the GARP/TGF-β/Smad pathway in PM2.5-exposed cells, potential EMT targets and major compounds were subjected to molecular docking analysis using Discovery Studio CDOCKER. The main extract of lentinan was selected for docking with key GARP targets, revealing that the ligands and receptors exhibited binding properties (Figure 6A). Proteins associated with the GARP/TGF-β/Smad pathway were detected through WB analysis 24 h after lentinan treatment. According to the results, the expression of the GARP, TGF-β1, and p-Smad2/3 proteins was significantly lower post-treatment compared to the PM2.5 exposure group (Figure 6B). Subsequently, GARP and TGF-β1 mRNA levels were detected using PCR, revealing that the mRNA expression levels of GARP and TGF-β1 were lower compared to those in the PM2.5-exposed group (Figure 6C,D). These findings suggest that lentinan inhibited the PM2.5-induced GARP/TGF-β/Smad pathway activation. Thus, it is demonstrated that Lentinan alleviated PM2.5 exposure-induced epithelial–mesenchymal transition in pulmonary epithelial cells by inhibiting the GARP/TGF-β/Smad pathway (Figure 7).

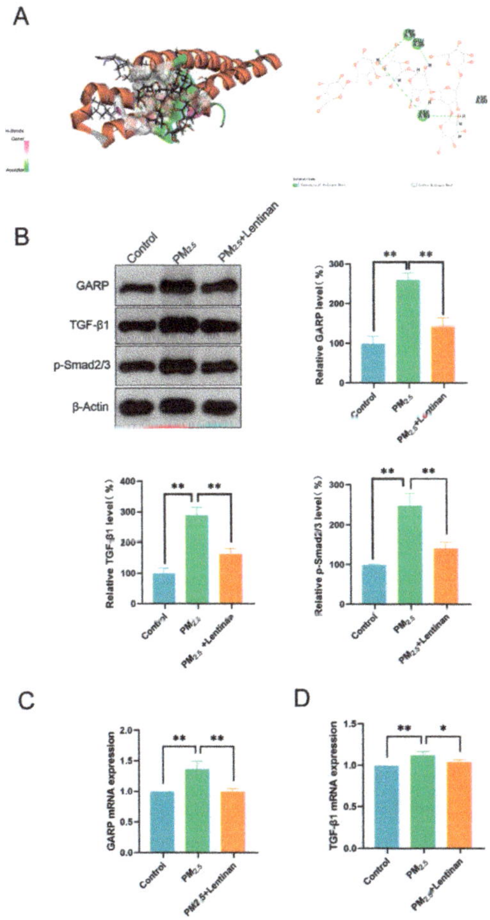


**Figure 6.** Lentinan inhibited the PM2.5-induced GARP/TGF-β/Smad pathway activation: (**A**) Docking of Lentinan with GARP; (**B**) WB analysis of GARP/TGF-β/Smad pathway-associated proteins; (**C**) PCR-detected relative GARP mRNA expression; and (**D**) PCR-detected relative TGF-β1 mRNA expression. *: $p < 0.05$, **: $p < 0.01$.

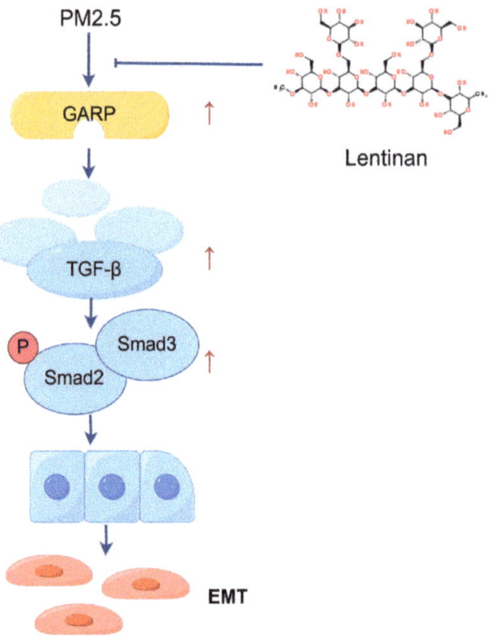


**Figure 7.** Possible mechanism of lentinan in alleviating the PM2.5-induced EMT process in Beas-2B cells. PM2.5 can upregulate GARP, activating TGF-β, thus promoting the phosphorylation of Smad2 and Smad3 and activating the GARP/TGF-β/Smad pathway, which, in turn, induces EMT in Beas-2B cells. Lentinan inhibited GARP production and GARP/TGF-β/Smad pathway activation, thus improving the PM2.5-induced EMT (Figdraw).

## 4. Discussion

Numerous studies have highlighted the crucial involvement of PM2.5 in triggering EMT, which promotes tissue remodeling, fibrosis, and metastasis [29,30]. Due to their small size and chemical composition, PM2.5 particles can penetrate deeply into the respiratory system, inducing OS [31], inflammation [32], and alterations in cellular signaling [33]. One of the key mechanisms through which PM2.5 induces EMT is via TGF-β signaling pathway activation. This pathway, often dysregulated by environmental pollutants such as PM2.5, promotes the expression of mesenchymal markers (e.g., N-Cadherin, vimentin) and suppresses epithelial markers (e.g., E-Cadherin), thus triggering EMT [34]. Therefore, PM2.5 exposure could drive EMT in various models of respiratory diseases such as COPD and asthma, as well as in cancer [35], contributing to airway fibrosis [36], lung damage [37], and tumor metastasis [38]. In other words, PM2.5 exposure could accelerate the progression of both respiratory diseases and cancer through EMT.

Our study reveals a previously unreported role of GARP in promoting EMT in relation to PM2.5 exposure. Notably, GARP has been largely studied in the context of immune modulation and TGF-β activation. Consequently, our findings on its role in EMT, particularly in respiratory cells and under conditions such as PM2.5 exposure, offer novel insights into its potential as a therapeutic target. Specifically, we found that GARP enhances TGF-β activation, which, in turn, induces the expression of EMT markers and facilitates the transition from an epithelial to a mesenchymal phenotype in lung ECs. This finding positions GARP as a novel molecular mediator of PM2.5-induced EMT, suggesting that targeting GARP could be an avenue to mitigating the deleterious effects of PM2.5 exposure in respiratory diseases and other related conditions.

To further elucidate the mechanisms by which GARP regulates PM2.5-induced EMT, it is essential to explore both Smad-dependent and Smad-independent pathways. GARP, as a key regulator of TGF-β activation, may influence the phosphorylation of Smad2 and Smad3, which are critical downstream effectors of the TGF-β signaling pathway. The activation of Smad2/3 can lead to the upregulation of transcription factors such as Snail, Twist, and ZEB1, which are known to promote EMT by repressing epithelial markers and enhancing mesenchymal markers [39]. Future studies should investigate whether GARP directly interacts with Smad proteins or if it modulates other signaling molecules that crosstalk with the TGF-β pathway, such as MAPK/ERK or PI3K/Akt. Additionally, the role of GARP in regulating non-canonical TGF-β signaling pathways, such as those involving RhoA or JNK, should be explored to provide a more comprehensive understanding of its regulatory mechanisms.

Moreover, the interaction between GARP and other cellular components, such as integrins or extracellular matrix proteins, could also play a role in PM2.5-induced EMT [40,41]. GARP may facilitate the activation of latent TGF-β by binding to integrins, which are known to be involved in the mechanical transduction of signals from the extracellular environment. This interaction could be particularly relevant in the context of PM2.5 exposure, as the physical properties of particulate matter may alter the mechanical forces within the lung tissue, thereby influencing EMT. Further research should aim to identify the specific integrins or other cell surface receptors that interact with GARP and determine how these interactions contribute to the activation of TGF-β and subsequent EMT.

Although GARP has been identified as a key player in PM2.5-induced EMT, it is noteworthy that other molecules and signaling pathways could also contribute to this process. Potential candidates include TGF-β receptors, Smad proteins, and TFs (such as Snail, Twist, and ZEB1), which are known to regulate EMT in various disease models. Furthermore, PM2.5 could activate the MAPK/ERK and PI3K/Akt pathways [42], which are involved in inflammation and cell survival, thus contributing to EMT. Therefore, targeting these molecules could provide alternative therapeutic avenues for alleviating the harmful effects of PM2.5 exposure.

Our findings also revealed that lentinan could alleviate PM2.5-induced EMT, a phenomenon attributable to its ability to inhibit the GARP signaling pathway and reduce OS. Lentinan could exert its effects through various mechanisms including inhibiting inflammation pathway activation [43], reducing Reactive Oxygen Species (ROS) production [44], and suppressing the expression of key Transcription Factors (TF) that regulate EMT (such as Snail and Twist). Additionally, lentinan may protect cells by chelating toxic metals present in PM2.5, thereby reducing their bioavailability and cellular toxicity. Polysaccharides have been shown to bind metal ions, which could prevent their interaction with cellular components. Future studies should explore whether lentinan's protective effects are partially mediated through this mechanism [45]. Nonetheless, hitherto, lentinan's molecular mechanism in protecting against PM2.5 exposure was unreported. Furthermore, the bioavailability of lentinan in vivo is an important consideration. Polysaccharides like lentinan may be degraded by gut microbiota into smaller oligosaccharides, which are more easily absorbed through the intestinal mucosa. This raises the possibility that the protective effects of lentinan observed in vitro may be mediated by its metabolites rather than the intact polysaccharide [46]. For example, β-1,3-oligosaccharides derived from polysaccharides have been shown to activate monocytes and release TNF-α, which may contribute to their anti-inflammatory and protective effects [47]. Future studies should explore the metabolic pathways of lentinan in vivo, its bioavailability, and compare the efficacy of polysaccharides and oligosaccharides in mitigating PM2.5-induced EMT.

In light of its findings, this study offers several valuable contributions to the medical field. First, it identifies GARP as a novel regulator of PM2.5-induced EMT, highlighting its involvement in TGF-β activation and its potential as a therapeutic target. Furthermore, it provides novel insights into the mechanisms through which lentinan can mitigate PM2.5-induced EMT, presenting a potentially natural therapeutic strategy for counteracting the adverse effects of air pollution on lung health. Overall, our study lays the groundwork for additional research into GARP-targeting therapies and natural compounds for respiratory disease treatment.

Despite its valuable insights regarding GARP's role in PM2.5-induced EMT, this study had certain limitations. For instance, the in vivo relevance of our findings in animal models of PM2.5 exposure remains to be fully established. This study was primarily based on in vitro cell models, and the translation of its findings to in vivo models could be challenging. Additionally, although our in vitro data suggest that GARP is crucially involved in EMT mediation, we did not explore the precise molecular mechanisms linking GARP activation to the TGF-β signaling pathway, necessitating additional research for a deeper mechanistic understanding of how GARP influences the Smad-dependent and Smad-independent pathways in response to PM2.5 exposure to validate its therapeutic potential. Moreover, we did not explore the long-term effects of lentinan treatment in chronic PM2.5 exposure models. This study did not explore the broader impact of GARP inhibition or lentinan treatment on the immune system, as well as the potential side effects. Finally, we have only provided preliminary insights into the mechanisms of EMT, necessitating further detailed molecular profiling and validation in animal models to confirm our findings and refine the potential therapeutic approaches.

Future studies should focus on elucidating the precise molecular mechanisms linking GARP activation to both Smad-dependent and Smad-independent pathways in response to PM2.5 exposure. Specifically, CRISPR/Cas9-mediated GARP knockout models and RNA-seq analysis could provide deeper insights into the regulatory networks involved. Additionally, in vivo studies using animal models of PM2.5 exposure are needed to validate the therapeutic potential of lentinan and GARP-targeting strategies. Furthermore, the synergistic effects of PM2.5 with other environmental pollutants, such as microplastics and nanoparticles, should be explored to better understand the broader implications of air pollution on lung health.

Beyond the molecular mechanisms explored herein, it is also essential to consider the broader implications of PM2.5-induced EMT regarding environmental health and disease prevention. Presently, PM2.5 exposure is a global concern due to its pervasiveness in urban areas, as well as its association with a range of respiratory and cardiovascular diseases. Therefore, understanding the molecular players involved in EMT, such as GARP, offers critical insights into the pathophysiology of air pollution-related diseases. Moreover, targeting GARP and other key regulators of EMT offers a promising avenue for developing novel therapeutic strategies, especially in the face of increasing pollution levels worldwide. Furthermore, natural compounds like lentinan, which exert protective effects against PM2.5-induced EMT, could serve as adjuncts to contemporary therapeutic options, offering a more holistic approach to combating the deleterious effects of air pollution. There is also a need to explore the potential synergistic effects of combining GARP inhibition agents with other pharmacological or lifestyle interventions in mitigating the adverse impacts of PM2.5 exposure on public health.

## 5. Conclusions

This article highlights the critical role of PM2.5 in EMT induction and the novel function of GARP in this process, as well as the potential therapeutic benefits of lentinan.

In conclusion, this study identifies GARP as a novel regulator of PM2.5-induced EMT and highlights the therapeutic potential of lentinan in mitigating this process. Our findings provide new insights into the molecular mechanisms underlying PM2.5-induced lung damage, and they lay the groundwork for future research into GARP-targeting therapies and natural compounds for the treatment of respiratory diseases. Moreover, we emphasize the need for further investigation into unresolved questions, the identification of additional therapeutic targets, and the in vivo validation of this study's findings. Overall, this study presents a step forward in understanding the molecular mechanisms underlying PM2.5-induced lung damage and lays the groundwork for future research into EMT-targeting therapeutic strategies for respiratory illnesses.

**Author Contributions:** Writing—original draft preparation, Z.W.; data curation, S.X.; conceptualization, B.B.; software, F.W.; methodology, S.Z. and X.W.; validation, Z.W. and Z.H.; formal analysis, Z.W.; investigation, Z.W.; resources, T.M.; writing—review and editing, T.M. and L.W.; supervision, S.Z. and X.W.; funding acquisition and project administration, T.M. All authors have read and agreed to the published version of the manuscript.

**Funding:** This research was funded by the Natural Science Foundation Project of Inner Mongolia Autonomous Region (2022QN08019) and the Key Project of Natural Sciences for Higher Education Institutions in the Inner Mongolia Autonomous Region (NJZZ21045).

**Institutional Review Board Statement:** Not applicable.

**Informed Consent Statement:** Not applicable.

**Data Availability Statement:** The data that support the findings of this study are available from the corresponding author upon reasonable request.

**Acknowledgments:** We would also like to thank everyone who worked so hard on this whole experiment.

**Conflicts of Interest:** The authors declare no conflicts of interest.

## References

1. Huang, J.; Deng, Y.; Tin, M.S.; Lok, V.; Ngai, C.H.; Zhang, L.; Lucero-Prisno, D.E.; Xu, W.; Zheng, Z.-J.; Elcarte, E.; et al. Distribution, Risk Factors, and Temporal Trends for Lung Cancer Incidence and Mortality: A Global Analysis. *Chest* **2022**, *161*, 1101–1111. [CrossRef] [PubMed]
2. Zaręba, Ł.; Piszczatowska, K.; Dżaman, K.; Soroczynska, K.; Motamedi, P.; Szczepański, M.J.; Ludwig, N. The Relationship between Fine Particle Matter (PM2.5) Exposure and Upper Respiratory Tract Diseases. *J. Pers. Med.* **2024**, *14*, 98. [CrossRef] [PubMed]
3. Behinaein, P.; Hutchings, H.; Knapp, T.; Okereke, I.C. The Growing Impact of Air Quality on Lung-Related Illness: A Narrative Review. *J. Thorac. Dis.* **2023**, *15*, 5055–5063. [CrossRef] [PubMed]
4. Xu, F.; Xu, A.; Guo, Y.; Bai, Q.; Wu, X.; Ji, S.-P.; Xia, R.-X. PM2.5 Exposure Induces Alveolar Epithelial Cell Apoptosis and Causes Emphysema through P53/Siva-1. *Eur. Rev. Med. Pharmacol. Sci.* **2020**, *24*, 3943–3950.
5. Yue, D.; Zhang, Q.; Zhang, J.; Liu, W.; Chen, L.; Wang, M.; Li, R.; Qin, S.; Song, X.; Ji, Y. Diesel Exhaust PM2.5 Greatly Deteriorates Fibrosis Process in Pre-Existing Pulmonary Fibrosis via Ferroptosis. *Environ. Int.* **2023**, *171*, 107706. [CrossRef]
6. Zhang, Y.; Jiang, M.; Xiong, Y.; Zhang, L.; Xiong, A.; Wang, J.; He, X.; Li, G. Integrated Analysis of ATAC-Seq and RNA-Seq Unveils the Role of Ferroptosis in PM2.5-Induced Asthma Exacerbation. *Int. Immunopharmacol.* **2023**, *125 Pt B*, 111209. [CrossRef]
7. Obeng, G.M.; Aram, S.A.; Agyei, D.; Saalidong, B.M. Exposure to Particulate Matter (PM2.5) and Volatile Organic Compounds (VOCs), and Self-Reported Health Symptoms among Fish Smokers: A Case Study in the Western Region of Ghana. *PLoS ONE* **2023**, *18*, e0283438. [CrossRef]
8. Wu, C.; Zhang, Y.; Wei, J.; Zhao, Z.; Norbäck, D.; Zhang, X.; Lu, C.; Yu, W.; Wang, T.; Zheng, X.; et al. Associations of Early-Life Exposure to Submicron Particulate Matter With Childhood Asthma and Wheeze in China. *JAMA Netw. Open* **2022**, *5*, e2236003. [CrossRef]
9. Zeng, X.; Xu, X.; Zheng, X.; Reponen, T.; Chen, A.; Huo, X. Heavy Metals in PM2.5 and in Blood, and Children's Respiratory Symptoms and Asthma from an e-Waste Recycling Area. *Environ. Pollut.* **2016**, *210*, 346–353. [CrossRef]

10. Amnuaylojaroen, T.; Parasin, N. Pathogenesis of PM2.5-Related Disorders in Different Age Groups: Children, Adults, and the Elderly. *Epigenomes* **2024**, *8*, 13. [CrossRef]
11. Firoozi, Z.; Shahi, A.; Mohammadisoleimani, E.; Afzali, S.; Mansoori, B.; Bahmanyar, M.; Mohaghegh, P.; Dastsooz, H.; Pezeshki, B.; Nikfar, G.; et al. CircRNA-Associated ceRNA Networks (circCeNETs) in Chronic Obstructive Pulmonary Disease (COPD). *Life Sci.* **2024**, *349*, 122715. [CrossRef] [PubMed]
12. Cochard, M.; Ledoux, F.; Landkocz, Y. Atmospheric Fine Particulate Matter and Epithelial Mesenchymal Transition in Pulmonary Cells: State of the Art and Critical Review of the in Vitro Studies. *J. Toxicol. Environ. Health B Crit. Rev.* **2020**, *23*, 293–318. [CrossRef] [PubMed]
13. Hou, W.; Hu, S.; Li, C.; Ma, H.; Wang, Q.; Meng, G.; Guo, T.; Zhang, J. Cigarette Smoke Induced Lung Barrier Dysfunction, EMT, and Tissue Remodeling: A Possible Link between COPD and Lung Cancer. *BioMed Res. Int.* **2019**, *2019*, 2025636. [CrossRef]
14. Wang, Y.; Liao, S.; Pan, Z.; Jiang, S.; Fan, J.; Yu, S.; Xue, L.; Yang, J.; Ma, S.; Liu, T.; et al. Hydrogen Sulfide Alleviates Particulate Matter-Induced Emphysema and Airway Inflammation by Suppressing Ferroptosis. *Free Radic. Biol. Med.* **2022**, *186*, 1–16. [CrossRef]
15. Xu, Z.; Ding, W.; Deng, X. PM2.5, Fine Particulate Matter: A Novel Player in the Epithelial-Mesenchymal Transition? *Front. Physiol.* **2019**, *10*, 1404. [CrossRef]
16. Liu, X.; Xu, D.; Liu, Z.; Li, Y.; Zhang, C.; Gong, Y.; Jiang, Y.; Xing, B. THBS1 Facilitates Colorectal Liver Metastasis through Enhancing Epithelial-Mesenchymal Transition. *Clin. Transl. Oncol.* **2020**, *22*, 1730–1740. [CrossRef]
17. Hu, C.; Xin, Z.; Sun, X.; Hu, Y.; Zhang, C.; Yan, R.; Wang, Y.; Lu, M.; Huang, J.; Du, X.; et al. Activation of ACLY by SEC63 Deploys Metabolic Reprogramming to Facilitate Hepatocellular Carcinoma Metastasis upon Endoplasmic Reticulum Stress. *J. Exp. Clin. Cancer Res.* **2023**, *42*, 108. [CrossRef]
18. Song, Y.; Chen, Y.; Cai, H.; Zhu, G.; Zeng, Y.; Abuduxukuer, Z.; Chen, K.; Wang, J.; Ye, L.; Jin, M. Lentinan Attenuates Allergic Airway Inflammation and Epithelial Barrier Dysfunction in Asthma via Inhibition of the PI3K/AKT/NF-κB Pathway. *Phytomedicine* **2024**, *134*, 155965. [CrossRef]
19. Zhang, Z.; Zha, Z.; Zhao, Z.; Liu, W.; Li, W. Lentinan Inhibits AGE-Induced Inflammation and the Expression of Matrix-Degrading Enzymes in Human Chondrocytes. *Drug Des. Dev. Ther.* **2020**, *14*, 2819–2829. [CrossRef]
20. Liu, Y.; Zhao, J.; Zhao, Y.; Zong, S.; Tian, Y.; Chen, S.; Li, M.; Liu, H.; Zhang, Q.; Jing, X.; et al. Therapeutic Effects of Lentinan on Inflammatory Bowel Disease and Colitis-Associated Cancer. *J. Cell. Mol. Med.* **2019**, *23*, 750–760. [CrossRef]
21. Qi, H.; Liu, Y.; Wang, N.; Xiao, C. Lentinan Attenuated the PM2.5 Exposure-Induced Inflammatory Response, Epithelial-Mesenchymal Transition and Migration by Inhibiting the PVT1/miR-199a-5p/Caveolin1 Pathway in Lung Cancer. *DNA Cell Biol.* **2021**, *40*, 683–693. [CrossRef] [PubMed]
22. Metelli, A.; Salem, M.; Wallace, C.H.; Wu, B.X.; Li, A.; Li, X.; Li, Z. Immunoregulatory Functions and the Therapeutic Implications of GARP-TGF-β in Inflammation and Cancer. *J. Hematol. Oncol.* **2018**, *11*, 24. [CrossRef] [PubMed]
23. Miyazono, K.; Katsuno, Y.; Koinuma, D.; Ehata, S.; Morikawa, M. Intracellular and Extracellular TGF-β Signaling in Cancer: Some Recent Topics. *Front. Med.* **2018**, *12*, 387–411. [CrossRef] [PubMed]
24. Metelli, A.; Wu, B.X.; Riesenberg, B.; Guglietta, S.; Huck, J.D.; Mills, C.; Li, A.; Rachidi, S.; Krieg, C.; Rubinstein, M.P.; et al. Thrombin Contributes to Cancer Immune Evasion via Proteolysis of Platelet-Bound GARP to Activate LTGF-β. *Sci. Transl. Med.* **2020**, *12*, eaay4860. [CrossRef]
25. Li, A.; Chang, Y.; Song, N.-J.; Wu, X.; Chung, D.; Riesenberg, B.P.; Velegraki, M.; Giuliani, G.D.; Das, K.; Okimoto, T.; et al. Selective Targeting of GARP-LTGFβ Axis in the Tumor Microenvironment Augments PD-1 Blockade via Enhancing CD8+ T Cell Antitumor Immunity. *J. Immunother. Cancer* **2022**, *10*, e005433. [CrossRef]
26. Hou, J.; Wang, X.; Su, C.; Ma, W.; Zheng, X.; Ge, X.; Duan, X. Reduced Frequencies of $Foxp3^+$ $GARP^+$ Regulatory T Cells in COPD Patients Are Associated with Multi-Organ Loss of Tissue Phenotype. *Respir. Res.* **2022**, *23*, 176. [CrossRef]
27. Nookala, S.; Mukundan, S.; Fife, A.; Alagarsamy, J.; Kotb, M. Heterogeneity in FoxP3- and GARP/LAP-Expressing T Regulatory Cells in an HLA Class II Transgenic Murine Model of Necrotizing Soft Tissue Infections by Group A Streptococcus. *Infect. Immun.* **2018**, *86*, e00432-18. [CrossRef]
28. Yang, T.; Gao, Y.; Shi, X.; Zhang, Q.; Ren, Q.; Fu, Y.; Li, H.; Wang, Y.; He, T.; He, M.; et al. Analysis of Atmospheric PM2.5 Composition and Source in an Industrial City in Northern China. *Chin. Rare Earths* **2023**, *44*, 113–122. (In Chinese)
29. Wang, Y.; Zhong, Y.; Hou, T.; Liao, J.; Zhang, C.; Sun, C.; Wang, G. PM2.5 Induces EMT and Promotes CSC Properties by Activating Notch Pathway in Vivo and Vitro. *Ecotoxicol. Environ. Saf.* **2019**, *178*, 159–167. [CrossRef]
30. Wang, Y.; Zhong, Y.; Zhang, C.; Liao, J.; Wang, G. PM2.5 Downregulates MicroRNA-139-5p and Induces EMT in Bronchiolar Epithelium Cells by Targeting Notch1. *J. Cancer* **2020**, *11*, 5758–5767. [CrossRef]
31. Liu, K.; Hua, S.; Song, L. PM2.5 Exposure and Asthma Development: The Key Role of Oxidative Stress. *Oxid. Med. Cell. Longev.* **2022**, *2022*, 3618806. [CrossRef] [PubMed]
32. Zou, W.; Liu, S.; Ye, D.; Bai, G.; Guo, M.; Sun, R.; Ran, P. PM2.5 Induces Lung Inflammation and Fibrosis via Airway Smooth Muscle Cell Expression of the Wnt5a/JNK Pathway. *J. Thorac. Dis.* **2023**, *15*, 6094–6105. [CrossRef] [PubMed]

33. Yu, H.; Lin, Y.; Zhong, Y.; Guo, X.; Lin, Y.; Yang, S.; Liu, J.; Xie, X.; Sun, Y.; Wang, D.; et al. Impaired AT2 to AT1 Cell Transition in PM2.5-Induced Mouse Model of Chronic Obstructive Pulmonary Disease. *Respir. Res.* **2022**, *23*, 70. [CrossRef] [PubMed]
34. Leilei, L.; Xue, S.; Yan, L.; Yuyuan, L.; Ying, W.; Wenke, Q.; Xuesong, Y.; Ming, L. PM2.5-Exposed Hepatocytes Induce Hepatic Stellate Cells Activation by Releasing TGF-B1. *Biochem. Biophys. Res. Commun.* **2021**, *569*, 125–131. [CrossRef]
35. Lin, C.-H.; Liu, W.-S.; Wan, C.; Wang, H.-H. Pentraxin 3 Mediates Early Inflammatory Response and EMT Process in Human Tubule Epithelial Cells Induced by PM2.5. *Int. Immunopharmacol.* **2022**, *112*, 109258. [CrossRef]
36. Zhao, C.; Pu, W.; Wazir, J.; Jin, X.; Wei, L.; Song, S.; Su, Z.; Li, J.; Deng, Y.; Wang, H. Long-Term Exposure to PM2.5 Aggravates Pulmonary Fibrosis and Acute Lung Injury by Disrupting Nrf2-Mediated Antioxidant Function. *Environ. Pollut.* **2022**, *313*, 120017. [CrossRef]
37. Wang, H.; Wang, G.; Meng, Y.; Liu, Y.; Yao, X.; Feng, C. Modified Guo-Min Decoction Ameliorates PM2.5-Induced Lung Injury by Inhibition of PI3K-AKT and MAPK Signaling Pathways. *Phytomedicine* **2024**, *123*, 155211. [CrossRef]
38. Chao, X.; Yi, L.; Lan, L.L.; Wei, H.Y.; Wei, D. Long-Term PM2.5 Exposure Increases the Risk of Non-Small Cell Lung Cancer (NSCLC) Progression by Enhancing Interleukin-17a (IL-17a)-Regulated Proliferation and Metastasis. *Aging* **2020**, *12*, 11579–11602. [CrossRef]
39. Hao, Y.; Long, Z.; Gu, X. Farrerol Suppresses Epithelial-Mesenchymal Transition in Hepatocellular Carcinoma via Suppression of TGF-B1/Smad2/3 Signaling. *Pathol. Res. Pract.* **2024**, *264*, 155719. [CrossRef]
40. Moreau, J.M.; Velegraki, M.; Bolyard, C.; Rosenblum, M.D.; Li, Z. Transforming Growth Factor-B1 in Regulatory T Cell Biology. *Sci. Immunol.* **2022**, *7*, eabi4613. [CrossRef]
41. Campbell, M.G.; Cormier, A.; Ito, S.; Seed, R.I.; Bondesson, A.J.; Lou, J.; Marks, J.D.; Baron, J.L.; Cheng, Y.; Nishimura, S.L. Cryo-EM Reveals Integrin-Mediated TGF-β Activation without Release from Latent TGF-β. *Cell* **2020**, *180*, 490–501.e16. [CrossRef] [PubMed]
42. Wang, Y.; Zhang, Y.; Li, Y.; Kou, X.; Xue, Z. Mechanisms of Biochanin A Alleviating PM2.5 Organic Extracts-Induced EMT of A549 Cells through the PI3K/Akt Pathway. *J. Nat. Prod.* **2022**, *85*, 2290–2301. [CrossRef] [PubMed]
43. Meng, M.; Huo, R.; Wang, Y.; Ma, N.; Shi, X.; Shen, X.; Chang, G. Lentinan Inhibits Oxidative Stress and Alleviates LPS-Induced Inflammation and Apoptosis of BMECs by Activating the Nrf2 Signaling Pathway. *Int. J. Biol. Macromol.* **2022**, *222 Pt B*, 2375–2391. [CrossRef] [PubMed]
44. Liu, H.; Liu, B.; Zhang, S.; Fan, M.; Ji, X.; Zhang, S.; Wang, Z.; Qiao, K. Lentinan Protects Caenorhabditis Elegans against Fluopyram-Induced Toxicity through DAF-16 and SKN-1 Pathways. *Ecotoxicol. Environ. Saf.* **2023**, *265*, 115510. [CrossRef]
45. Yap, P.G.; Gan, C.Y. Optimized Extraction and Characterization of Ramie Leaf Polysaccharides Using Deep Eutectic Solvent and Microwave: Antioxidant, Metal Chelation, and UV Protection Properties. *Int. J. Biol. Macromol.* **2024**, *282 Pt 3*, 136927. [CrossRef]
46. Yu, L.; Gao, Y.; Ye, Z.; Duan, H.; Zhao, J.; Zhang, H.; Narbad, A.; Tian, F.; Zhai, Q.; Chen, W. Interaction of Beta-Glucans with Gut Microbiota: Dietary Origins, Structures, Degradation, Metabolism, and Beneficial Function. *Crit. Rev. Food Sci. Nutr.* **2024**, *64*, 9884–9909. [CrossRef]
47. Jiang, Y.; Chang, Z.; Xu, Y.; Zhan, X.; Wang, Y.; Gao, M. Advances in Molecular Enzymology of β-1,3-Glucanases: A Comprehensive Review. *Int. J. Biol. Macromol.* **2024**, *279 Pt 3*, 135349. [CrossRef]

toxics

MDPI

Article

# A Multi-Omics Study of Neurodamage Induced by Growth-Stage Real-Time Air Pollution Exposure in Mice via the Microbiome–Gut–Brain Axis

Zijun Yang [1], Yi Zhang [2], Shanshan Ran [1], Jingyi Zhang [1], Fei Tian [1], Hui Shi [1], Shengtao Wei [1], Xiuxiu Li [3], Xinyue Li [1], Yonggui Gao [1], Guang Jia [2], Hualiang Lin [1], Zhangjian Chen [2,*] and Zilong Zhang [1,*]

1 Department of Epidemiology, School of Public Health, Sun Yat-sen University, Guangzhou 510080, China; yangzj39@mail2.sysu.edu.cn (Z.Y.); ranshsh@mail2.sysu.edu.cn (S.R.); zhangjy563@mail2.sysu.edu.cn (J.Z.); tianf8@mail2.sysu.edu.cn (F.T.); shih39@mail2.sysu.edu.cn (H.S.); weisht3@mail2.sysu.edu.cn (S.W.); lixy856@mail2.sysu.edu.cn (X.L.); gaoyg5@mail2.sysu.edu.cn (Y.G.); linhualiang@mail.sysu.edu.cn (H.L.)

2 Department of Occupational and Environmental Health Sciences, School of Public Health, Peking University, Beijing 100191, China; 2411110207@pku.edu.cn (Y.Z.); jiaguangjia@bjmu.edu.cn (G.J.)

3 Department of Science and Education, Nanshan Maternity & Child Healthcare Hospital of Shenzhen, Shenzhen 518067, China; lixiuxiu1103@163.com

* Correspondence: zhangjianchen@pku.edu.cn (Z.C.); zhangzilong@mail.sysu.edu.cn (Z.Z.)

**Abstract:** Air pollution has been widely recognized as a risk factor for neurological disorders, and the gut microbiome may play a mediating role. However, current evidence remains limited. In this study, a mouse model was employed with continuous exposure to real-time air pollution from conception to late adolescence. Effects of growth-stage air pollution exposure on the gut microbiome, host metabolites, and brain tissue were assessed. Pathological damage in the hippocampus and cortex was observed. Fecal metagenomic sequencing revealed alterations in both compositions and functions of the gut microbiome. Metabolic disturbances in unsaturated fatty acids and glycerophospholipids were identified in the intestine, serum, and brain tissues, with significant changes in metabolites (e.g., gamma-linolenic acid, alpha-linolenic acid, docosahexaenoic acid (DHA), phosphatidylethanolamine (PE), phosphatidylcholine (PC) and phosphatidylserine (PS). Serum levels of the pro-inflammatory mediator leukotriene C4 were also elevated. Correlation analysis identified a group of different gut microbiome species that were associated with host metabolites. Furthermore, mediation analysis showed that intestinal and serum metabolites mediated the associations between the key gut microbiome and brain microbiome. These findings indicate that the metabolic crosstalk in the gut–brain axis mediates the neuronal damage in mice induced by growth-stage air pollution exposure, potentially through pathways involving lipid metabolism and inflammation.

**Keywords:** air pollution; growth-stage; multi-omics; microbiome–gut–brain axis; neuronal damage

## 1. Introduction

Air pollution, especially fine particulate matter ($PM_{2.5}$), has been widely recognized as a major threat to public health [1]. In recent years, the potential effects of air pollution on the nervous system have gained increasing attention [2,3]. A growing number of epidemiological studies have shown that exposure to air pollution during early life (e.g., pregnancy and infancy) is associated with increased risks of autism spectrum disorder (ASD), attention deficit hyperactivity disorder (ADHD), and other neurodevelopmental disorders (NDDs) [4–6], a group of diseases that not only seriously affect children's cognition, behavior, and social abilities, but also have profound impacts on lifelong mental health and socioeconomics. However, a remaining question is that the specific mechanisms by which early-life air pollution exposure causes neurodevelopmental harm are largely unclear. A better understanding of these mechanisms is imperative for the development of effective interventions against NDDs.

In recent years, the description of the microbiome–gut–brain axis (MGBA) has provided a new theoretical perspective for understanding how environmental exposure, including air pollution, affects the nervous system [7]. The MGBA is a complex signaling network through which the gut microbiome interacts with the central nervous system via neural, immune, endocrine, and metabolic pathways. It is hypothesized that the gut microbiome can influence brain development and function as well as behaviors of the host by modulating immune responses, producing metabolites (e.g., fatty acids, neurotransmitter precursors), activating vagal nerve signals, and affecting neuroendocrine pathways [7,8]. Both the gut microbiome and the nervous system undergo critical development in growth stages, especially the early-life stage, and the MGBA plays an important role in maintaining neurodevelopmental homeostasis [9,10]. Studies have shown that air pollution, particularly $PM_{2.5}$, significantly alters the diversity and function of the gut microbiome [11,12]. Furthermore, alterations in the microbiome induced by air pollution may further disrupt the nervous system [13–15]. However, the exact mechanisms by which the gut microbiome affects brain development following exposure to air pollution are largely unknown.

Metabolites, as both intermediates and endpoints of biological processes, can directly reflect biological disturbances within the body. Changes in brain metabolism are closely related to the pathogenesis of neurological diseases, including NDDs [16]. Previous studies have shown that air pollution could impact brain metabolism and gene expression, contributing to disease pathogenesis [17,18]. Moreover, brain metabolites are also influenced by the cross-talk of the MGBA [19]. Therefore, metabolites may be a key mechanism linking air pollution and the nervous system via the MGBA. However, such a hypothesis has not been examined yet.

In recent years, advances in integrated multi-omics techniques including metagenomics, metabolomics, and transcriptomics, provide a more comprehensive approach to study air pollution's impact on the gut microbiome and various organ systems. In the present study, a mouse model was employed to systematically investigate the health impact of growth stage air pollution exposure on brain development and the potential mediating effect of the gut microbiome, with a multi-omics approach incorporating gut metagenomics, metabolomics, and transcriptomics. The main aim was to reveal the role of the MGBA in the associations between air pollution exposure, neural damage in offspring, and the underlying mechanisms, which can inform the development of intervention strategies for NDDs.

## 2. Materials and Methods

### 2.1. Animals and Study Design

The present study used 6-week-old male and female C57BL/6 mice (average weight: 20 g for males and 18 g for females) purchased from the Peking University Health Science Center Laboratory Animal Center (Beijing, China). A total of 24 female mice and 12 male mice were randomly assigned to either the filtered air group (FA, as the control) or the real-world air pollution exposure group (Exp). After a one-week adaptation, males were housed individually, while females were housed according to their group. A three-day mating period was set, and two females were placed in the same cage with one male each night. Once the females became pregnant, they were assigned to either the exposure or control group for the subsequent exposure experiment. The start of embryonic development (E0.5) was determined when a vaginal plug was observed. After birth, the offspring mice were weaned on postnatal day 21 (PND 21), and continued to be housed in cages exposed to air pollution or filtered air until late adolescence. To avoid litter effects, one mouse per litter was selected in subsequent experiments. The mice were euthanized after reaching adulthood (10 weeks), and samples of feces, intestine, serum, and brain tissues were collected. Fecal samples were used for metagenomic sequencing, intestine samples were used for untargeted metabolomics and transcriptomics analysis, serum samples were used for untargeted metabolomics analysis, and brain tissue samples were used for untargeted metabolomics and transcriptomics analysis. The detailed experimental procedure is shown in Figure 1. In this study, the mice were housed in an environment with a 12 h light/dark cycle, at a temperature of 20–25 °C, with relative humidity maintained at 40–70%, and provided with standard chow and clean drinking water. The study protocol was approved by the Institutional Animal Care and Use Committee of Peking University Health Science Center (protocol code BCJD0130, approval date: 29 April 2023).

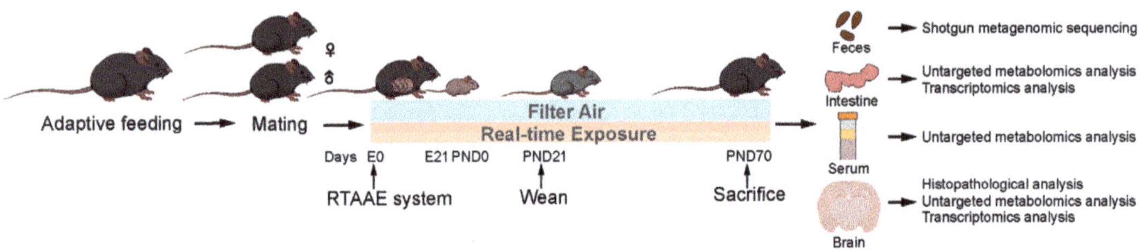


**Figure 1.** Schematic diagram depicting growth-stage real-time air pollution exposure of mice, as well as sample collection and testing conducted on the offspring mice. E: Embryonic day; PND: Postnatal day; RTAAE: real-time ambient air pollution exposure.

### 2.2. Real-Time Ambient Air Pollution Exposure (RTAAE) System

To simulate real-time environmental air pollution exposure, a whole-body RTAAE system was established. Detailed information about the RTAAE system, including the monitoring system, has been provided in our previous studies [20–22]. Briefly, the individual ventilated cages (IVCs) for the FA group were fitted with high-efficiency particulate air (HEPA) filters to supply clean air, while the IVCs for the exposed group had the filters removed and replaced with retention devices, allowing particles smaller than 2.5 μm to enter. The RTAAE system was set up 10 m above ground, and approximately 200 m from the North Fourth Ring Road in Beijing, an area with high traffic volume. According to our previous study [21], $PM_{2.5}$ and $O_3$ were the primary pollutants in the exposure cages. Composition analysis showed that $PM_{2.5}$ mainly contained metal elements such as Fe, Na, and Ca, and the main water-soluble substances were $NH_4^+$ and $Ca^{2+}$. In this study, the concentrations of air pollutants in the system were continuously monitored throughout the study. In particular, $PM_{2.5}$ was collected using a BUCK LP-5 air sampling pump (AP Buck Inc., Orlando, FL, USA) with 37 mm quartz fiber filters at a flow rate of 1.70 L/min, and the concentration was determined by gravimetric analysis. $O_3$ concentration ($[O_3]_{8\ h,max}$) was measured using a Two Technology 220 Model real-time ozone concentration detector (2B Technologies, Boulder, CO, USA). Meanwhile, background air pollution (i.e., ambient air pollution) concentrations were obtained from the Olympic Sports Center Monitoring Station of the Beijing Environmental Protection Monitoring Center (approximately 4.5 km away from the study site) (http://www.bjmemc.com.cn/, URL accessed from 1 June to 30 September 2023).

### 2.3. Histopathological Analysis

Mice were euthanized after reaching adulthood, and brain tissues were immediately collected. The tissues were first immersed in 4% paraformaldehyde solution for fixation for at least 24 h, followed by paraffin embedding. Sections with a thickness of 4 μm from the prefrontal cortex and hippocampus were prepared and mounted on glass slides. The sections were then stained with hematoxylin and eosin (H&E). Finally, the slides were observed and analyzed using a Pannoramic MIDI digital slide scanner (3DHISTECH, Hungary) and digital slide viewing software (CaseViewer 2.4).

### 2.4. Gut Microbiome Assessment by Shotgun Metagenomic Sequencing

Fresh fecal samples (0.5 g, approximately four pellets) were collected from mice at early adulthood, and then rapidly frozen in liquid nitrogen and stored at −80 °C until metagenomic sequencing. First, genomic DNA was extracted from fecal samples using the E.Z.N.A.® Stool DNA Kit D4015 (Omega, Norcross, GA, USA) following the manufacturer' s instructions. The extracted DNA was assessed for purity and integrity using agarose gel electrophoresis (AGE) and quantified using a Qubit fluorometer (Thermo Fisher Scientific, Waltham, MA, USA). High-quality DNA was fragmented to ~350 bp, followed by end repair, A-tailing, adapter ligation, purification, and PCR amplification to construct sequencing libraries. Libraries passing quality control were sequenced on the Illumina PE150 platform (Illumina Inc., San Diego, CA, USA). Preprocessed sequencing data were assembled into contigs using MEGAHIT software (version 1.0.3). Assembly quality was assessed using SOAP2.21 to ensure data reliability. Gene prediction was performed using Prokka software (version 1.14.5) to identify functional genes in each metagenomic dataset. CD-HIT software (version 4.8.1) was used to remove redundant genes, yielding a set of non-redundant Uniq Genes. For gene abundance analysis, Salmon software (version 1.10.1) was used to calculate the transcripts per million (TPM) values of each gene and normalize them to obtain relative abundance. Functional annotation of non-redundant Uniq Genes was performed by comparing protein sequences to multiple databases, including the NCBI non-redundant protein database (NR, version 20170730). Taxonomic classification of Uniq Genes was determined by mapping NR-annotated genes to specific taxonomic ranks (kingdom, phylum, class, order, family, genus, species). The last common ancestor (LCA) method was applied to gene abundance data to estimate taxonomic abundance at various levels. Species abundance was calculated as the sum of all gene abundances assigned to that species. Finally, DEGseq R package (version 1.56.1) was used for differential analysis, with screening criteria of fold change ≥2 and FDR Q-value < 0.01 to identify differentially expressed genes under different conditions. $\alpha$-Diversity indices (Shannon, Chao 1, Observed species, Simpson, ACE) were calculated using the Qiime (version 1.8.0) to evaluate gut microbiome richness and diversity. $\beta$-diversity was analyzed using Bray–Curtis distance, and differences in microbiome composition were evaluated through non-metric multidimensional scaling (NMDS) in the "vegan" R package (version 2.6-3). The linear discriminant analysis effect size (LEfSe) method was applied to identify significantly different microbes between groups from the phylum to species level. Microbes were classified and ranked based on their linear discriminant analysis (LDA) scores. Benjamini–Hochberg (BH) correction was performed to adjust for multiple testing and control the false discovery rate.

### 2.5. Untargeted Metabolomics Analysis

Liquid chromatography-mass spectrometry (LC-MS) was used for untargeted metabolomic analysis. After euthanasia, intestine, brain tissue, and serum samples were rapidly collected, flash-frozen in liquid nitrogen, and stored at −80 °C for subsequent metabolite extraction. Internal standard A0 was prepared by dissolving 10 mg of reserpine and 10 mg of chloramphenicol in 10 mL of acetonitrile at a concentration of 1 mg/mL. Then, 1 mL of internal standard A0 was diluted to 0.1 mg/mL to prepare internal standard A. Subsequently, 500 µL of internal standard A was added to 50 mL of acetonitrile to prepare solvent B. For serum samples, 50 µL of serum was mixed with 200 µL of solvent B. For intestine and brain tissue samples, 50 mg of tissue was homogenized with 200 µL of solvent B using liquid nitrogen grinding. Samples were centrifuged at 12,000 rpm for 10 min at 4 °C. The acetonitrile supernatant was collected, and 100 µL was used for polar metabolite analysis. Additionally, individual samples were pooled at a 1:1:1 ratio, and 10 µL was used to prepare a quality control (QC) sample. Next, samples were analyzed using the UPLC-Synapt XS system (Waters Corp., Milford, CT, USA). Ultra-performance liquid chromatography (UPLC) separation was performed using an HSS T3 column. Mobile phase A consisted of 0.1% formic acid in water, while mobile phase B contained 0.1% formic acid in acetonitrile. The flow rate was 0.4 mL/min, with a gradient elution from 98% A/2% B to 2% A/98% B. Separated samples were analyzed using the Synapt XS high-resolution mass spectrometer in positive and negative ion modes. The mass range was set to 50–1200 Da, with data acquired in MSE/DDA mode. The spray voltage was 2.0 kV, with a source temperature of 120 °C and a desolvation temperature of 450 °C. Raw data were converted to mzML format using MSConvertGUI software (version 3.0.24212-8361512) and imported into MS-DIAL software (version 4.24) for peak extraction, matching, and identification. Metabolites were identified by comparing with cationic and anionic standard databases in MS-Dial-based mass spectral libraries. Metabolite names were further confirmed using INCHIKEY and the Human Metabolome Database (HMDB, https://hmdb.ca, URL accessed on 20 October 2024). An unpaired Student's $t$-test was used to analyze differences between groups. An orthogonal partial least squares discriminant analysis (OPLS-DA) model was constructed, and metabolites with VIP > 1 and $p < 0.05$ were selected as key differential metabolites. Enrichment and pathway analyses were performed using the MetaboAnalyst 6.0 platform (https://www.metaboanalyst.ca/, URL accessed on 20 October 2024), with pathway analysis based on the Kyoto Encyclopedia of Genes and Genomes (KEGG) database.

### 2.6. Transcriptomics Analysis

Intestinal and brain tissues were used for transcriptomics analysis. Total RNA was extracted using TRIzol® reagent (Thermo Fisher Scientific, Carlsbad, CA, USA). RNA quality was assessed with ND-2000 (NanoDrop Technologies, Wilmington, DE, USA). and a 5300 Bioanalyzer (Agilent Technologies, Santa Clara, CA, USA, and only samples with OD260/280 = 1.8–2.2 and RQN $\geq$ 6.5 were selected for sequencing. RNA purification, reverse transcription, library construction, and sequencing were performed according to standard protocols. First, mRNA was enriched using Oligo(dT) magnetic beads, fragmented, and then used for double-stranded cDNA synthesis, end repair, phosphorylation, and adapter ligation to construct sequencing libraries. After library quantification, paired-end sequencing (PE150) was performed on the NovaSeq X Plus platform (Illumina, San Diego, CA, USA). Sequencing data were processed using fastp for quality control, removing low-quality reads. The cleaned reads were aligned to the mouse reference genome (GRCm38/mm10) using HISAT2, followed by transcriptome assembly and gene expression quantification with StringTie. Differential expression analysis was performed using DESeq2 with $|\log_2 FC| \geq 1$ and FDR Q-value < 0.05 as the criteria for defining differentially expressed genes (DEGs). KEGG pathway enrichment analysis of DEGs was conducted using Python's scipy package (version 1.13.1).

*2.7. Statistical Analysis*

Data were presented as mean ± standard deviation (x ± SD). Group comparisons were performed using Student's *t*-test or ANOVA for normally distributed data and the Wilcoxon rank-sum test or Kruskal–Wallis test for non-normally distributed data. Spearman correlation analysis was used to assess the relationships among the microbiome, intestinal metabolites, serum metabolites and brain metabolites. Mediation analysis was performed to assess whether intestinal and serum metabolites mediated the relationship between gut microbiome and brain metabolic changes. The proportion mediated was calculated as the ratio of indirect effects to total effects, quantifying the contribution of intestinal and serum metabolites. Mediation analyses were conducted using the "mediation" package (version 4.5.0) in R (version 4.4.2). Statistical analyses and data visualization were conducted using GraphPad Prism (version 9) and R (version 4.4.2). Statistical significance was set at $p < 0.05$. False discovery rate (FDR) correction for multiple comparisons was performed using the Benjamini–Hochberg (BH) method. Q-values were used for FDR adjustment in metagenomic and transcriptomic analyses.

## 3. Results

*3.1. Level of Air Pollutants in the Exposure System*

Figure S1 shows the distribution of the concentrations of $PM_{2.5}$ and $[O_3]_{8\ h,max}$ over the study period. The mean weekly concentration of $PM_{2.5}$ was 12.56 μg/m$^3$ inside the system and 24.41 μg/m$^3$ in the ambient environment. The corresponding concentrations of $[O3]_{8\ h,max}$ were 105.49 μg/m$^3$ and 135.76 μg/m$^3$, respectively. In the filtered air group, the concentrations of $PM_{2.5}$ and $O_3$ were below the limits of detection (LODs) of 0.5 μg/m$^3$ and 0.1 ppb, respectively.

*3.2. Effects of Air Pollution Exposure on the Hippocampus and Cortex*

Histopathological analysis revealed that growth-stage exposure to air pollution caused disorganized cell arrangement, neuronal shrinkage, necrosis, and edema in the hippocampal CA1 and CA3 regions of offspring mice. Additionally, the cortical tissue exhibited neuronal nuclear loss and edema (Figure 2).

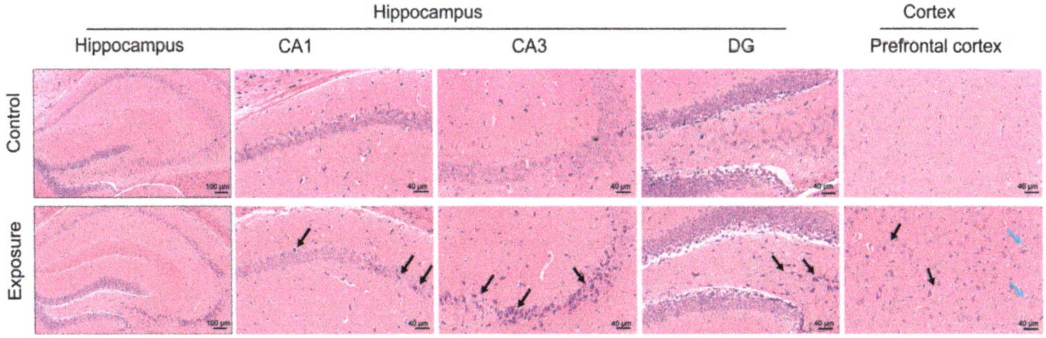


**Figure 2.** Pathological changes in the hippocampus and cortex following growth-stage air pollution exposure. Images of H&E staining in the hippocampus (scale bar = 100 μm), as well as pathological sections of the CA1, CA3, and DG regions of the hippocampus (scale bar = 40 μm), and cortical sections (scale bar = 40 μm). Black arrows indicate shrunken cytoplasm, reduced cell volume, and irregular shape; blue arrows highlight edema in pyramidal cells, characterized by cell swelling and pale cytoplasm.

To further examine metabolic alterations in the hippocampus and cortex, untargeted metabolomics analysis was conducted. OPLS-DA analysis (Figure 3A) was performed, and VIP scores were calculated for each metabolite based on their contribution to group separation (Figure S2). Using a VIP threshold > 1 and $p < 0.05$, 11 significantly altered metabolites were identified in the hippocampus and cortex of exposed mice (Figure 3B). A heatmap of key differential metabolites is presented in Figure 3C. KEGG pathway topological analysis (Figure 3D) identified significant disruptions in glycerophospholipid metabolism, glycosylphosphatidylinositol (GPI)-anchor biosynthesis, and unsaturated fatty acid biosynthesis in the exposed group. Key metabolites included PE(P-16:0/22:6(4Z,7Z,10Z,13Z,16Z,19Z)), lysophosphatidylcholine (LysoPC) (17:0/0:0), and arachidic acid (Figure 3E). To investigate potential sex differences, separate analyses were performed for male and female mice. Significant metabolic alterations were still observed in both sexes following exposure. Differentially altered metabolites were primarily associated with pathways such as purine metabolism, pyrimidine metabolism, glycerophospholipid metabolism, linoleic acid metabolism, and unsaturated fatty acid biosynthesis (Figure S3).

To assess molecular alterations in the hippocampus and cortex, RNA sequencing was performed. Under the criteria of $|\log_2(FC)| > 1$ and Q-value < 0.05, a total of 198 significantly upregulated genes and 98 downregulated genes were identified (Figure 3F). KEGG enrichment analysis (Figure 3G) revealed significant enrichment in neural pathways (e.g., neuroactive ligand–receptor interaction, synaptic vesicle cycle), lipid metabolism pathways (e.g., PPAR signaling, phospholipase D signaling), and inflammatory pathways (e.g., NOD-like receptor signaling). A total of 34 key differentially expressed genes were identified in these pathways, including Gabrq, Brs3, Gzma, C3, Ltb4r1, Pck1, Acox2, Angptl4, Avpr1a, Dgkk, and Agt. Collectively, metabolomics and transcriptomics results indicate that air pollution exposure during growth stages significantly alters lipid metabolism pathways, including glycerophospholipid metabolism and unsaturated fatty acid biosynthesis, as well as pathways related to neuro-communication and inflammation in the brain.

### 3.3. Alterations in the Gut Microbiome Induced by Air Pollution Exposure

NMDS analysis revealed some differences in the microbiome community structure between the exposed and control groups following exposure to air pollution (Figure 4A). Compositions of the microbiome at the phylum and genus levels are depicted in Figure 4B,C. No significant differences were found in the $\alpha$-diversity indices between the two groups ($p > 0.05$) (Table 1). LEfSe analysis revealed 35 taxa with an LDA score greater than 3, among which 15 taxa were more highly expressed in the control group, while 20 taxa were more highly expressed in the exposed group ($P_{FDR} < 0.05$) (Figure 4D). The relative abundance heatmap of the microbiome in the samples is shown in Figure S4. KEGG pathway enrichment analysis of differentially expressed genes from metagenomic sequencing showed significant enrichment in lipid metabolism pathways in the exposed mice (Figure 4E). Both male and female mice exhibited changes in the microbiome structure and lipid-related functional alterations following exposure (Figure S5).

**Table 1.** Alpha diversity indices of gut microbiome.

| Characteristics | Control (Mean ± SD) | Exposure (Mean ± SD) | $t$ | $p$ |
|---|---|---|---|---|
| Shannon index | 6.50 ± 0.42 | 6.62 ± 0.27 | −0.73 | 0.479 |
| Chao1 | 33,650.24 ± 18,032.92 | 34,495.96 ± 16,589.99 | −0.11 | 0.914 |
| Observed species | 8378.50 ± 696.35 | 8805.20 ± 579.11 | −1.49 | 0.154 |
| Simpson index | 0.97 ± 0.01 | 0.96 ± 0.01 | 0.32 | 0.754 |
| ACE index | 9255.11 ± 890.40 | 9704.75 ± 569.13 | −1.35 | 0.198 |

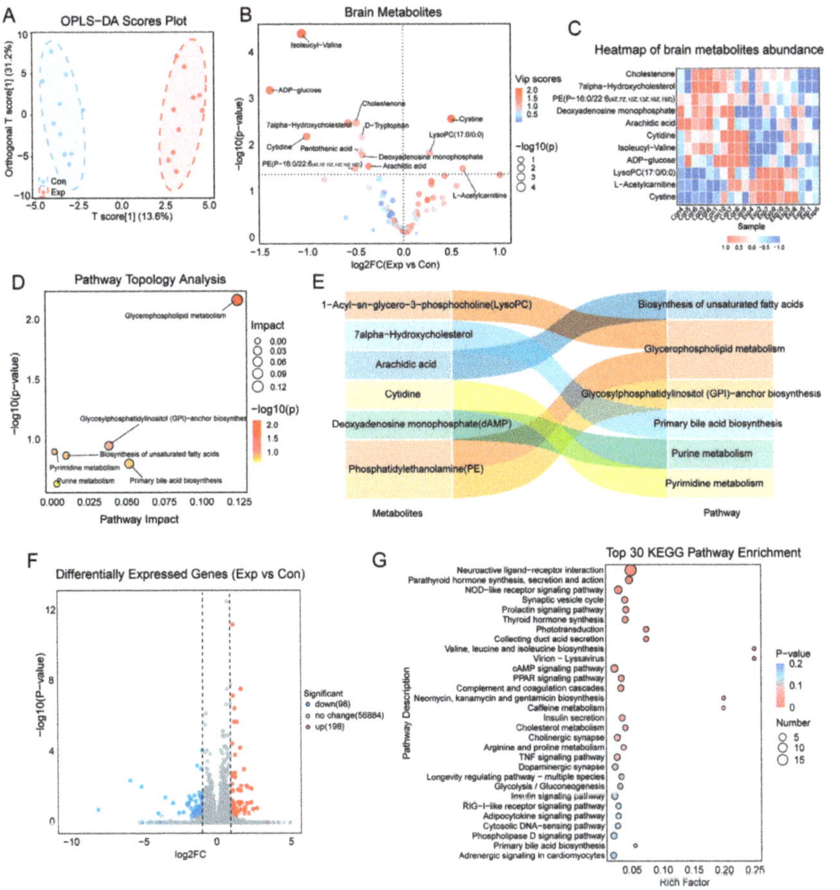


**Figure 3.** Alterations in metabolomics and transcriptomics in the hippocampus and cortex following growth-stage air pollution exposure. (**A**) OPLS-DA scores plot. (**B**) Volcano plot of brain metabolites, with the names of the top 13 metabolites based on VIP scores labeled. (**C**) Heatmap of brain metabolites abundance. (**D**) Topological analysis of differential metabolites in the KEGG pathway. (**E**) The correlations between differential metabolites and pathways. (**F**) Differentially expressed genes (DEGs): blue dots represent downregulated genes, red dots represent upregulated genes. (**G**) KEGG enrichment of DEGs: the y-axis represents enriched pathways, the x-axis shows the enrichment factor, circle size reflects gene count, and color indicates pathway $p$-values. Metabolomics: $n = 10$ per group. Transcriptomics: $n = 6$ per group.

### *3.4. Metabolomic and Transcriptomic Alterations in the Intestine*

OPLS-DA results from untargeted metabolomics analysis on intestine tissues are shown in Figure 5A. Based on the differential contributions, VIP scores for each metabolite were obtained (Figure S6). Under the screening thresholds of VIP > 1 and $p < 0.05$, 34 metabolites that were significantly different in the intestines of the two groups were identified (Figure 5B). The sample expression heatmap of key differential metabolites is shown in Figure 5C. KEGG pathway topological analysis (Figure 5D) showed that in the exposed group, significant changes occurred in pathways related to unsaturated fatty acid biosynthesis, alpha-linolenic acid metabolism, glycerophospholipid metabolism, pyrimidine metabolism, linoleic acid metabolism, and sphingolipid metabolism. In the separate sex analyses, similar results were also observed (Figure S7). Key differential metabolites included alpha-linolenic acid, DHA, gamma-linolenic acid, PC (16:0/18:1(9Z)), PE (P-18:0/20:4(5Z,8Z,11Z,14Z)), stearic acid and N-Acylsphingosine (Figure 5E).

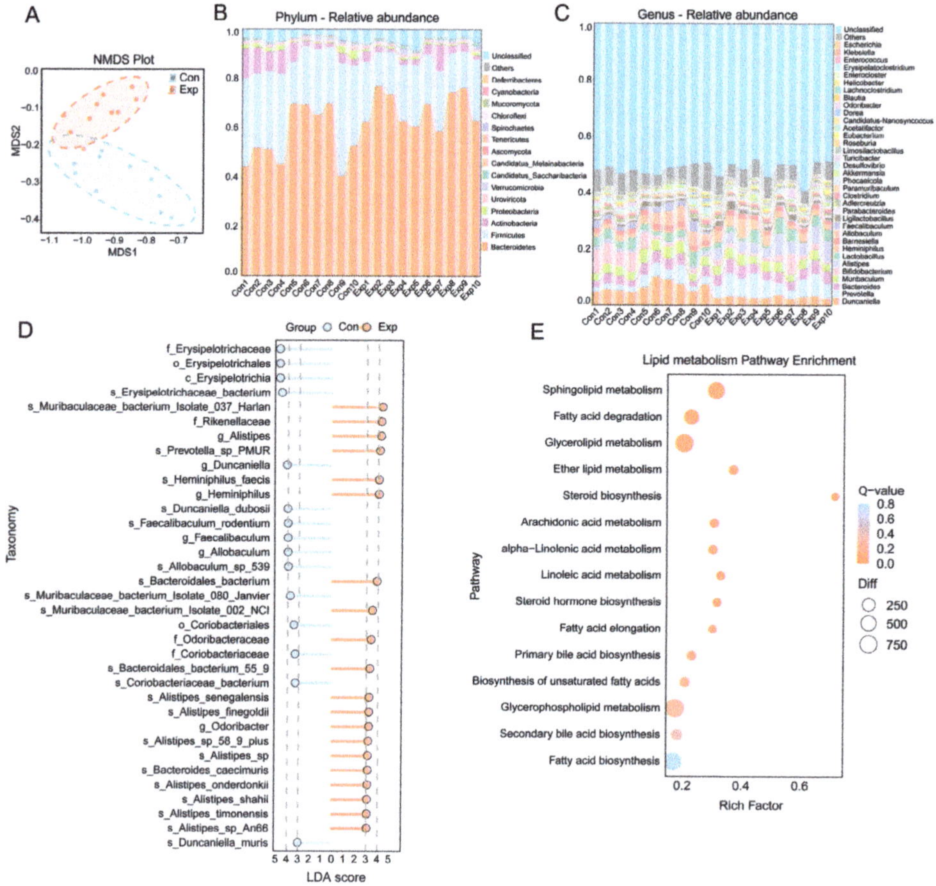


**Figure 4.** Effect of growth-stage air pollution exposure on gut microbiome, revealed by metagenomic sequencing. (**A**) NMDS plot of gut microbiome. (**B**,**C**) Relative abundance of microbiome at the phylum and genus levels for the samples. (**D**) Differential bacterial taxa identified by LEfSe analysis (Kruskal–Wallis test, $P_{FDR} < 0.05$ with Benjamini–Hochberg correction) with LDA scores $\geq 3$. (**E**) KEGG enrichment of DEGs. The y-axis represents enriched pathways, the x-axis shows the enrichment factor, circle size reflects gene count, and color indicates pathway Q-values. $n = 10$ per group.

In transcriptome analysis, a total of 425 significantly upregulated genes and 138 downregulated genes were identified (Figure 5F) using the criteria of $|\log_2(FC)| > 1$ and Q-value < 0.05. KEGG enrichment analysis indicated significant enrichment in pathways related to unsaturated fatty acid biosynthesis, including linoleic acid metabolism, arachidonic acid metabolism, alpha-linolenic acid metabolism, and the PPAR signaling pathway (Figure 5G). Key differential genes included Cyp3a13, Cyp2e1, Cyp3a25, Pla2g12b, Ggt1, Aloxe3, Acaa1b, Plin5, Me3, Hmgcs2, and Plin1. Taken together, metabolomics and transcriptomics results indicate that growth-stage air pollution exposure significantly alters unsaturated fatty acid biosynthesis, alpha-linolenic acid metabolism, and glycerophospholipid metabolism in the mouse intestine.

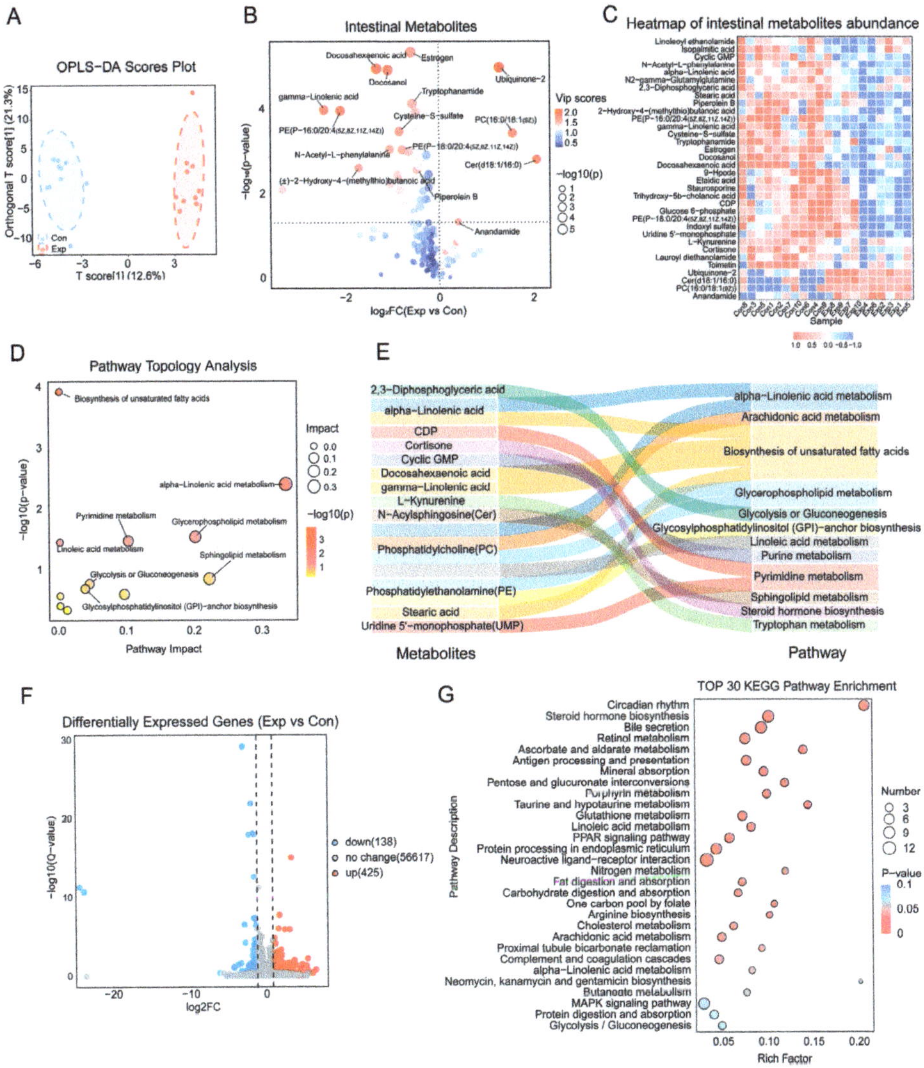

**Figure 5.** Metabolomic and transcriptomic alterations in the intestine. (**A**) OPLS-DA scores plot. (**B**) Volcano plot of intestinal metabolites, with the names of the top 15 metabolites based on VIP scores labeled. (**C**) Heatmap of intestinal metabolites abundance. (**D**) Topological analysis of differential metabolites in the KEGG pathway. (**E**) Correlations between differential metabolites and pathways. (**F**) Differentially expressed genes (DEGs): blue dots represent downregulated genes, red dots represent upregulated genes. (**G**) KEGG enrichment of DEGs: the y-axis represents enriched pathways, the x-axis shows the enrichment factor, circle size reflects gene count, and color indicates pathway $p$-values. Metabolomics: $n = 10$ per group. Transcriptomics: $n = 6$ per group.

*3.5. Serum Metabolomic Alterations*

The OPLS DA results from the untargeted metabolomics analysis of serum, including the VIP scores for metabolites, are shown in Figure 6A and Figure S8. Under the screening criteria of VIP > 1 and $p < 0.05$, 38 significantly different metabolites were identified in the serum of exposed and control mice (Figure 6B). The sample expression heatmap of key differential metabolites is shown in Figure 6C. KEGG pathway topological analysis (Figure 6D) showed significant changes in sphingolipid metabolism, unsaturated fatty acid biosynthesis, glycerophospholipid metabolism, arachidonic acid metabolism, linolenic acid metabolism and arachidonic acid metabolism in the exposed group. Key differential metabolites included sphinganine, sphingosine, gamma-linolenic acid, oleic acid, palmitic acid, PC (16:0/20:4(5Z,8Z,11Z,14Z)), PC (16:0/18:1(9Z)), LysoPC (18:1(9Z)/0:0), PS (18:1(11Z)/20:0), and leukotriene C4 (Figure 6E). Further analysis revealed a significant increase in saturated fatty acids (oleic acid, palmitic acid) and the pro-inflammatory mediator leukotriene C4 in the exposed group, whereas sphingolipid metabolites (sphinganine and sphingosine), unsaturated fatty acid (gamma-linolenic acid), and lipid metabolites (PC(16:0/20:4(5Z,8Z,11Z,14Z)), PC(16:0/18:1(9Z)), LysoPC(18:1(9Z)/0:0), PS(18:1(11Z)/20:0)) were significantly reduced. As leukotriene C4, a metabolite of the arachidonic acid pathway, is a potent pro-inflammatory mediator, its upregulation may indicate systemic inflammation [23]. In the separate sex analyses, similar results were also observed (Figure S9). The findings about serum metabolic changes suggest that air pollution exposure during growth stages may disrupt lipid-related metabolic pathways (e.g., unsaturated fatty acid, phospholipid, and sphingolipid metabolism), trigger systemic inflammation, and impair physiological homeostasis.

### *3.6. Correlation Between the Gut Microbiome and Host Metabolome*

Spearman correlation analysis revealed significant associations between key intestinal metabolites and differences in the microbiome ($P_{FDR} < 0.05$) (Figure 7A). For example, some microbes (e.g., *Alistipes.sp*, g_*Faecalibaculum*, *s_Coriobacteriaceae_bacterium* and *f_Erysipelotrichaceae*) were significantly associated with lipid-related metabolites (e.g., PE(P−16:0/20:4(5Z,8Z,11Z,14Z)), PC(16:0/18:1(9Z)), PS(18:1(11Z)/20:0), ceramide (Cer) (d18:1/16:0), DHA and gamma−Linolenic acid) ($P_{FDR} < 0.05$). Significant associations between gut microbiome and serum metabolites were also observed ($P_{FDR} < 0.05$) (Figure 7B). Notably, *Alistipes.sp* and *s_Bacteroidales_caecimuris* were positively correlated with the pro-inflammatory metabolite leukotriene C4 in serum ($P_{FDR} < 0.05$), but negatively correlated with sphinganine, sphingosine, gamma-linolenic acid, PS, PC and LysoPC ($P_{FDR} < 0.05$). Conversely, *s_Coriobacteriaceae_bacterium* and *o_Coriobacteriales* exhibited a negative correlation with leukotriene C4 ($P_{FDR} < 0.05$) and a positive correlation with these metabolites ($P_{FDR} < 0.05$).

Additionally, several intestinal and serum metabolites were significantly correlated with metabolic changes in the brain, including PE (P−16:0/22:6(4Z,7Z,10Z,13Z,16Z,19Z)), Arachidic acid, LysoPC (17:0/0:0), and Cystine ($P_{FDR} < 0.05$) (Figure 7C,D).

### *3.7. Mediating Role of Intestinal and Serum Metabolites*

Mediation analysis was conducted to explore the mediating effects of intestinal and serum metabolites in the relationship between differentially abundant microbiome (with LDA scores greater than 3) and brain metabolic changes. The results revealed that intestinal and serum metabolites mediated the effects of microbial taxa on different brain metabolites (proportion mediated: 9.5–99.6%, $p < 0.05$) (Table S1). Specifically, 13 metabolites (intestinal Cer(d18:1/16:0) and Ubiquinone-2, serum metabolites such as PS(18:1(11Z)/20:0), Sphingosine, gamma-Linolenic acid, Leukotriene C4, esterase, dimyristoylphosphatidylcholine, 16-Hydroxyhexadecanoic acid, Phenyllactic acid, arachidoyl ethanolamide, palmitoylethanolamide, phenyllactic acid, and heptadecanoic acid) mediated the influence of 22 key microbial taxa (*f_Coriobacteriaceae*, *f_Rikenellaceae*, *o_Coriobacteriales*, *g_Duncaniella*, *g_Alistipes*, *g_Heminiphilus*, *g_Allobaculum*, *s_Muribaculaceae_bacterium_Isolate_037_Harlan*, *s_Bacteroidales_bacterium*, *s_Bacteroidales_bacterium_55_9*, *s_Coriobacteriaceae_bacterium*, *s_Alistipes_sp_58_9_plus*, *s_Alistipes_sp*, *s_Bacteroides_caecimuris*, *s_Duncaniella_dubosii*, *s_Alistipes_senegalensis*, *s_Alistipes_onderdonkii*, *s_Allobaculum_sp_539*, *s_Alistipes_finegoldii*, *s_Alistipes_shahii*, *s_Alistipes_timonensis*, *s_Alistipes_sp_An66*) on brain LysoPC(17:0/0:0) and brain_PE(P-16:0/22:6(4Z,7Z,10Z,13Z,16Z,19Z)) metabolic changes (proportion mediated: 32.7–98.7%, $p < 0.05$) (Table 2).

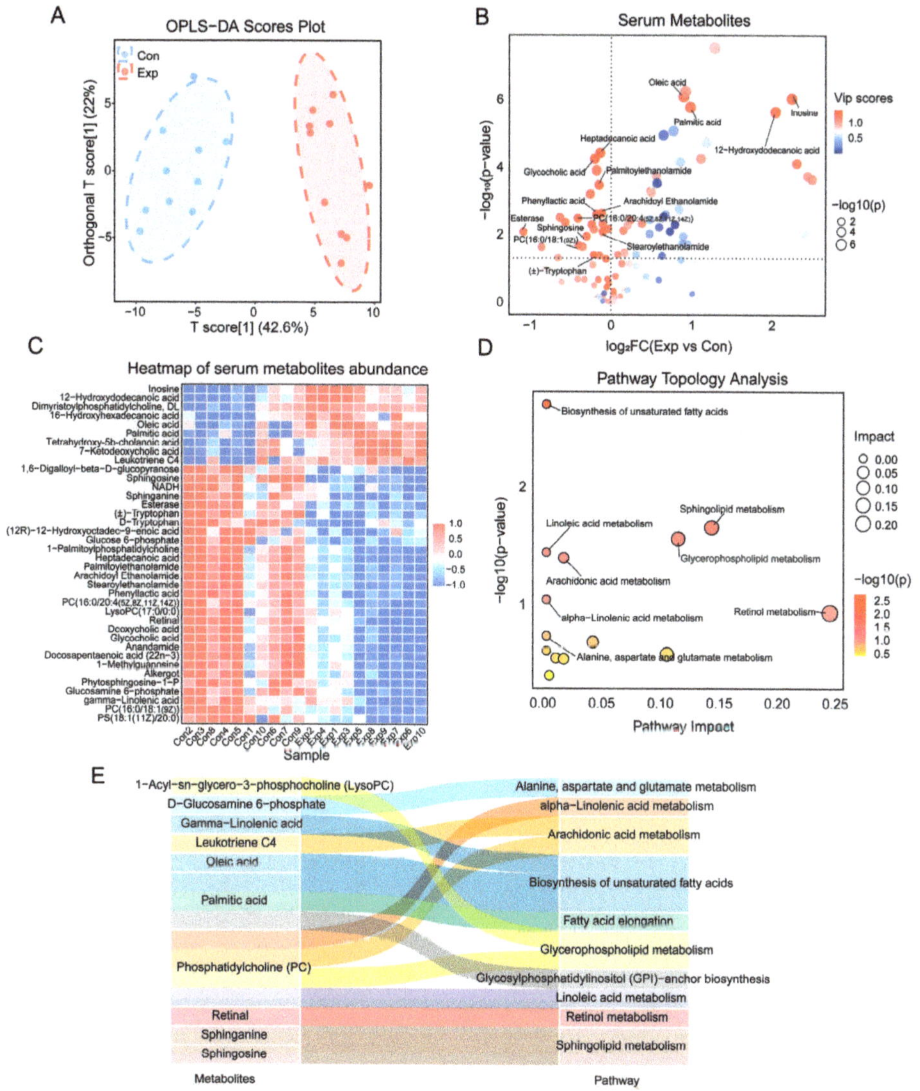


**Figure 6.** Metabolomic alterations in serum. (**A**) OPLS-DA scores plot. (**B**) Volcano plot of serum metabolites, with the names of the top 15 metabolites based on VIP scores labeled. (**C**) Heatmap of serum metabolites abundance. (**D**) Topological analysis of differential metabolites in the KEGG pathway. (**E**) Correlations between differential metabolites and pathways.

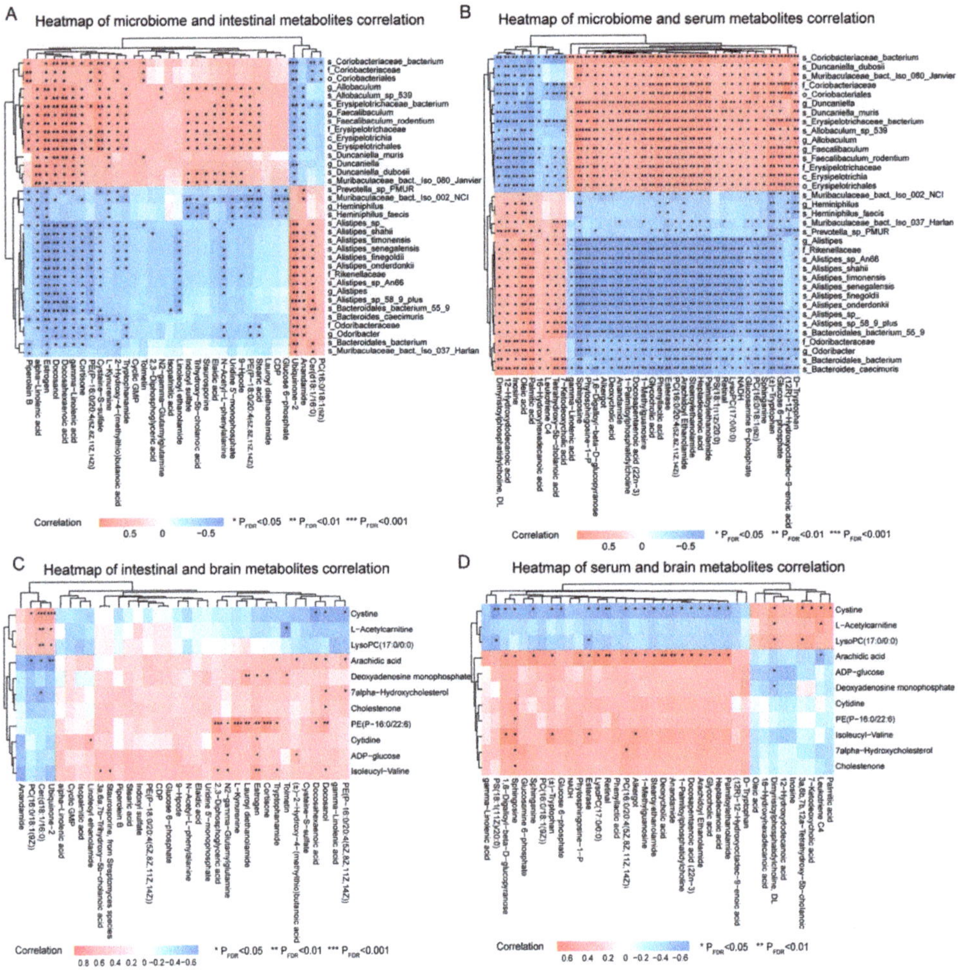


**Figure 7.** Correlation between the gut microbiome and host metabolome. (**A**) Heatmap of Spearman correlation analysis between differential taxa identified by LEfSe analysis (LDA $\geq$ 3) and differential intestinal metabolites. (**B**) Heatmap of Spearman correlation analysis between differentially identified taxa (LDA $\geq$ 3) from LEfSe analysis and differential serum metabolites. (**C**) Heatmap of Spearman correlation analysis between different intestinal metabolites and different brain metabolites. (**D**) Heatmap of Spearman correlation analysis between different serum metabolites and different brain metabolites. $n$ = 10 per group. $P_{FDR}$ indicates the $p$-value adjusted using the Benjamini–Hochberg method. * $P_{FDR} < 0.05$, ** $P_{FDR} < 0.01$, *** $P_{FDR} < 0.001$.

**Table 2.** Mediation analysis of the microbiome and brain lipid-related metabolites.

| Outcome Indicator | Exposure | Mediators | Indirect Effect (95% CI) | Proportion Mediated (%) |
|---|---|---|---|---|
| brain_LysoPC (17:0/0:0) | s__Muribaculaceae_bacterium_Isolate_037_Harlan_ | intestinal_Cer(d18:1/16:0) | 0.493 (0.106, 1.136) | 75.4 |
| | s__Muribaculaceae_bacterium_Isolate_037_Harlan_ | serum_Esterase | 0.377 (0.083, 0.792) | 57.8 |

**Table 2.** *Cont.*

| Outcome Indicator | Exposure | Mediators | Indirect Effect (95% CI) | Proportion Mediated (%) |
|---|---|---|---|---|
| | s__Muribaculaceae_bacterium_Isolate_037_Harlan_ | serum_PS(18:1(11Z)/20:0) | 0.332 (0.015, 0.882) | 50.8 |
| | s__Bacteroidales_bacterium | intestinal_Cer(d18:1/16:0) | 0.485 (0.073, 1.11) | 77.3 |
| | s__Bacteroidales_bacterium | serum_Esterase | 0.368 (0.076, 0.763) | 58.7 |
| | s__Bacteroidales_bacterium | serum_PS(18:1(11Z)/20:0) | 0.343 (0.068, 0.833) | 54.6 |
| | s_Bacteroidales_bacterium | serum_gamma-Linolenic acid | 0.283 (0.011, 0.736) | 45.2 |
| | o__Coriobacteriales | serum_PS(18:1(11Z)/20:0) | −0.102 (−0.23, −0.021) | 46.9 |
| | f__Coriobacteriaceae | serum_PS(18:1(11Z)/20:0) | −0.104 (−0.242, −0.022) | 46.6 |
| | s__Bacteroidales_bacterium_55_9 | serum_Esterase | 0.112 (0.004, 0.275) | 90.1 |
| | s__Bacteroidales_bacterium_55_9 | serum_16-Hydroxyhexadecanoic acid | 0.041 (0.003, 0.172) | 32.7 |
| | s__Coriobacteriaceae_bacterium | serum_PS(18:1(11Z)/20:0) | −0.064 (−0.189, −0.011) | 72.7 |
| | s__Alistipes_sp_58_9_plus | serum_Dimyristoylphosphatidylcholine | 0.074 (0.004, 0.148) | 66.2 |
| | s__Alistipes_sp_ | serum_Leukotriene C4 | 0.097 (0.007, 0.213) | 78.8 |
| | s__Bacteroides_caecimuris | intestinal_Cer(d18:1/16:0) | 0.271 (0.042, 0.554) | 98.4 |
| | s__Bacteroides_caecimuris | serum_Esterase | 0.228 (0.045, 0.576) | 83 |
| | s__Bacteroides_caecimuris | intestinal_Ubiquinone-2 | 0.164 (0.017, 0.395) | 59.7 |
| | s__Bacteroides_caecimuris | serum_PS(18:1(11Z)/20:0) | 0.216 (0.064, 0.477) | 78.4 |
| | s__Bacteroides_caecimuris | serum_Leukotriene C4 | 0.132 (0.01, 0.326) | 48 |
| | s__Bacteroides_caecimuris | serum_gamma-Linolenic acid | 0.134 (0.006, 0.415) | 48.9 |
| brain_PE(P−16:0/22:6(4Z,7Z,10Z,13Z,16Z,19Z)) | f__Rikenellaceae | serum_Arachidoyl Ethanolamide | −0.138 (−0.322, −0.014) | 87.6 |
| | f__Rikenellaceae | serum_Heptadecanoic acid | −0.142 (−0.365, −0.018) | 89.8 |
| | f__Rikenellaceae | serum_Palmitoylethanolamide | −0.133 (−0.309, −0.028) | 84.1 |
| | g_Alistipes | serum_Arachidoyl Ethanolamide | −0.128 (−0.288, −0.003) | 94.3 |
| | g_Alistipes | serum_Palmitoylethanolamide | −0.122 (−0.288, −0.01) | 90.2 |
| | g__Duncaniella | serum_Phenyllactic acid | 0.207 (0.032, 0.48) | 51.6 |
| | g__Duncaniella | serum_Sphingosine | 0.397 (0.002, 1.091) | 98.7 |
| | g_Heminiphilus | serum_Phenyllactic acid | −0.11 (−0.237, −0.01) | 52.3 |
| | s__Duncaniella_dubosii | serum_Phenyllactic acid | 0.114 (0.008, 0.248) | 37.1 |
| | g_Allobaculum | serum_Phenyllactic acid | 0.032 (0.005, 0.061) | 55.4 |
| | s_Allobaculum_sp_539 | serum_Phenyllactic acid | 0.032 (0.01, 0.059) | 74.1 |
| | s__Alistipes_senegalensis | serum_Arachidoyl Ethanolamide | −0.113 (−0.256, −0.007) | 72.9 |
| | s_Alistipes_finegoldii | serum_Arachidoyl Ethanolamide | −0.099 (−0.231, −0.003) | 69.5 |
| | s_Alistipes_finegoldii | serum_Heptadecanoic acid | −0.101 (−0.226, −0.002) | 70.9 |
| | s__Alistipes_onderdonkii | serum_Arachidoyl Ethanolamide | −0.1 (−0.257, −0.02) | 74 |
| | s__Alistipes_onderdonkii | serum_Heptadecanoic acid | −0.103 (−0.238, −0.001) | 75.8 |
| | s__Alistipes_shahii | serum_Heptadecanoic acid | −0.147 (−0.329, −0.022) | 86.4 |
| | s__Alistipes_timonensis | serum_Palmitoylethanolamide | −0.096 (−0.223, −0.007) | 63.7 |
| | s__Alistipes_sp_An66 | serum_Arachidoyl Ethanolamide | −0.1 (−0.24, −0.003) | 78.1 |

## 4. Discussion

To our knowledge, this is among the first studies to integrate gut metagenomics, metabolomics, and transcriptomics techniques to comprehensively examine the neurological impact of growth-stage air pollution exposure and the mediating effects of the gut microbiome. This study demonstrated that exposure to real-time ambient air pollution during growth stages induced damage in the hippocampus and cortex of offspring mice, along with alterations in brain glycerophospholipid metabolism. Additionally, changes in the gut microbiome and lipid metabolism, unsaturated fatty acid metabolism, and inflammatory signaling pathways across multiple organs were observed. Such changes partially mediated the detrimental effects of air pollution on the nervous system.

Growth stage is a crucial period for neurodevelopment, and epidemiological studies have shown that exposure to air pollution during pregnancy and the postnatal period can impact the neurodevelopment of offspring [4,6,24–26]. Using a whole-body real-time exposure system to simulate real-world environmental conditions, the present study revealed that exposure to ambient air pollution during growth stages induced pathological changes in the cortical and hippocampal regions of mouse brain tissue, including disordered cell arrangement, neuronal damage, and edema. This is generally consistent with previous studies [17,27].

Although previous studies have clearly revealed the direct toxic effects (e.g., cognitive dysfunction and pathological changes) of air pollution on the central nervous system (CNS) [28–30], the exact mechanisms by which air pollution leads to neural injury remain largely unclear. The MGBA axis interaction may be a key mechanism involved. Previous studies have demonstrated that air pollution, including $PM_{2.5}$, $NO_2$, and $O_3$, significantly alters the composition and function of the gut microbiome [31–33]. In this study, growth-stage exposure to air pollution significantly altered gut microbiome composition in mice. In particular, metagenomic analysis revealed that in the exposed group, the relative abundance of *s_Muribaculaceae_bacterium_Isolate_037_Harlan_*, *f_Rikenellaceae*, *g_Alistipes*, *s_Prevotella_sp_PMUR* increased, while *f_Erysipelotrichaceae*, *s_Erysipelotrichaceae_bacterium*, *g_Duncaniell* and *s_Duncaniella_dubosii* decreased. Previous studies have shown that these microbial taxa are closely linked to the health and disease status of the host and may have impacts on host metabolism and immune homeostasis. For example, studies have indicated that *Alistipes* is closely associated with colitis, and it is also linked to stress and depression [34,35]. These microbial changes may have profound effects on host metabolism and immune homeostasis, which could in turn impact brain development and function.

Evidence from both humans and animals has shown that air pollution can lead to metabolic disruptions [18,36], and changes in brain metabolism play a key role in the pathogenesis of neurological diseases [16]. At the same time, metabolites are key mediators for the interactions between the microbiome and host in the framework of MGBA. This study indicates that the changes in the gut microbiome induced by air pollution exposure are closely related to the host's metabolites. In addition to pathological damage in brain tissue, metabolomic analysis further revealed significant alterations in glycerophospholipid metabolism pathways. Such alterations were also observed in the intestine and serum. Meanwhile, functional analysis of the gut microbiome also revealed significant alterations in lipid-related metabolic pathways in different taxa, suggesting that lipid metabolism may play an important role. Furthermore, our mediation analysis suggests that intestinal and serum metabolites may mediate the impact of the microbiome on brain lipid metabolites (e.g., PE and PC), linked to glycerophospholipid metabolism. Therefore, these findings suggest that glycerophospholipid metabolism may represent an important altered cross-talk pathway in the microbiome–gut–brain axis, contributing to neurodamage caused by air pollution exposure during the growth stage.

Previous evidence from human and animal studies has also shown that air pollution, particularly $PM_{2.5}$, leads to disruptions in glycerophospholipid and sphingolipid metabolism [18,36]. Glycerophospholipids are major components of eukaryotic cell membranes, with PC and PE being the most abundant [37]. PC constitutes approximately 95% of total choline in most tissues, while PE is the second most abundant glycerophospholipid in cell membranes [37]. Other minor phospholipids, such as phosphatidylinositol (PI) and PS, are also involved in the structure of biological membranes. Glycerophospholipid metabolism is particularly important in the central nervous system, as it is a major component of neuronal membranes and myelin sheaths, maintaining neuronal stability and membrane fluidity [38]. Previous research has indicated that glycerophospholipid metabolism is disrupted in Alzheimer's disease (AD) patients and AD mouse models [19,39]. The gastrointestinal tract is the primary source of glycerophospholipids for brain neural membranes [40]. Recent studies have shown that disruptions in glycerophospholipid metabolism are closely associated with the microbiome–gut–brain axis in depression patients [41,42]. Therefore, disruptions in glycerophospholipid metabolism may be a key mechanism underlying neural dysfunction and could serve as an important metabolite in the gut–brain axis. In the present study, transcriptomic analysis of brain tissue further revealed that air pollution exposure activated several neuro-related pathways, particularly neuroactive ligand–receptor interactions, synaptic vesicle cycling, and phospholipase D signaling pathways, which may be related to changes in membrane fluidity and neuronal signal transmission. Notably, changes in the expression of Avpr1a (vasopressin receptor 1A), Dgkk (diacylglycerol kinase K), and Agt (angiotensinogen) were closely linked to glycerophospholipid metabolism. These genes may influence the stability of brain cell membranes and neuronal signal transmission. Additionally, changes in the expression of Gabrq (GABA receptor q subunit) and Chrna6 (nicotinic acetylcholine receptor $\alpha$6 subunit) could further affect neurotransmitter function and alter neuronal signal transmission. In summary, our findings suggest that air pollution may disrupt brain homeostasis and impair neural function by altering glycerophospholipid metabolism and related signaling pathways, with the gut–brain axis playing a key role in this process.

Notably, significant alterations in the unsaturated fatty acid biosynthesis pathway were also observed in the intestine, serum, and brain tissue in the present study. Mediation analysis suggests that these changes in intestine and serum partially mediated the alterations in brain lipids. Specifically, significant alterations in several fatty acids were observed in the intestine, serum, and brain, including alpha-linolenic acid, gamma-linolenic acid, DHA, oleic acid, palmitic acid, and arachidonic acid. These metabolites play crucial roles in immune regulation, lipid balance, and neural health. For instance, DHA, alpha-linolenic acid, and gamma-linolenic acid are involved in regulating inflammation and oxidative stress [43–46]. Fatty acids are essential components of lipids, and changes in fatty acid levels are closely linked to alterations in brain lipid metabolism. Also, transcriptomic analysis further revealed changes in PPAR signaling pathways, linoleic acid metabolism, and arachidonic acid metabolism in the intestine. Key differentially expressed genes, such as Acaa1b (acetyl-CoA carboxylase 1B), which is critical for fatty acid synthesis, may affect lipid metabolism and function in both the body and brain [47]. Additionally, Pla2g12b, a member of the phospholipase A2 family involved in lipid metabolism, particularly in the hydrolysis of phospholipids, may influence brain lipid metabolism by regulating lipid distribution and transport [48]. Therefore, the biosynthesis of unsaturated fatty acids may be an important pathway in the microbiome–gut–brain metabolic cross-talk.

The role of inflammation in neurological diseases has gained increasing attention, with inflammation being a crucial component of the MGBA. Studies have shown that dysregulation of the inflammatory response is closely associated with various neurological diseases, such as ASD, AD, and Parkinson's disease (PD) [49]. This study found that growth-stage exposure to air pollution significantly increased Leukotriene C4 levels in serum, a potent pro-inflammatory mediator, suggesting that air pollution may trigger a systemic inflammatory response. Transcriptomic analysis of brain tissue revealed that exposure activated several inflammation-related signaling pathways, including NOD-like receptor signaling. Metabolomic analysis revealed significant changes in inflammation-related metabolites in the intestine and serum of the exposed group, particularly DHA, alpha-linolenic acid, and gamma-linolenic acid. The decrease in these anti-inflammatory omega-3 fatty acids may weaken immune defense and contribute to the elevated systemic inflammation triggered by air pollution [44,50]. Furthermore, mediation analysis suggests that Leukotriene C4 in the serum mediates the effect of the key differential bacterium *s_Bacteroides_caecimuris* on brain LysoPC levels. Therefore, the disruption of unsaturated fatty acid levels and systemic inflammation induced by air pollution are closely related, potentially leading to brain lipid dysregulation and neuroinflammation, further exacerbating neuronal damage.

This study reveals that exposure to air pollution during the growth stage in mice leads to dysregulation of fatty acid metabolism, abnormal lipid metabolites, and inflammation in multiple organs (such as the intestine and brain), suggesting that environmental factors may affect neurodevelopment by disrupting the MGBA. While fecal microbiome transplantation shows potential for improving neurodevelopmental disorders like autism, precise intervention strategies targeting specific strains or metabolic molecules are still needed. Through multi-omics integration, the study identifies mechanisms by which the gut microbiome, the intestine, and the brain interact through lipid metabolism to regulate neurodevelopment, highlighting their potential as therapeutic targets.

This study has several strengths. First, a whole-body exposure system was used to simulate real-time exposure conditions, offering a more realistic approximation of air pollution exposure. Second, a multi-omics approach was employed to investigate the effects of air pollution exposure during the growth stage on multiple organs and omics in offspring, allowing for a more comprehensive analysis. However, several limitations should be noted. First, as our exposure model simulates real-world conditions with air pollution as a complex mixture, it is challenging to differentiate the effects of individual pollutants, particularly $PM_{2.5}$ and ozone. Second, this study only assessed changes in the microbiome and host metabolites, along with their mediating relationships. Future studies should explore more on the specific microbial strains affecting neurodamage through metabolic pathways. Third, metabolite selection based solely on OPLS-DA VIP scores (VIP > 1) and *p*-values ($p < 0.05$) may increase false-positive risks. Future studies should consider refining the analytical approach to improve the reliability and robustness of results. Fourth, further validation was not conducted using in vitro experiments with cell lines. Future research is encouraged to validate our findings and to shed light on the relevant molecular mechanisms.

## 5. Conclusions

In conclusion, our study demonstrates that growth-stage exposure to air pollution induces neurodamage in mice, potentially via the crosstalk mechanism of the MGBA, and dysregulation of multi-organ lipid metabolism, unsaturated fatty acid metabolism, and systemic inflammation are the potential pathways involved. These findings provide novel insights into the mechanisms underlying growth-stage air pollution-related neuronal damage.

**Supplementary Materials:** The following supporting information can be downloaded at: https://www.mdpi.com/article/10.3390/toxics13040260/s1. Figure S1: Mass concentration in the ambient air and exposure chambers of $PM_{2.5}$ and ozone; Figure S2: Top 30 VIP scores of brain metabolites; Figure S3: Sex-specific metabolic alterations in the hippocampus and cortex following growth-stage air pollution exposure; Figure S4: Heatmap of gut microbiome abundance; Figure S5: Sex-specific alterations in microbiome structure and function; Figure S6: Top 30 VIP scores of intestinal metabolites; Figure S7: Sex-specific metabolomic and transcriptomic alterations in the intestine; Figure S8: Top 30 VIP scores of serum metabolites; Figure S9: Sex-specific metabolomic alterations in serum; Table S1: The mediation analysis for microbiome and brain metabolites.

**Author Contributions:** Conceptualization, Z.C. and Z.Z.; Data curation, Z.Y.; Formal analysis, Z.Y., Y.Z., S.R., J.Z., F.T., H.S., X.L. (Xiuxiu Li), X.L. (Xinyue Li) and Y.G.; Funding acquisition, H.L. and Z.Z.; Investigation, Z.Y., Y.Z., S.R., J.Z., F.T., H.S., S.W., X.L. (Xiuxiu Li), X.L. (Xinyue Li) and Y.G.; Methodology, Z.Y. and Y.Z.; Project administration, Z.Z.; Resources, S.W., G.J., H.L. and Z.C.; Software, Z.Y.; Validation, Z.Y., Y.Z. and S.R.; Visualization, Z.Y.; Writing—original draft, Z.Y.; Writing—review and editing, Z.Y., Y.Z., S.R., J.Z., F.T., H.S., S.W., X.L. (Xiuxiu Li), X.L. (Xinyue Li), Y.G., G.J., H.L., Z.C. and Z.Z. All authors have read and agreed to the published version of the manuscript.

**Funding:** The present study was supported by the National Natural Science Foundation of China (NO. 82203988), the Guangdong Basic and Applied Basic Research Foundation (NO. 2022A1515010695 and NO. 2024A1515010465), the Science and Technology Program of Guangzhou (NO. 2023A04J2071) and the Fundamental Research Funds for the Central Universities of Sun Yat-sen University (NO. 23qnpy107).

**Institutional Review Board Statement:** The animal study protocol was approved by the Institutional Animal Care and Use Committee of Peking University Health Science Center (protocol code BCJD0130, approval date: 29 April 2023).

**Informed Consent Statement:** Not applicable.

**Data Availability Statement:** The datasets used and/or analyzed during the current study are available from the corresponding author on reasonable request.

**Acknowledgments:** We are grateful to all the staff involved in this work.

**Conflicts of Interest:** The authors declare no competing interests.

## Abbreviations

Acox2: Acyl-CoA Oxidase 2; ADHD, Attention-Deficit/Hyperactivity Disorder; Agt, Angiotensinogen; Aloxe3, Arachidonate Lipoxygenase 3; Angptl4, Angiopoietin-like 4; ASD, Autism Spectrum Disorder; Avpr1a, Arginine Vasopressin Receptor 1A; Brs3, Bombesin-like Receptor 3; C3, Complement Component 3; CA, Cornu Ammonis; Ca, Calcium; $Ca^{2+}$, Calcium Ion; Cer, Ceramide; Chrna6, Cholinergic Receptor Nicotinic Alpha 6 Subunit; CNS, Central Nervous System; Cyp2e1, Cytochrome P450 Family 2 Subfamily E Member 1; Cyp3a13, Cytochrome P450 Family 3 Subfamily A Member 13; Cyp3a25, Cytochrome P450 Family 3 Subfamily A Member 25; DEGs, Differentially Expressed Genes; DHA, Docosahexaenoic Acid; DG, Dentate Gyrus; E, Embryonic Day; Exp, Exposure; FA, Filtered Air; Fe, Iron; FDR, False Discovery Rate; f, Family; Gabrq, Gamma-Aminobutyric Acid Type A Receptor Subunit Theta; g, Genus; Ggt1, Gamma-Glutamyltransferase 1; GPI, Glycosylphosphatidylinositol; Gzma, Granzyme A; HEPA, High-Efficiency Particulate Air; HMDB, Human Metabolome Database; Hmgcs2, 3-Hydroxy-3-Methylglutaryl-CoA Synthase 2; IVCs, Individually Ventilated Cages; KEGG, Kyoto Encyclopedia of Genes and Genomes; LC-MS, Liquid Chromatography-Mass Spectrometry; LDA, Linear Discriminant Analysis; LEfSe, Linear Discriminant Analysis Effect Size; Ltb4r1, Leukotriene B4 Receptor 1; LysoPC, Lysophosphatidylcholine; Me3, Methylation Level 3; MGBA, Microbiome–Gut–Brain Axis; Na, Sodium; $NH^{4+}$, Ammonium Ion; NDDs, Neurodevelopmental Disorders; NMDS, Non-metric Multidimensional Scaling; $NO_2$, Nitrogen Dioxide; NOD-like, Nucleotide-binding Oligomerization Domain-like; o, Order; $O_3$, Ozone;

OPLS-DA, Orthogonal Partial Least Squares Discriminant Analysis; p, Phylum; Pck1, Phosphoenolpyruvate Carboxykinase 1; PC, Phosphatidylcholine; PE, Phosphatidylethanolamine; Pla2g12b, Phospholipase A2 Group XII B; Plin1, Perilipin 1; Plin5, Perilipin 5; $PM_{2.5}$, Fine Particulate Matter; PND, Postnatal Day; PPAR, Peroxisome Proliferator-Activated Receptor; PS, Phosphatidylserine; QC, Quality Control; Q-value, Adjusted *p*-value Controlling for False Discovery Rate; RTAAE, Real-Time Ambient Air Exposure; s, Species; UPLC, Ultra-Performance Liquid Chromatography; VIP score, Variable Importance in Projection Score.

## References


1. Cohen, A.J.; Brauer, M.; Burnett, R.; Anderson, H.R.; Frostad, J.; Estep, K.; Balakrishnan, K.; Brunekreef, B.; Dandona, L.; Dandona R.; et al. Estimates and 25-Year Trends of the Global Burden of Disease Attributable to Ambient Air Pollution: An Analysis of Data from the Global Burden of Diseases Study 2015. *Lancet* **2017**, *389*, 1907–1918. [CrossRef] [PubMed]
2. Costa, L.G.; Cole, T.B.; Dao, K.; Chang, Y.-C.; Coburn, J.; Garrick, J.M. Effects of Air Pollution on the Nervous System and Its Possible Role in Neurodevelopmental and Neurodegenerative Disorders. *Pharmacol. Ther.* **2020**, *210*, 107523. [CrossRef]
3. Murata, H.; Barnhill, L.M.; Bronstein, J.M. Air Pollution and the Risk of Parkinson's Disease: A Review. *Mov. Disord.* **2022**, *37*, 894–904. [CrossRef] [PubMed]
4. Castagna, A.; Mascheroni, E.; Fustinoni, S.; Montirosso, R. Air Pollution and Neurodevelopmental Skills in Preschool- and School-Aged Children: A Systematic Review. *Neurosci. Biobehav. Rev.* **2022**, *136*, 104623. [CrossRef]
5. Chun, H.; Leung, C.; Wen, S.W.; McDonald, J.; Shin, H.H. Maternal Exposure to Air Pollution and Risk of Autism in Children: A Systematic Review and Meta-Analysis. *Environ. Pollut.* **2020**, *256*, 113307. [CrossRef]
6. Pagalan, L.; Bickford, C.; Weikum, W.; Lanphear, B.; Brauer, M.; Lanphear, N.; Hanley, G.E.; Oberlander, T.F.; Winters, M. Association of Prenatal Exposure to Air Pollution with Autism Spectrum Disorder. *JAMA Pediatr.* **2019**, *173*, 86–92. [CrossRef]
7. Morais, L.H.; Schreiber, H.L.; Mazmanian, S.K. The Gut Microbiota-Brain Axis in Behaviour and Brain Disorders. *Nat. Rev. Microbiol.* **2021**, *19*, 241–255. [CrossRef]
8. Wang, Q.; Yang, Q.; Liu, X. The Microbiota-Gut-Brain Axis and Neurodevelopmental Disorders. *Protein Cell* **2023**, *14*, 762–775. [CrossRef]
9. Borre, Y.E.; O'Keeffe, G.W.; Clarke, G.; Stanton, C.; Dinan, T.G.; Cryan, J.F. Microbiota and Neurodevelopmental Windows: Implications for Brain Disorders. *Trends Mol. Med.* **2014**, *20*, 509–518. [CrossRef]
10. Desbonnet, L.; Clarke, G.; Traplin, A.; O'Sullivan, O.; Crispie, F.; Moloney, R.D.; Cotter, P.D.; Dinan, T.G.; Cryan, J.F. Gut Microbiota Depletion from Early Adolescence in Mice: Implications for Brain and Behaviour. *Brain Behav. Immun.* **2015**, *48*, 165–173. [CrossRef]
11. Guilloteau, E.; Coll, P.; Lu, Z.; Djouina, M.; Cazaunau, M.; Waxin, C.; Bergé, A.; Caboche, S.; Gratien, A.; Al Marj, E.; et al. Murine in Utero Exposure to Simulated Complex Urban Air Pollution Disturbs Offspring Gut Maturation and Microbiota during Intestinal Suckling-to-Weaning Transition in a Sex-Dependent Manner. *Part. Fibre Toxicol.* **2022**, *19*, 41. [CrossRef]
12. Xie, S.; Zhang, C.; Zhao, J.; Li, D.; Chen, J. Exposure to Concentrated Ambient PM2.5 (CAPM) Induces Intestinal Disturbance via Inflammation and Alternation of Gut Microbiome. *Environ. Int.* **2022**, *161*, 107138. [CrossRef]
13. Li, T.; Fang, J.; Tang, S.; Du, H.; Zhao, L.; Wang, Y.; Deng, F.; Liu, Y.; Du, Y.; Cui, L.; et al. PM2.5 Exposure Associated with Microbiota Gut-Brain Axis: Multi-Omics Mechanistic Implications from the BAPE Study. *Innovation* **2022**, *3*, 100213. [CrossRef] [PubMed]
14. Yi, W.; Ji, Y.; Gao, H.; Pan, R.; Song, J.; He, Y.; Li, Y.; Wu, Y.; Yan, S.; Liang, Y.; et al. Effects of Urban Particulate Matter on Gut Microbiome and Partial Schizophrenia-like Symptoms in Mice: Evidence from Shotgun Metagenomic and Metabolomic Profiling. *Sci. Total Environ.* **2023**, *857*, 159305. [CrossRef] [PubMed]
15. Zhu, X.; Xia, Y.; Wang, H.; Shi, L.; Yin, H.; Gu, M.; Yan, F. PM2.5 Induced Neurotoxicity through Unbalancing Vitamin B12 Metabolism by Gut Microbiota Disturbance. *Gut Microbes* **2023**, *15*, 2267186. [CrossRef] [PubMed]
16. Dumas, M.-E.; Davidovic, L. Metabolic Profiling and Phenotyping of Central Nervous System Diseases: Metabolites Bring Insights into Brain Dysfunctions. *J. Neuroimmune Pharmacol.* **2015**, *10*, 402–424. [CrossRef]
17. Cole, T.B.; Chang, Y.-C.; Dao, K.; Daza, R.; Hevner, R.; Costa, L.G. Developmental Exposure to Diesel Exhaust Upregulates Transcription Factor Expression, Decreases Hippocampal Neurogenesis, and Alters Cortical Lamina Organization: Relevance to Neurodevelopmental Disorders. *J. Neurodev. Disord.* **2020**, *12*, 41. [CrossRef]
18. Nassan, F.L.; Wang, C.; Kelly, R.S.; Lasky-Su, J.A.; Vokonas, P.S.; Koutrakis, P.; Schwartz, J.D. Ambient PM2.5 Species and Ultrafine Particle Exposure and Their Differential Metabolomic Signatures. *Environ. Int.* **2021**, *151*, 106447. [CrossRef]
19. Akyol, S.; Ugur, Z.; Yilmaz, A.; Ustun, I.; Gorti, S.K.K.; Oh, K.; McGuinness, B.; Passmore, P.; Kehoe, P.G.; Maddens, M.E.; et al. Lipid Profiling of Alzheimer's Disease Brain Highlights Enrichment in Glycerol(Phospho)Lipid, and Sphingolipid Metabolism. *Cells* **2021**, *10*, 2591. [CrossRef]

20. Xu, J.; Zhang, Q.; Su, Z.; Liu, Y.; Yan, T.; Zhang, Y.; Wang, T.; Wei, X.; Chen, Z.; Hu, G.; et al. Genetic Damage and Potential Mechanism Exploration under Different Air Pollution Patterns by Multi-Omics. *Environ. Int.* **2022**, *170*, 107636. [CrossRef]
21. Xu, J.; Liu, Y.; Zhang, Q.; Su, Z.; Yan, T.; Zhou, S.; Wang, T.; Wei, X.; Chen, Z.; Hu, G.; et al. DNA Damage, Serum Metabolomic Alteration and Carcinogenic Risk Associated with Low-Level Air Pollution. *Environ. Pollut.* **2022**, *297*, 118763. [CrossRef] [PubMed]
22. Yan, T.; Wang, W.; Xia, J.; Jia, J.; Xu, J.; Dan, M.; Zhou, S.; Niu, P.; Gong, S.; Chen, Z.; et al. Exposure to the Real Ambient Air Pollutants Alters the Composition of Nasal Mucosa Bacteria in the Rat Model. *Chemosphere* **2022**, *287*, 132269. [CrossRef] [PubMed]
23. Funk, C.D. Prostaglandins and Leukotrienes: Advances in Eicosanoid Biology. *Science* **2001**, *294*, 1871–1875. [CrossRef]
24. Guxens, M.; Garcia-Esteban, R.; Giorgis-Allemand, L.; Forns, J.; Badaloni, C.; Ballester, F.; Beelen, R.; Cesaroni, G.; Chatzi, L.; de Agostini, M.; et al. Air Pollution during Pregnancy and Childhood Cognitive and Psychomotor Development: Six European Birth Cohorts. *Epidemiology* **2014**, *25*, 636–647. [CrossRef] [PubMed]
25. Holm, S.M.; Balmes, J.R.; Gunier, R.B.; Kogut, K.; Harley, K.G.; Eskenazi, B. Cognitive Development and Prenatal Air Pollution Exposure in the CHAMACOS Cohort. *Environ. Health Perspect.* **2023**, *131*, 37007. [CrossRef]
26. Ni, Y.; Loftus, C.T.; Szpiro, A.A.; Young, M.T.; Hazlehurst, M.F.; Murphy, L.E.; Tylavsky, F.A.; Mason, W.A.; LeWinn, K.Z.; Sathyanarayana, S.; et al. Associations of Pre- and Postnatal Air Pollution Exposures with Child Behavioral Problems and Cognitive Performance: A U.S. Multi-Cohort Study. *Environ. Health Perspect.* **2022**, *130*, 67008. [CrossRef]
27. Zhang, T.; Zheng, X.; Wang, X.; Zhao, H.; Wang, T.; Zhang, H.; Li, W.; Shen, H.; Yu, L. Maternal Exposure to PM2.5 during Pregnancy Induces Impaired Development of Cerebral Cortex in Mice Offspring. *Int. J. Mol. Sci.* **2018**, *19*, 257. [CrossRef]
28. Allen, J.L.; Liu, X.; Pelkowski, S.; Palmer, B.; Conrad, K.; Oberdörster, G.; Weston, D.; Mayer-Pröschel, M.; Cory-Slechta, D.A. Early Postnatal Exposure to Ultrafine Particulate Matter Air Pollution: Persistent Ventriculomegaly, Neurochemical Disruption, and Glial Activation Preferentially in Male Mice. *Environ. Health Perspect.* **2014**, *122*, 939–945. [CrossRef]
29. Liu, F.; Liu, C.; Liu, Y.; Wang, J.; Wang, Y.; Yan, B. Neurotoxicity of the Air-Borne Particles: From Molecular Events to Human Diseases. *J. Hazard. Mater.* **2023**, *457*, 131827. [CrossRef]
30. Fonken, L.K.; Xu, X.; Weil, Z.M.; Chen, G.; Sun, Q.; Rajagopalan, S.; Nelson, R.J. Air Pollution Impairs Cognition, Provokes Depressive-like Behaviors and Alters Hippocampal Cytokine Expression and Morphology. *Mol. Psychiatry* **2011**, *16*, 987–995. [CrossRef]
31. Mutlu, E.A.; Comba, I.Y.; Cho, T.; Engen, P.A.; Yazıcı, C.; Soberanes, S.; Hamanaka, R.B.; Niğdelioğlu, R.; Meliton, A.Y.; Ghio, A.J.; et al. Inhalational Exposure to Particulate Matter Air Pollution Alters the Composition of the Gut Microbiome. *Environ. Pollut.* **2018**, *240*, 817–830. [CrossRef] [PubMed]
32. Wang, W.; Zhou, J.; Chen, M.; Huang, X.; Xie, X.; Li, W.; Cao, Q.; Kan, H.; Xu, Y.; Ying, Z. Exposure to Concentrated Ambient PM2.5 Alters the Composition of Gut Microbiota in a Murine Model. *Part. Fibre Toxicol.* **2018**, *15*, 17. [CrossRef] [PubMed]
33. Liu, Y.; Wang, T.; Si, B.; Du, H.; Liu, Y.; Waqas, A.; Huang, S.; Zhao, G.; Chen, S.; Xu, A. Intratracheally Instillated Diesel PM2.5 Significantly Altered the Structure and Composition of Indigenous Murine Gut Microbiota. *Ecotoxicol. Environ. Saf.* **2021**, *210*, 111903. [CrossRef] [PubMed]
34. Naseribafrouei, A.; Hestad, K.; Avershina, E.; Sekelja, M.; Linløkken, A.; Wilson, R.; Rudi, K. Correlation between the Human Fecal Microbiota and Depression. *Neurogastroenterol. Motil.* **2014**, *26*, 1155–1162. [CrossRef]
35. Parker, B.J.; Wearsch, P.A.; Veloo, A.C.M.; Rodriguez-Palacios, A. The Genus Alistipes: Gut Bacteria with Emerging Implications to Inflammation, Cancer, and Mental Health. *Front. Immunol.* **2020**, *11*, 906. [CrossRef]
36. Li, R.; Wang, Y.; Hou, B.; Lam, S.M.; Zhang, W.; Chen, R.; Shui, G.; Sun, Q.; Qiang, G.; Liu, C. Lipidomics Insight into Chronic Exposure to Ambient Air Pollution in Mice. *Environ. Pollut.* **2020**, *262*, 114668. [CrossRef]
37. Guido, M.E.; Monjes, N.M.; Wagner, P.M.; Salvador, G.A. Circadian Regulation and Clock-Controlled Mechanisms of Glycerophospholipid Metabolism from Neuronal Cells and Tissues to Fibroblasts. *Mol. Neurobiol.* **2022**, *59*, 326–353. [CrossRef]
38. Mochel, F. Lipids and Synaptic Functions. *J. Inherit. Metab. Dis.* **2018**, *41*, 1117–1122. [CrossRef]
39. Qian, X.; Hai, W.; Chen, S.; Zhang, M.; Jiang, X.; Tang, H. Multi-Omics Data Reveals Aberrant Gut Microbiota-Host Glycerophospholipid Metabolism in Association with Neuroinflammation in APP/PS1 Mice. *Gut Microbes* **2023**, *15*, 2282790. [CrossRef]
40. Zheng, P.; Wu, J.; Zhang, H.; Perry, S.W.; Yin, B.; Tan, X.; Chai, T.; Liang, W.; Huang, Y.; Li, Y.; et al. The Gut Microbiome Modulates Gut-Brain Axis Glycerophospholipid Metabolism in a Region-Specific Manner in a Nonhuman Primate Model of Depression. *Mol. Psychiatry* **2021**, *26*, 2380–2392. [CrossRef]
41. Tian, T.; Mao, Q.; Xie, J.; Wang, Y.; Shao, W.-H.; Zhong, Q.; Chen, J.-J. Multi-Omics Data Reveals the Disturbance of Glycerophospholipid Metabolism Caused by Disordered Gut Microbiota in Depressed Mice. *J. Adv. Res.* **2022**, *39*, 135–145. [CrossRef]
42. Xie, J.; Zhong, Q.; Wu, W.-T.; Chen, J.-J. Multi-Omics Data Reveals the Important Role of Glycerophospholipid Metabolism in the Crosstalk between Gut and Brain in Depression. *J. Transl. Med.* **2023**, *21*, 93. [CrossRef] [PubMed]
43. Kim, H.-Y.; Huang, B.X.; Spector, A.A. Molecular and Signaling Mechanisms for Docosahexaenoic Acid-Derived Neurodevelopment and Neuroprotection. *Int. J. Mol. Sci.* **2022**, *23*, 4635. [CrossRef]

44. Ferreira, I.; Falcato, F.; Bandarra, N.; Rauter, A.P. Resolvins, Protectins, and Maresins: DHA-Derived Specialized pro-Resolving Mediators, Biosynthetic Pathways, Synthetic Approaches, and Their Role in Inflammation. *Molecules* **2022**, *27*, 1677. [CrossRef]
45. Sergeant, S.; Rahbar, E.; Chilton, F.H. Gamma-Linolenic Acid, Dihommo-Gamma Linolenic, Eicosanoids and Inflammatory Processes. *Eur. J. Pharmacol.* **2016**, *785*, 77–86. [CrossRef] [PubMed]
46. Kim, O.Y.; Song, J. Important Roles of Linoleic Acid and α-Linolenic Acid in Regulating Cognitive Impairment and Neuropsychiatric Issues in Metabolic-Related Dementia. *Life Sci.* **2024**, *337*, 122356. [CrossRef] [PubMed]
47. Dave, A.; Park, E.-J.; Kumar, A.; Parande, F.; Beyoğlu, D.; Idle, J.R.; Pezzuto, J.M. Consumption of Grapes Modulates Gene Expression, Reduces Non-Alcoholic Fatty Liver Disease, and Extends Longevity in Female C57BL/6J Mice Provided with a High-Fat Western-Pattern Diet. *Foods* **2022**, *11*, 1984. [CrossRef]
48. Thierer, J.H.; Foresti, O.; Yadav, P.K.; Wilson, M.H.; Moll, T.O.C.; Shen, M.-C.; Busch-Nentwich, E.M.; Morash, M.; Mohlke, K.L.; Rawls, J.F.; et al. Pla2g12b Drives Expansion of Triglyceride-Rich Lipoproteins. *Nat. Commun.* **2024**, *15*, 2095. [CrossRef]
49. Xu, J.; Ma, C.; Hua, M.; Li, J.; Xiang, Z.; Wu, J. CNS and CNS Diseases in Relation to Their Immune System. *Front. Immunol.* **2022**, *13*, 1063928. [CrossRef]
50. Simopoulos, A.P. Omega-3 Fatty Acids in Inflammation and Autoimmune Diseases. *J. Am. Coll. Nutr.* **2002**, *21*, 495–505. [CrossRef]

toxics

MDPI

Article

# Associations of Urinary Perchlorate, Nitrate, and Thiocyanate with Female Infertility and Mediation of Obesity: Insights from NHANES 2013–2018

Lan Zhang, Yuhe Peng, Yue Song, Yu Zhang, Qi Qin, Mengya Ying, Yiyun Bi and Ping Yin *

Department of Epidemiology and Biostatistics, School of Public Health, Tongji Medical College, Huazhong University of Science and Technology, Wuhan 430030, China; calva_lan@163.com (L.Z.); p2yu303@163.com (Y.P.); m202275511@hust.edu.cn (Y.S.); zhangyu81717@163.com (Y.Z.); m202275593@hust.edu.cn (Q.Q.); ymy199661@163.com (M.Y.); byy112ybb@163.com (Y.B.)

* Correspondence: ping_y@hust.edu.cn

**Abstract:** Classified as endocrine disrupting chemicals (EDCs), perchlorate, nitrate, and thiocyanate have been implicated with obesity and reproductive disorders. This study used three cycles of the National Health and Nutrition Examination Survey (NHANES 2013–2018); 813 women of reproductive age were finally included. We used multivariable logistic regression to analyze the associations between the three anions and obesity and infertility. Subsequently, we performed mediation analysis to explore the potential mediating effect of obesity on infertility in association with anion exposure. Increased concentrations of perchlorate and nitrate showed inverse correlations with the risk of obesity (OR = 0.73, 95% CI: 0.55–0.96; OR = 0.59, 95% CI: 0.40–0.87). Perchlorate was negatively associated with infertility (OR = 0.68, 95% CI: 0.51–0.91), and obesity was a mediator in association between perchlorate and infertility. These findings suggest that women of reproductive age may be protected from obesity and infertility by exposure to perchlorate and nitrate, with obesity acting as a moderating factor in the observed association. This study provides a valuable understanding of the complex links between environmental contaminants, obesity, and reproductive health, and identifies potential strategies to reduce the risk of infertility and improve women's health.

**Keywords:** perchlorate; nitrate; thiocyanate; female infertility; obesity; mediation

## 1. Introduction

Female infertility, defined as the inability to achieve pregnancy after 12 months or more of regular, unprotected sexual intercourse [1], influences 5.8% to 8.1% women in the US, and is increasing year over year [2,3]. This condition not only profoundly impacts women's reproductive and cardiovascular health, but also exerts significant social and psychological effects on individuals, families, and society, making it a critical public health issue [4,5].

Obesity is defined by the World Health Organization (WHO) as having a body mass index (BMI) greater than 30 kg/m$^2$, a condition that affects approximately 800 million people worldwide [6,7]. Obesity rates continue to rise globally every year [8]. About 42% adults in the US are identified as having obesity [9], with the prevalence among women of reproductive age reaching 23% [10]. Obesity in women can lead to a number of reproductive problems, including menstrual irregularities, endometrial abnormalities, and infertility. Additionally, women with obesity are more susceptible to pregnancy complications, including hypertension and gestational diabetes [11,12].



https://doi.org/10.3390/toxics13010015

In the United States, perchlorate, thiocyanate, and nitrate in food and the environment are regulated by the Environmental Protection Agency (EPA) and the Food and Drug Administration (FDA). Numerous studies have confirmed that perchlorate, nitrate, and thiocyanate are common environmental endocrine disruptors with significant health impacts [13–15]. Perchlorate is widely used in military and industrial sectors, including aerospace, fireworks, and explosives, with environmental exposure mainly through contaminated food and drinking water [16]. Nitrate is widely used in agriculture and food preservation, with dietary intake, particularly from contaminated leafy vegetables and processed foods, being the primary source of exposure [17,18]. Thiocyanate, a cyanide metabolite, is mainly found in cruciferous vegetables (such as broccoli and kale), leafy greens, and dairy products, with tobacco exposure also being a major source [19,20]. Studies have emphasized that the levels of perchlorate, nitrate and thiocyanate in urine can serve as indicators of previous bodily exposure [21]. These three anions are known to disrupt thyroid function by competitively inhibiting iodine uptake at the sodium iodide symporter, thereby exerting endocrine-disrupting effects [22,23]. Research indicated that endocrine disruption caused by thyroid hormone dysfunction affects the hypothalamic–pituitary–ovarian (HPO) axis, thereby influencing female reproduction [24]. Previous biomonitoring reports showed higher exposure to perchlorate, nitrate, and thiocyanate in women. These reports underscore the need for further investigation into the specific risks posed by these chemicals, particularly in relation to reproductive health and endocrine function [25].

Previous studies have shown negative associations between urinary nitrate and obesity, while thiocyanate showed the opposite effect [26]. Obesity can disrupt the HPO axis through mechanisms such as insulin resistance and increased androgen production, potentially leading to infertility and negatively affecting women's reproductive capacity [27]. Based on these findings, we hypothesize that obesity may mediate the relationship between perchlorate, nitrate, thiocyanate, and infertility. Previous studies have confirmed the association between these anions and the risk of metabolic disorders [28–32]; some studies found that perchlorate was associated with increasing birthweight, while exposure to the baby food and breastfed infants were not associated with adverse outcomes [33–35]. These studies suggest that perchlorate may have effects on reproductive health, but the specific association remains unclear. Additionally, the extent to which obesity mediates this association remains largely unexplored, requiring further investigation into the associations between EDCs and obesity and infertility.

This cross-sectional study used data from the National Health and Nutrition Examination Survey (NHANES). We explored the association between perchlorate, nitrate, and thiocyanate and obesity and infertility among women of reproductive age in the United States. Additionally, we performed stratified analyses based on age, marital status, alcohol consumption, and obesity to further investigate the relationship between exposure to these endocrine disruptors and infertility. Finally, we performed mediation analysis to assess the indicator effect of obesity in these associations, providing valuable epidemiological insights for future mechanistic research.

## 2. Materials and Methods

### 2.1. Study Design

This cross-sectional study used data combined from three cycles of NHANES: 2013–2014, 2015–2016, and 2017–2018. Conducted by the National Center for Health Statistics (NCHS) of the Centers for Disease Control and Prevention, NHANES employed a complex multistage probability sampling design to select a representative sample of the U.S. civilian, non-institutionalized population for assessing the health and nutritional status of American children and adults. Participants provided multiple biological samples during physical examinations, including blood and urine, which were used to analyze the associations between environmental exposures and health outcomes. The NHANES protocol was reviewed and approved by the NCHS Research Ethics Review Board, all participants signed informed written consent.

A total of 29,400 participants were included. Participants were excluded based on the following criteria: (1) males (N = 14,452); (2) age under 20 or over 45 years (N = 11,093); (3) participants who completed only the interview portion (N = 155); (4) pregnant or breast-feeding women (N = 318); (5) history of hysterectomy (N = 140); (6) bilateral oophorectomy (N = 1); (7) missing urinary perchlorate, nitrate, or thiocyanate measurements (N = 2197); and (8) incomplete covariate or outcome data (N = 232). Finally, 813 participants were included. Details are presented in Figure 1.

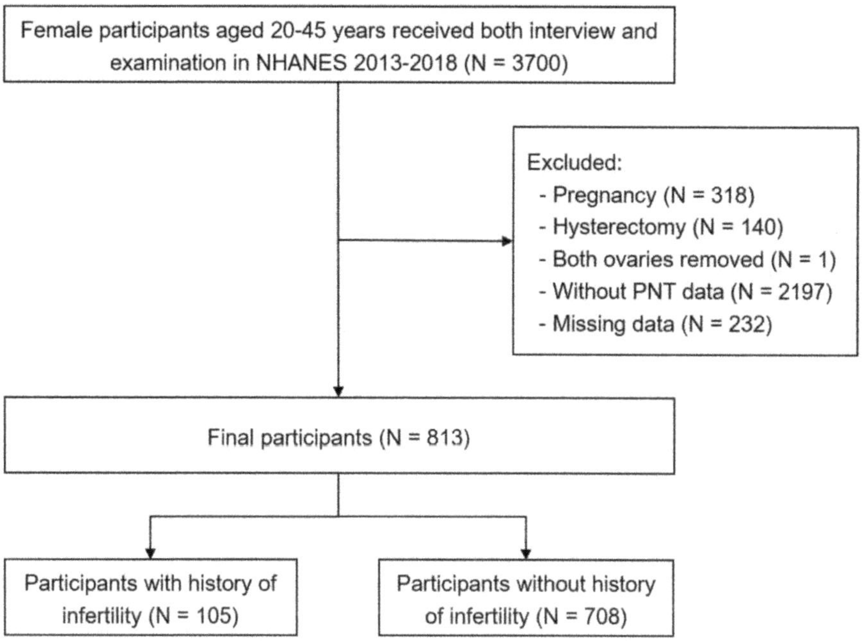


**Figure 1.** Flowchart for this study. NHANES, National Health and Nutrition Examination Survey; PNT, perchlorate, nitrate, and thiocyanate.

### 2.2. Exposure Ascertainment

Trained survey personnel collected 250 mL random urine samples from participants following standardized procedures outlined in the NHANES laboratory procedures manual. The urine samples were initially processed and preserved under suitable conditions (−20 °C or −30 °C). Perchlorate, nitrate, and thiocyanate concentrations in the urine samples were quantified using ion chromatography and electrospray tandem mass spectrometry. Chromatographic separation was conducted with an IonPac AS16 column using sodium hydroxide as the eluent. The detection limits (LOD) were 0.05 ng/mL for urinary perchlorate, 700 ng/mL for urinary nitrate, and 20 ng/mL for urinary thiocyanate. Analyte concentrations below the LOD were assigned a value of the square root of LOD/2. Further methodological details are provided in the NHANES laboratory methods manual.

### 2.3. Outcome Ascertainment

Infertility was assessed using responses from two questions in reproductive health questionnaire: (1) "Have you ever tried to get pregnant for at least a year without becoming pregnant?" and (2) "Have you ever seen a doctor or other healthcare provider because you were unable to get pregnant?" Individuals who answered "yes" to either question were classified as having infertility, while those who answered "no" were assigned to the control group. To ensure the accuracy and completeness of the data, participants who refused to answer or were unsure were excluded from the analysis.

### 2.4. Mediator Ascertainment

Obesity may serve as a mediator in the association between perchlorate, nitrate, thiocyanate, and infertility, and was therefore treated as a mediator variable in this study. BMI data were collected through physical examinations, and calculated by dividing weight (kg) by height squared ($m^2$). According to WHO standards, participants with a BMI of $\geq$30 kg/$m^2$ were classified as obese.

### 2.5. Covariates

The covariates included in the analysis included age (continuous variable), race/ethnicity (non-Hispanic White, non-Hispanic Black, and Others), education level (less than high school, high school or equivalent, and above high school), economic status (low, middle, and high income), alcohol consumption (yes and no), smoking status (yes and no), marital status (living alone and cohabitating), physical activity (sedentary, insufficient, moderate, and high), diabetes (yes and no), hypertension (yes and no), regularity of menstrual cycles (yes and no), use of contraceptive pills (yes and no), and use of female hormone medication (yes and no).

Covariate information was gathered through interviews or questionnaires. Economic status was categorized by the poverty–income ratio (PIR), PIR < 1.3 was considered poverty, PIR 1.3–3.5 was considered normal, and PIR > 3.5 was considered wealthy. Consuming more than 12 alcoholic drinks in the past year was considered alcohol consumption. Smoking was characterized as having smoked more than 100 cigarettes. Marital status was classified based on whether the participant lived with a partner; those who were married or cohabitating were classified as cohabitating [36]. According to weekly leisure-time metabolic equivalent (MET) minutes, physical activity was divided into four groups by 500 and 1000 min [37].

### 2.6. Statistical Analysis

General characteristics were presented as mean (standard deviation, SD), median (interquartile range, IQR) or number (percentage) where appropriate. Continuous variables between groups were compared using the Student's $t$-test and the Mann–Whitney U test. Categorical variables were compared between the infertility and non-infertility groups using Chi-square or Fisher's exact tests. To adjust for differences in urine dilution, perchlorate, nitrate, and thiocyanate were adjusted for urinary creatinine prior to analysis (urinary perchlorate: μg/g creatinine; urinary nitrate and thiocyanate: mg/g creatinine) [23]. Creatinine-adjusted urinary perchlorate, nitrate, and thiocyanate were log-transformed to normalize their distribution. We used Spearman correlation analysis to assess the correlation between the three anions. The associations between three anions and outcomes, as well as the odds ratios (OR) and corresponding 95% confidence intervals (95% CI) were examined using multivariable logistic regression models. Several models were established: In Model 1, we adjusted for age and race, we further adjusted demographic factors such as education level and economic status in Model 2, and Model 3 additionally adjusted for diabetes, hypertension, menstrual cycle regularity, contraceptive use, and use of female hormone medications. The analysis accounted for the complex, multistage probability design of NHANES by incorporating appropriate sample weights, in accordance with NHANES analytic guidelines. Stratified analyses were also performed based on age (20–35, 36–45), marital status (living alone, cohabitating), alcohol consumption (yes and no), and obesity (yes and no). Finally, we used the R package "lavaan" to perform mediation analysis.

Additionally, we performed some sensitivity analyses to validate our findings. First, we conducted multivariable logistic regression without applying NHANES weights (sensitivity analysis i). Second, based on Model 3, we further adjusted for perchlorate, nitrate, and thiocyanate simultaneously, in addition to the covariates already included in Model 3 (sensitivity analysis ii). Third, instead of adjusting analyte concentrations for creatinine, we adjusted it as a covariate in Model 3 (sensitivity analysis iii). Fourth, participants with missing covariate data were not excluded; instead, multiple imputation was used to account for missing values (sensitivity analysis iv). Finally, we repeated the analysis after excluding extreme values from the top and bottom 1% (sensitivity analysis v).

All data analyses were used R version 4.3.3, and a bilateral $p$-value of $<0.05$ was regarded as indicative of statistical significance.

## 3. Results

### 3.1. Characteristics of Participants

Table 1 shows the baseline characteristics of the participants. A total of 813 reproductive-aged women from the United States were included in this study, with 105 participants (12.9%) diagnosed with infertility. Participants in the infertility group were older ($p = 0.001$), with a higher proportion living alone (74.3%). The prevalence of obesity (60.0%), diabetes (7.6%), and hypertension (24.8%) was similarly higher in infertility group. The three anions were detected above the detection limit in more than 99% of participants. After adjusted by urine creatine, perchlorate levels showed a statistically significant difference between the infertility and control groups ($p = 0.008$). The three anions were significantly correlated ($p < 0.001$); details are shown in Figure S1.

**Table 1.** Baseline characteristics of the participants.

| Characteristics | All Participants (N = 813) | Infertility Status | | $p$ Value |
|---|---|---|---|---|
| | | Non Infertility (N = 708) | Infertility (N = 105) | |
| Age [years, Mean (SD)] | 33.0 (7.4) | 32.7 (7.5) | 35.1 (6.9) | 0.001 [a] |
| Race/ethnicity [No. (%)] | | | | 0.417 [c] |
| White | 281 (34.6) | 248 (35.0) | 33 (31.4) | |
| Black | 170 (20.9) | 143 (20.2) | 27 (25.7) | |
| Others | 362 (44.5) | 317 (44.8) | 45 (42.9) | |
| Education level [No. (%)] | | | | 0.313 [c] |
| Less than high school | 113 (13.9) | 100 (14.1) | 13 (12.4) | |
| High school graduate or equivalent | 163 (20.0) | 147 (20.8) | 16 (15.2) | |
| Above high school | 537 (66.1) | 461 (65.1) | 76 (72.4) | |
| Marital status [No. (%)] | | | | <0.001 [c] |
| Living without partner | 466 (57.3) | 388 (54.8) | 78 (74.3) | |
| Married/living with partner | 347 (42.7) | 320 (45.2) | 27 (25.7) | |
| Economic status [No. (%)] | | | | 0.700 [c] |
| Poverty | 285 (35.1) | 247 (34.9) | 38 (36.2) | |
| Normal | 300 (36.9) | 265 (37.4) | 35 (33.3) | |
| Wealthy | 228 (28.0) | 196 (27.7) | 32 (30.5) | |

**Table 1.** *Cont.*

| Characteristics | All Participants | Infertility Status | | p Value |
|---|---|---|---|---|
| | | Non Infertility | Infertility | |
| | (N = 813) | (N = 708) | (N = 105) | |
| Alcohol consumption [No. (%)] | | | | 0.669 [c] |
| No | 306 (37.6) | 264 (37.3) | 42 (40.0) | |
| Yes | 507 (62.4) | 444 (62.7) | 63 (60.0) | |
| Smoke status [No. (%)] | | | | 0.467 [c] |
| No | 563 (69.2) | 494 (69.8) | 69 (65.7) | |
| Yes | 250 (30.8) | 214 (30.2) | 36 (34.3) | |
| Physical activity [No. (%)] | | | | 0.686 [c] |
| Sedentary | 348 (42.8) | 299 (42.2) | 49 (46.7) | |
| Insufficient | 119 (14.6) | 102 (14.4) | 17 (16.2) | |
| Moderate | 93 (11.4) | 82 (11.6) | 11 (10.5) | |
| High | 253 (31.1) | 225 (31.8) | 28 (26.7) | |
| Obesity [No. (%)] | | | | <0.001 [c] |
| No | 471 (57.9) | 429 (60.6) | 42 (40.0) | |
| Yes | 342 (42.1) | 279 (39.4) | 63 (60.0) | |
| Diabetes [No. (%)] | | | | 0.045 [c] |
| No | 783 (96.3) | 686 (96.9) | 97 (92.4) | |
| Yes | 30 (3.7) | 22 (3.1) | 8 (7.6) | |
| Hypertension [No. (%)] | | | | 0.002 [c] |
| No | 697 (85.7) | 618 (87.3) | 79 (75.2) | |
| Yes | 116 (14.3) | 90 (12.7) | 26 (24.8) | |
| Menstrual cycle regularity [No. (%)] | | | | 0.197 [c] |
| No | 743 (91.4) | 651 (91.9) | 92 (87.6) | |
| Yes | 70 (8.6) | 57 (8.1) | 13 (12.4) | |
| Contraceptive pills [No. (%)] | | | | 0.330 [c] |
| No | 238 (29.3) | 212 (29.9) | 26 (24.8) | |
| Yes | 575 (70.7) | 496 (70.1) | 79 (75.2) | |
| Female hormones [No. (%)] | | | | 0.378 [c] |
| No | 786 (96.7) | 686 (96.9) | 100 (95.2) | |
| Yes | 27 (3.3) | 22 (3.1) | 5 (4.8) | |
| Urine Perchlorate [ug/g Cr, median (IQR)] | 2.45 (1.54, 4.09) | 2.52 (1.56, 4.32) | 2.07 (1.30, 3.52) | 0.008 [b] |
| Urine Nitrate [mg/g Cr, median (IQR)] | 45.77 (34.43, 67.56) | 46.08 (34.24, 67.36) | 45.51 (35.90, 72.44) | 0.918 [b] |
| Urine Thiocyanate [mg/g Cr, median (IQR)] | 1.18 (0.63, 2.42) | 1.19 (0.62, 2.43) | 1.10 (0.65, 2.40) | 0.988 [b] |

Abbreviation: Cr: creatinine. [a]: Student's *t*-test was used for normally distributed continuous variables. [b]: Mann–Whitney U test was used for the skewed variables. [c]: Chi-square test was used for categorical variables.

### 3.2. Associations Between Perchlorate, Nitrate, and Thiocyanate Exposures and Obesity

The association between the three anions and obesity are summarized in Table 2. In Model 1, both urinary perchlorate (OR = 0.70; 95% CI: 0.53, 0.93; $p = 0.017$) and urinary nitrate (OR = 0.60; 95% CI: 0.40, 0.90; $p = 0.018$) were negatively associated with obesity for each unit increase in ln-transformed concentrations. Participants in the highest quartile of perchlorate and nitrate had a lower risk of obesity than the lowest quartile (perchlorate OR = 0.50; 95% CI: 0.27, 0.91; $p = 0.028$; nitrate OR = 0.45; 95% CI: 0.24, 0.84; $p = 0.018$). After adjusting for covariates in Models 2 and 3, the associations of perchlorate and nitrate with a reduced risk of obesity remained statistically significant. However, we did not find any significant association between thiocyanate and obesity in this study.

**Table 2.** Associations between perchlorate, nitrate, and thiocyanate exposures and obesity.

| Exposures | | Ln-Transformed OR (95% CI), *p* Value | Q1 OR (95% CI) *p* Value | Q2 OR (95% CI) *p* Value | Q3 OR (95% CI) *p* Value | Q4 OR (95% CI) *p* Value | *p* Trend |
|---|---|---|---|---|---|---|---|
| Perchlorate | Model 1 | 0.70 (0.53–0.93) 0.017 | 1 [Reference] Ref. | 0.87 (0.50–1.51) 0.620 | 0.66 (0.38–1.15) 0.152 | 0.50 (0.27–0.91) 0.028 | 0.016 |
| | Model 2 | 0.73 (0.55–0.96) 0.031 | 1 [Reference] Ref. | 0.88 (0.51–1.54) 0.660 | 0.72 (0.41–1.27) 0.266 | 0.53 (0.30–0.96) 0.045 | 0.032 |
| | Model 3 | 0.73 (0.55–0.96) 0.032 | 1 [Reference] Ref. | 0.86 (0.50–1.48) 0.598 | 0.74 (0.42–1.29) 0.295 | 0.54 (0.30–0.96) 0.045 | 0.037 |
| Nitrate | Model 1 | 0.60 (0.40–0.90) 0.018 | 1 [Reference] Ref. | 0.83 (0.48–1.47) 0.533 | 0.85 (0.48–1.52) 0.597 | 0.45 (0.24–0.84) 0.018 | 0.016 |
| | Model 2 | 0.61 (0.40–0.92) 0.024 | 1 [Reference] Ref. | 0.85 (0.51–1.40) 0.525 | 0.93 (0.55–1.56) 0.775 | 0.46 (0.24–0.86) 0.020 | 0.023 |
| | Model 3 | 0.59 (0.40–0.87) 0.013 | 1 [Reference] Ref. | 0.88 (0.55–1.42) 0.610 | 1.00 (0.58–1.71) 0.999 | 0.45 (0.24–0.83) 0.016 | 0.029 |
| Thiocyanate | Model 1 | 1.01 (0.86–1.20) 0.880 | 1 [Reference] Ref. | 0.84 (0.55–1.30) 0.445 | 0.74 (0.42–1.29) 0.296 | 1.10 (0.67–1.80) 0.716 | 0.799 |
| | Model 2 | 0.91 (0.77–1.07) 0.268 | 1 [Reference] Ref. | 0.87 (0.57–1.34) 0.539 | 0.82 (0.47–1.42) 0.478 | 0.88 (0.55–1.39) 0.582 | 0.526 |
| | Model 3 | 0.92 (0.77–1.11) 0.398 | 1 [Reference] Ref. | 0.90 (0.59–1.37) 0.630 | 0.82 (0.46–1.46) 0.515 | 0.92 (0.56–1.51) 0.741 | 0.646 |

Abbreviation: OR: odds ratio, CI: confidence intervals; Q: quartile. Model 1 was adjusted for age and race. Model 2 further controlled for education level, marital status, economic status, alcohol consumption, smoke status, and physical activity. Model 3 further controlled for diabetes, hypertension, menstrual cycle regularity, contraceptive pills, and female hormones.

### 3.3. Associations Between Perchlorate, Nitrate, and Thiocyanate Exposures and Infertility

Table 3 presents the association between the three anions and infertility. In Model 1, each unit increase in urinary perchlorate (ln-transformed) was negatively associated with infertility (OR = 0.66; 95% CI: 0.50, 0.88; $p = 0.007$). Participants in the highest quartile of perchlorate had a significantly lower risk of infertility than the lowest quartile (OR = 0.46; 95% CI: 0.23, 0.94; $p = 0.040$). After adjusting for demographic factors, perchlorate remained negatively associated with infertility, both for each unit increase and for the highest quartile concentration. In the Model 3, each unit increase in log-transformed urinary perchlorate remained significantly associated with infertility (OR = 0.68; 95% CI: 0.51, 0.91; $p = 0.016$), and the highest quartile had a lower risk of infertility (OR = 0.45; 95% CI: 0.23, 0.90; $p = 0.034$), with a linear trend observed ($p = 0.013$). Results were largely consistent with the main analysis in sensitivity analyses (Table S1).

Figure 2 shows the results of subgroup analysis. Higher levels of perchlorate were negatively associated with infertility in most subgroups, consistent with the primary findings. Specifically, each unit increase in perchlorate was associated with a lower risk of infertility in the 36–45 age group (OR = 0.51; 95% CI: 0.31, 0.82; $p = 0.012$), the cohabitating group (OR = 0.60; 95% CI: 0.41, 0.87; $p = 0.013$), the middle-income group (OR = 0.61; 95% CI: 0.39, 0.95; $p = 0.039$), the alcohol consumption group (OR = 0.60; 95% CI: 0.43, 0.85; $p = 0.008$), the smoking group (OR = 0.63; 95% CI: 0.41, 0.96; $p = 0.043$), and the non-obese group (OR = 0.50; 95% CI: 0.33, 0.75; $p = 0.003$).

**Table 3.** Associations between perchlorate, nitrate, and thiocyanate exposures and infertility.

| Exposure | | Ln-Transformed OR (95% CI), *p* Value | Q1 OR (95% CI) *p* Value | Q2 OR (95% CI) *p* Value | Q3 OR (95% CI) *p* Value | Q4 OR (95% CI) *p* Value | *p* Trend |
|---|---|---|---|---|---|---|---|
| Perchlorate | Model 1 | 0.66 (0.50–0.88) 0.007 | 1 [Reference] Ref. | 1.23 (0.61–2.47) 0.571 | 0.86 (0.43–1.72) 0.678 | 0.46 (0.23–0.94) 0.040 | 0.015 |
| | Model 2 | 0.65 (0.48–0.86) 0.006 | 1 [Reference] Ref. | 1.34 (0.67–2.69) 0.420 | 0.85 (0.42–1.73) 0.655 | 0.46 (0.22–0.94) 0.042 | 0.015 |
| | Model 3 | 0.68 (0.51–0.91) 0.016 | 1 [Reference] Ref. | 1.32 (0.64–2.72) 0.453 | 0.85 (0.42–1.72) 0.653 | 0.45 (0.23–0.90) 0.034 | 0.013 |

**Table 3.** *Cont.*

| Exposure | | Ln-Transformed OR (95% CI), *p* Value | Q1 OR (95% CI) *p* Value | Q2 OR (95% CI) *p* Value | Q3 OR (95% CI) *p* Value | Q4 OR (95% CI) *p* Value | *p* Trend |
|---|---|---|---|---|---|---|---|
| Nitrate | Model 1 | 0.97 (0.67–1.39) 0.858 | 1 [Reference] Ref. | 1.31 (0.63–2.69) 0.476 | 0.80 (0.40–1.59) 0.526 | 1.03 (0.48–2.20) 0.944 | 0.763 |
| | Model 2 | 0.91 (0.63–1.32) 0.627 | 1 [Reference] Ref. | 1.21 (0.59–2.47) 0.606 | 0.72 (0.36–1.43) 0.350 | 0.86 (0.40–1.85) 0.699 | 0.455 |
| | Model 3 | 1.02 (0.68–1.53) 0.930 | 1 [Reference] Ref. | 1.26 (0.62–2.56) 0.534 | 0.78 (0.40–1.53) 0.471 | 1.02 (0.43–2.41) 0.973 | 0.796 |
| Thiocyanate | Model 1 | 0.95 (0.77–1.17) 0.610 | 1 [Reference] Ref. | 1.48 (0.68–3.21) 0.330 | 0.98 (0.49–1.97) 0.954 | 0.91 (0.46–1.79) 0.784 | 0.410 |
| | Model 2 | 0.85 (0.67–1.07) 0.177 | 1 [Reference] Ref. | 1.32 (0.62–2.82) 0.484 | 0.84 (0.42–1.68) 0.624 | 0.62 (0.31–1.22) 0.174 | 0.089 |
| | Model 3 | 0.88 (0.67–1.16) 0.372 | 1 [Reference] Ref. | 1.54 (0.69–3.46) 0.301 | 0.89 (0.42–1.89) 0.765 | 0.70 (0.33–1.47) 0.353 | 0.188 |

Abbreviation: OR: odds ratio, CI: confidence intervals; Q: quartile. Model 1 was adjusted for age and race. Model 2 further controlled for education level, marital status, economic status, alcohol consumption, smoke status, and physical activity. Model 3 further controlled for diabetes, hypertension, menstrual cycle regularity, contraceptive pills, and female hormones.

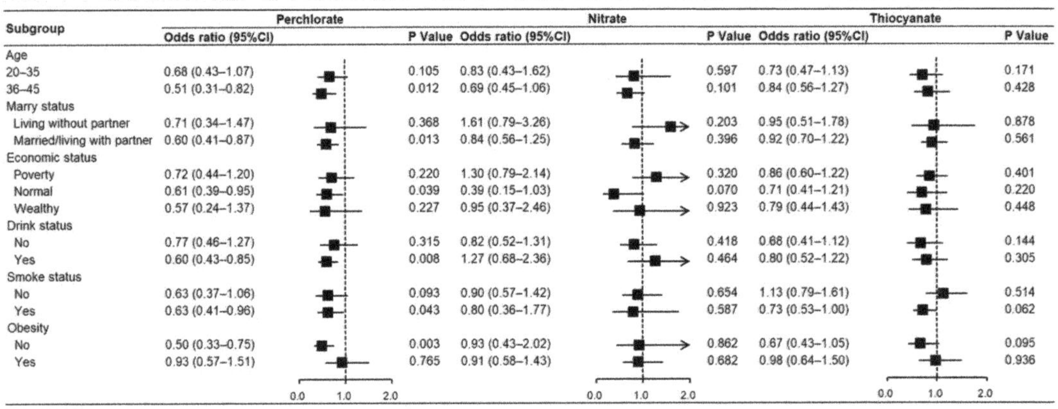


**Figure 2.** Subgroup analysis of three anions and infertility. Models were adjusted for age (continuous variable), education level, marital status, economic status, alcohol consumption, smoke status, physical activity, diabetes, hypertension, menstrual cycle regularity, contraceptive pills, and female hormones.

### *3.4. Mediation Analysis for Association of Perchlorate with Infertility*

Figure 3 presents the results of mediation analyses. As shown in Figure 3, perchlorate was negatively associated with infertility (total effect: −0.042; 95% CI: −0.057, −0.027; $p = 0.004$). Obesity was identified as a significant mediator in this association, accounting for 19.28% of the mediating effect (mediation effect: −0.008; 95% CI: −0.011, −0.005; $p = 0.005$).

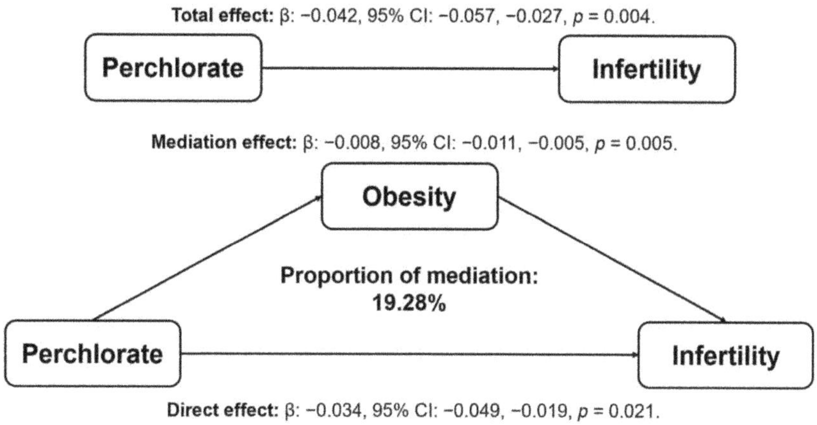


**Figure 3.** Mediation analysis for associations between perchlorate and infertility. Model was adjusted for age (continuous variable), education level, marital status, economic status, alcohol consumption, smoke status, physical activity, diabetes, hypertension, menstrual cycle regularity, contraceptive pills, and female hormones.

## 4. Discussion

This study investigated the associations of perchlorate, nitrate, and thiocyanate with obesity and infertility in women of reproductive age, as well as the role of obesity as a mediator in the association between perchlorate and infertility. Our results suggest that perchlorate and nitrate were negatively associated with obesity, and perchlorate was also negatively associated with infertility. Mediation analysis further showed that obesity mediated the association between perchlorate and infertility, with a mediation effect of 19.28%.

We found that exposure to perchlorate and nitrate was negatively associated with obesity in women of reproductive age, consistent with findings from previous studies conducted in US adults and children [34,38]. Similarly, other research has reported that perchlorate, nitrate, and thiocyanate was associated with lower waist circumference and BMI in girls [39]. One study found an interesting result that perchlorate was negatively associated with LDL-C elevation [40]. Another study found that perchlorate and thiocyanate were associated with metabolic syndrome, which is contrary to the results of this study [13]. However, the causal relationship between these anions and obesity in women remains unclear, with thyroid function being a possible underlying mechanism. Thyroid hormones regulate many cellular processes involved in resting energy expenditure and basal metabolism [41], and can influence both the total amount and distribution of adipose tissue [42]. Current evidence indicates that higher exposures to perchlorate and nitrate are associated with elevated serum thyroid-stimulating hormone (TSH) levels and lower serum thyroid hormone (TH) levels [23,43]. Additionally, elevated perchlorate levels have been associated with increased sensitivity to central thyroid hormones [44]. Nevertheless, it remains uncertain whether changes in TSH or other thyroid hormones are a cause or consequence of obesity.

We also found that perchlorate was negatively associated with infertility in reproductive-aged women, an effect that may be mediated though thyroid function. Thyroid disease is a common endocrine disorder for reproductive-aged women [45], and affects female reproductive health in several ways, including modulating the HPO axis, regulating the effects of prolactin and leptin on gonadotropin-releasing hormone (GnRH), and altering binding proteins that affect the bioavailability of sex steroids [24,46–49]. In the 1950s, perchlorate was widely used as a treatment for thyroid dysfunction [50–52]. Perchlorate can inhibit the thyroid gland's ability to take up iodine, which is used to normalize thyroid function in patients with hypothyroidism [53], and has also been used to treat hyperthyroidism [54]. Thus, perchlorate exposure may reduce the risk of infertility by improving thyroid function. The mechanisms by which perchlorate influences infertility are likely to be complex, with obesity potentially playing a critical role in reducing infertility risk. Obesity can adversely affect female reproductive health by disrupting the HPO axis and promoting ovarian androgen production [35,55]. Our study identified a significant mediating effect of obesity in the relationship between perchlorate exposure and infertility, suggesting that obesity management may be a key pathway through which perchlorate exposure helps to reduce the risk of infertility.

Our study has several strengths. First, to our knowledge, this is the first study to investigate the association between exposure to perchlorate, nitrate, and thiocyanate and obesity among reproductive-aged women. Second, it is also the first to investigate the association between these three anions and female infertility. Third, by considering obesity as a mediating variable in the association between these anions and infertility, we offer a novel perspective on infertility treatment strategies. However, this study has some limitations. First, the cross-sectional design of the NHANES data limits our ability to establish causal relationships between the three anions, obesity, and infertility. Second, exposures were assessed using a single urine sample, which may not fully capture the participants' true exposure levels over time. However, the single-spot urine samples of these anions have shown considerable temporal reliability, making their urine concentrations reliable biomarkers [56,57]. Finally, although we adjusted for several infertility-related risk factors, residual confounding by unmeasured variables may still be present.

## 5. Conclusions

In conclusion, our study found negative associations between perchlorate and nitrate and obesity in women of reproductive age in the US, as well as a negative association between perchlorate and infertility. The inverse association between perchlorate and infertility appears to be mediated by obesity. These findings provide new insights into the health risk assessment of perchlorate, nitrate, and thiocyanate exposure, while offering a novel perspective on strategies for managing female infertility. Further research is needed to confirm these findings and to elucidate the underlying mechanisms.

**Supplementary Materials:** The following supporting information can be downloaded at: https://www.mdpi.com/article/10.3390/toxics13010015/s1, Figure S1: Spearman correlations among perchlorate, nitrate, and thiocyanate; Table S1: Associations between perchlorate, nitrate, thiocyanate exposures and infertility (sensitivity analysis i–v).

**Author Contributions:** L.Z.: Writing—Original Draft, Conceptualization, Methodology, Software, Formal Analysis, Investigation, Data Curation; Y.P.: Methodology, Software, Investigation, Data Curation; Y.S.: Validation, Visualization; Y.Z.: Supervision; Q.Q.: Validation, Visualization; M.Y.: Validation, Visualization; Y.B.: Validation, Visualization; P.Y.: Writing—Review and Editing, Supervision, Project Administration, Funding Acquisition. All authors have read and agreed to the published version of the manuscript.

**Funding:** This study was supported by funds from the National Natural Science Foundation of China (No. 82173628).

**Institutional Review Board Statement:** Ethical clearance for the survey protocols (protocol numbers: #2011-17, #2005-06, and #2018-01) were obtained from the Ethics Review Board of the National Center for Health Statistics.

**Informed Consent Statement:** Written informed consent was secured from all participants at the time of their recruitment into the survey.

**Data Availability Statement:** The original datasets supporting the analysis are publicly available on the NHANES website (https://www.cdc.gov/nchs/nhanes (accessed on 1 September 2024)). The analysis datasets and programming code are accessible from the corresponding author and will be provided if reasonably requested.

**Conflicts of Interest:** The authors declare no conflicts of interest.

## References

1. Carson, S.A.; Kallen, A.N. Diagnosis and Management of Infertility: A Review. *JAMA* **2021**, *326*, 65–76. [CrossRef] [PubMed]
2. Snow, M.; Vranich, T.M.; Perin, J.; Trent, M. Estimates of Infertility in the United States: 1995–2019. *Fertil. Steril.* **2022**, *118*, 560–567. [CrossRef]
3. Wang, Y.; Wang, W.; Li, H.; Du, Q. Trends in the Burden of Female Infertility among Adults Aged 20–49 Years during 1990–2019: An Analysis of Data from the Global Burden of Disease Study 2019. *BMJ Open* **2024**, *14*, e084755. [CrossRef]
4. Nichols, A.R.; Rifas-Shiman, S.L.; Switkowski, K.M.; Zhang, M.; Young, J.G.; Hivert, M.-F.; Chavarro, J.E.; Oken, E. History of Infertility and Midlife Cardiovascular Health in Female Individuals. *JAMA Netw. Open* **2024**, *7*, e2350424. [CrossRef] [PubMed]
5. Cox, C.M.; Thoma, M.E.; Tchangalova, N.; Mburu, G.; Bornstein, M.J.; Johnson, C.L.; Kiarie, J. Infertility Prevalence and the Methods of Estimation from 1990 to 2021: A Systematic Review and Meta-Analysis. *Hum. Reprod. Open* **2022**, *2022*, hoac051. [CrossRef] [PubMed]
6. Yárnoz-Esquiroz, P.; Olazarán, L.; Aguas-Ayesa, M.; Perdomo, C.M.; García-Goñi, M.; Silva, C.; Fernández-Formoso, J.A.; Escalada, J.; Montecucco, F.; Portincasa, P.; et al. "Obesities": Position Statement on a Complex Disease Entity with Multifaceted Drivers. *Eur. J. Clin. Investig.* **2022**, *52*, e13811. [CrossRef] [PubMed]
7. WHO. Acceleration Plan to Stop Obesity. Available online: https://www.who.int/publications/i/item/9789240075634 (accessed on 23 October 2024).
8. Ferrari, A.J.; Santomauro, D.F.; Aali, A.; Abate, Y.H.; Abbafati, C.; Abbastabar, H.; Abd ElHafeez, S.; Abdelmasseh, M.; Abd-Elsalam, S.; Abdollahi, A.; et al. Global Incidence, Prevalence, Years Lived with Disability (YLDs), Disability-Adjusted Life-Years (DALYs), and Healthy Life Expectancy (HALE) for 371 Diseases and Injuries in 204 Countries and Territories and 811 Subnational Locations, 1990–2021: A Systematic Analysis for the Global Burden of Disease Study 2021. *Lancet* **2024**, *403*, 2133–2161. [CrossRef]
9. Elmaleh-Sachs, A.; Schwartz, J.L.; Bramante, C.T.; Nicklas, J.M.; Gudzune, K.A.; Jay, M. Obesity Management in Adults: A Review. *JAMA* **2023**, *330*, 2000–2015. [CrossRef]
10. Vahratian, A. Prevalence of Overweight and Obesity among Women of Childbearing Age: Results from the 2002 National Survey of Family Growth. *Matern. Child Health J.* **2009**, *13*, 268–273. [CrossRef]
11. Wu, B.; Shabanova, V.; Taylor, S.; Hawley, N.L. Pre-Pregnancy BMI, Rate of Gestational Weight Gain, and Preterm Birth among US Pacific Islander Individuals. *Obesity* **2024**, *32*, 798–809. [CrossRef] [PubMed]
12. Knight, M.; Kurinczuk, J.J.; Spark, P.; Brocklehurst, P. UK Obstetric Surveillance System Extreme Obesity in Pregnancy in the United Kingdom. *Obstet. Gynecol.* **2010**, *115*, 989–997. [CrossRef] [PubMed]
13. Guo, X.; Wu, B.; Hu, W.; Wang, X.; Su, W.; Meng, J.; Lowe, S.; Zhao, D.; Huang, C.; Liang, M.; et al. Associations of Perchlorate, Nitrate, and Thiocyanate with Metabolic Syndrome and Its Components among US Adults: A Cross-Sectional Study from NHANES. *Sci. Total Environ.* **2023**, *879*, 163083. [CrossRef]
14. Serrano-Nascimento, C.; Nunes, M.T. Perchlorate, nitrate, and thiocyanate: Environmental relevant NIS-inhibitors pollutants and their impact on thyroid function and human health. *Front. Endocrinol.* **2022**, *13*, 995503. [CrossRef]
15. Poulsen, R.; Cedergreen, N.; Hayes, T.; Hansen, M. Nitrate: An Environmental Endocrine Disruptor? A Review of Evidence and Research Needs. *Environ. Sci. Technol.* **2018**, *52*, 3869–3887. [CrossRef] [PubMed]
16. Yao, Y.; He, G.-Y.; Wu, X.-J.; Wang, C.-P.; Luo, X.-B.; Zhao, Y.; Long, Y. Association between Environmental Exposure to Perchlorate, Nitrate, and Thiocyanate and Serum α-Klotho Levels among Adults from the National Health and Nutrition Examination Survey (2007–2014). *BMC Geriatr.* **2022**, *22*, 740. [CrossRef]
17. Sindelar, J.J.; Milkowski, A.L. Human Safety Controversies Surrounding Nitrate and Nitrite in the Diet. *Nitric Oxide.* **2012**, *26*, 259–266. [CrossRef]
18. Kalaycıoğlu, Z.; Erim, F.B. Nitrate and Nitrites in Foods: Worldwide Regional Distribution in View of Their Risks and Benefits. *J. Agric. Food Chem.* **2019**, *67*, 7205–7222. [CrossRef] [PubMed]
19. Felker, P.; Bunch, R.; Leung, A.M. Concentrations of thiocyanate and goitrin in human plasma, their precursor concentrations in brassica vegetables, and associated potential risk for hypothyroidism. *Nutr. Rev.* **2016**, *74*, 248–258. [CrossRef]
20. Willemin, M.-E.; Lumen, A. Thiocyanate: A Review and Evaluation of the Kinetics and the Modes of Action for Thyroid Hormone Perturbations. *Crit. Rev. Toxicol.* **2017**, *47*, 537–563. [CrossRef] [PubMed]

21. Zhao, H.; Chen, X.; Ni, J.; Fang, L.; Chen, Y.; Ma, Y.; Cai, G.; Pan, F. Associations of Perchlorate, Nitrate, and Thiocyanate Exposure with Arthritis and Inflammation Indicators in Young and Middle-Aged Adults, NHANES 2005–2016. *Front. Immunol.* **2024**, *15*, 1318737. [CrossRef] [PubMed]
22. Waugh, D.T. Fluoride Exposure Induces Inhibition of Sodium/Iodide Symporter (NIS) Contributing to Impaired Iodine Absorption and Iodine Deficiency: Molecular Mechanisms of Inhibition and Implications for Public Health. *Int. J. Environ. Res. Public Health* **2019**, *16*, 1086. [CrossRef] [PubMed]
23. King, L.; Wang, Q.; Xia, L.; Wang, P.; Jiang, G.; Li, W.; Huang, Y.; Liang, X.; Peng, X.; Li, Y.; et al. Environmental Exposure to Perchlorate, Nitrate and Thiocyanate, and Thyroid Function in Chinese Adults: A Community-Based Cross-Sectional Study. *Environ. Int.* **2023**, *171*, 107713. [CrossRef]
24. Concepción-Zavaleta, M.J.; Coronado-Arroyo, J.C.; Quiroz-Aldave, J.E.; Concepción-Urteaga, L.A.; Paz-Ibarra, J. Thyroid Dysfunction and Female Infertility. A Comprehensive Review. *Diabetes Metab. Syndr.* **2023**, *17*, 102876. [CrossRef] [PubMed]
25. National Center for Environmental Health. Fourth National Report on Human Exposure to Environmental Chemicals. Fourth National Report on Human Exposure to Environmental Chemicals. Updated Tables March 2021. Available online: https://stacks.cdc.gov/view/cdc/105345 (accessed on 16 December 2024).
26. Zhu, F.; Huang, M.; Jiao, J.; Zhuang, P.; Mao, L.; Zhang, Y. Environmental Exposure to Perchlorate, Nitrate, and Thiocyanate in Relation to Obesity: A Population-Based Study. *Environ. Int.* **2019**, *133*, 105191. [CrossRef] [PubMed]
27. Broughton, D.E.; Moley, K.H. Obesity and Female Infertility: Potential Mediators of Obesity's Impact. *Fertil. Steril.* **2017**, *107*, 840–847. [CrossRef] [PubMed]
28. Li, L.; Yang, X. The Essential Element Manganese, Oxidative Stress, and Metabolic Diseases: Links and Interactions. *Oxid. Med. Cell Longev.* **2018**, *2018*, 7580707. [CrossRef] [PubMed]
29. Lefranc, C.; Friederich-Persson, M.; Palacios-Ramirez, R.; Nguyen Dinh Cat, A. Mitochondrial oxidative stress in obesity: Role of the mineralocorticoid receptor. *J. Endocrinol.* **2018**, *238*, R143–R159. [CrossRef] [PubMed]
30. Alvares, T.S.; Oliveira, G.V.; Volino-Souza, M.; Conte-Junior, C.A.; Murias, J.M. Effect of dietary nitrate ingestion on muscular performance: A systematic review and meta-analysis of randomized controlled trials. *Crit. Rev. Food Sci. Nutr.* **2022**, *62*, 5284–5306. [CrossRef]
31. Liu, G.; Zong, G.; Dhana, K.; Hu, Y.; Blount, B.C.; Morel-Espinosa, M.; Sun, Q. Exposure to Perchlorate, Nitrate and Thiocyanate, and Prevalence of Diabetes Mellitus. *Int. J. Epidemiol.* **2017**, *46*, 1913–1923. [CrossRef]
32. Xu, D.; Zhu, X.; Xie, X.; Huang, C.; Fang, X.; Yin, T. Concurrent Dietary Intake to Nitrate, Thiocyanate, and Perchlorate Is Negatively Associated with Hypertension in Adults in the USA. *Environ. Sci. Pollut. Res. Int.* **2023**, *30*, 17573–17584. [CrossRef]
33. Rubin, R.; Pearl, M.; Kharrazi, M.; Blount, B.C.; Miller, M.D.; Pearce, E.N.; Valentin-Blasini, L.; DeLorenze, G.; Liaw, J.; Hoofnagle, A.N.; et al. Maternal perchlorate exposure in pregnancy and altered birth outcomes. *Environ. Res.* **2017**, *158*, 72–81. [CrossRef] [PubMed]
34. Li, M.; Xiao, M.; Xiao, Q.; Chen, Y.; Guo, Y.; Sun, J.; Li, R.; Li, C.; Zhu, Z.; Qiu, H.; et al. Perchlorate and chlorate in breast milk, infant formulas, baby supplementary food and the implications for infant exposure. *Environ. Int.* **2022**, *158*, 106939. [CrossRef] [PubMed]
35. Leung, A.M.; Braverman, L.E.; He, X.; Schuller, K.E.; Roussilhes, A.; Jahreis, K.A.; Pearce, E.N. Environmental perchlorate and thiocyanate exposures and infant serum thyroid function. *Thyroid* **2012**, *22*, 938–943. [CrossRef] [PubMed]
36. Zhong, J.; Zhang, Y.; Zhu, K.; Li, R.; Zhou, X.; Yao, P.; Franco, O.H.; Manson, J.E.; Pan, A.; Liu, G. Associations of Social Determinants of Health with Life Expectancy and Future Health Risks among Individuals with Type 2 Diabetes: Two Nationwide Cohort Studies in the UK and USA. *Lancet Healthy Longev.* **2024**, *5*, e542–e551. [CrossRef] [PubMed]
37. Zhou, H.-L.; Su, G.-H.; Zhang, R.-Y.; Di, D.-S.; Wang, Q. Association of Volatile Organic Compounds Co-Exposure with Bone Health Indicators and Potential Mediators. *Chemosphere* **2022**, *308*, 136208. [CrossRef] [PubMed]
38. Jiang, Q.; Li, Q. Association of Environmental Exposure to Perchlorate, Nitrate, and Thiocyanate with Overweight/Obesity and Central Obesity among Children and Adolescents in the United States of America Using Data from the National Health and Nutrition Examination Survey (NHANES) 2005–2016. *New Dir. Child. Adolesc. Dev.* **2022**, *2022*, 107–122. [CrossRef]
39. Mervish, N.A.; Pajak, A.; Teitelbaum, S.L.; Pinney, S.M.; Windham, G.C.; Kushi, L.H.; Biro, F.M.; Valentin-Blasini, L.; Blount, B.C.; Wolff, M.S.; et al. Thyroid Antagonists (Perchlorate, Thiocyanate, and Nitrate) and Childhood Growth in a Longitudinal Study of U.S. Girls. *Environ. Health Perspect.* **2016**, *124*, 542–549. [CrossRef] [PubMed]
40. Shi, M.; Zhu, X.; Cheang, I.; Zhu, Q.; Guo, Q.; Liao, S.; Gao, R.; Li, X. Associations of thiocyanate, nitrate, and perchlorate exposure with dyslipidemia: A cross-sectional, population-based analysis. *Environ. Sci. Pollut. Res. Int.* **2023**, *30*, 17217–17225. [CrossRef]
41. McAninch, E.A.; Bianco, A.C. Thyroid Hormone Signaling in Energy Homeostasis and Energy Metabolism. *Ann. N. Y. Acad. Sci.* **2014**, *1311*, 77–87. [CrossRef]
42. Prats-Puig, A.; Sitjar, C.; Ribot, R.; Calvo, M.; Clausell-Pomés, N.; Soler-Roca, M.; Soriano-Rodríguez, P.; Osiniri, I.; Ros-Miquel, M.; Bassols, J.; et al. Relative Hypoadiponectinemia, Insulin Resistance, and Increased Visceral Fat in Euthyroid Prepubertal Girls with Low-Normal Serum Free Thyroxine. *Obesity* **2012**, *20*, 1455–1461. [CrossRef] [PubMed]

43. Babić Leko, M.; Gunjača, I.; Pleić, N.; Zemunik, T. Environmental Factors Affecting Thyroid-Stimulating Hormone and Thyroid Hormone Levels. *Int. J. Mol. Sci.* **2021**, *22*, 6521. [CrossRef] [PubMed]
44. King, L.; Huang, Y.; Li, T.; Wang, Q.; Li, W.; Shan, Z.; Yin, J.; Chen, L.; Wang, P.; Dun, C.; et al. Associations of Urinary Perchlorate, Nitrate and Thiocyanate with Central Sensitivity to Thyroid Hormones: A US Population-Based Cross-Sectional Study. *Environ. Int.* **2022**, *164*, 107249. [CrossRef]
45. Strikić Đula, I.; Pleić, N.; Babić Leko, M.; Gunjača, I.; Torlak, V.; Brdar, D.; Punda, A.; Polašek, O.; Hayward, C.; Zemunik, T. Epidemiology of Hypothyroidism, Hyperthyroidism and Positive Thyroid Antibodies in the Croatian Population. *Biology* **2022**, *11*, 394. [CrossRef]
46. Brown, R.S.E.; Khant Aung, Z.; Phillipps, H.R.; Barad, Z.; Lein, H.-J.; Boehm, U.; Szawka, R.E.; Grattan, D.R. Acute Suppression of LH Secretion by Prolactin in Female Mice Is Mediated by Kisspeptin Neurons in the Arcuate Nucleus. *Endocrinology* **2019**, *160*, 1323–1332. [CrossRef] [PubMed]
47. Christen, T.; Trompet, S.; Noordam, R.; van Klinken, J.B.; van Dijk, K.W.; Lamb, H.J.; Cobbaert, C.M.; den Heijer, M.; Jazet, I.M.; Jukema, J.W.; et al. Sex Differences in Body Fat Distribution Are Related to Sex Differences in Serum Leptin and Adiponectin. *Peptides* **2018**, *107*, 25–31. [CrossRef] [PubMed]
48. Petrine, J.C.P.; Franci, C.R.; Del Bianco-Borges, B. Leptin Actions through the Nitrergic System to Modulate the Hypothalamic Expression of the Kiss1 mRNA in the Female Rat. *Brain Res.* **2020**, *1728*, 146574. [CrossRef] [PubMed]
49. Doufas, A.G.; Mastorakos, G. The Hypothalamic-Pituitary-Thyroid Axis and the Female Reproductive System. *Ann. N. Y. Acad. Sci.* **2000**, *900*, 65–76. [CrossRef]
50. Godley, A.F.; Stanbury, J.B. Preliminary Experience in the Treatment of Hyperthyroidism with Potassium Perchlorate. *J. Clin. Endocrinol. Metab.* **1954**, *14*, 70–78. [CrossRef] [PubMed]
51. Lisco, G.; Accardo, G.; Pupilli, C.; Malandrino, P.; De Geronimo, V.; Triggiani, V. Perchlorates in the Treatment of Hyperthyroidism and Thyrotoxicosis: A Comprehensive Review. *Endocrine* **2024**, *85*, 1–10. [CrossRef] [PubMed]
52. Leung, A.M.; Pearce, E.N.; Braverman, L.E. Perchlorate, Iodine and the Thyroid. *Best Pract. Res. Clin. Endocrinol. Metab.* **2010**, *24*, 133–141. [CrossRef] [PubMed]
53. Martino, E.; Mariotti, S.; Aghini-Lombardi, F.; Lenziardi, M.; Morabito, S.; Baschieri, L.; Pinchera, A.; Braverman, L.; Safran, M. Short Term Administration of Potassium Perchlorate Restores Euthyroidism in Amiodarone Iodine-Induced Hypothyroidism. *J. Clin. Endocrinol. Metab.* **1986**, *63*, 1233–1236. [CrossRef]
54. Martino, E.; Aghini-Lombardi, F.; Mariotti, S.; Lenziardi, M.; Baschieri, L.; Braverman, L.E.; Pinchera, A. Treatment of Amiodarone Associated Thyrotoxicosis by Simultaneous Administration of Potassium Perchlorate and Methimazole. *J. Endocrinol. Investig.* **1986**, *9*, 201–207. [CrossRef] [PubMed]
55. Rachoń, D.; Teede, H. Ovarian Function and Obesity--Interrelationship, Impact on Women's Reproductive Lifespan and Treatment Options. *Mol. Cell Endocrinol.* **2010**, *316*, 172–179. [CrossRef]
56. Ucal, Y.; Sahin, O.N.; Serdar, M.; Blount, B.; Kumru, P.; Muhcu, M.; Eroglu, M.; Akin-Levi, C.; Keles, Z.Z.Y.; Turam, C.; et al. Exposure to Perchlorate in Lactating Women and Its Associations With Newborn Thyroid Stimulating Hormone. *Front. Endocrinol.* **2018**, *9*, 348. [CrossRef]
57. Mervish, N.; Blount, B.; Valentin-Blasini, L.; Brenner, B.; Galvez, M.P.; Wolff, M.S.; Teitelbaum, S.L. Temporal variability in urinary concentrations of perchlorate, nitrate, thiocyanate and iodide among children. *J. Expo. Sci. Environ. Epidemiol.* **2012**, *22*, 212–218. [CrossRef] [PubMed]

*toxics*

MDPI

*Article*

# Associations of Environmental Pollutant Mixtures and Red Blood Cell Folate Concentrations: A Mixture Analysis of the U.S. Adult Population Based on NHANES Data, 2007–2016

**Michael Mascari [1], Katherine Reeves [1], Raji Balasubramanian [1], Zhenhua Liu [2], Nasser Laouali [3] and Youssef Oulhote [4,*]**

[1] Department of Epidemiology and Biostatistics, School of Public Health & Health Sciences, University of Massachusetts Amherst, Amherst, MA 01003, USA; mmascari@umass.edu (M.M.); kwreeves@umass.edu (K.R.); rbalasub@schoolph.umass.edu (R.B.)

[2] Department of Nutrition, School of Public Health & Health Sciences, University of Massachusetts Amherst, Amherst, MA 01003, USA; zliu@nutrition.umass.edu

[3] Faculty of Medical Sciences, Mohammed VI Polytechnic University, Benguerir 43150, Morocco; nasser.laouali@um6p.ma

[4] Department of Environmental Medicine and Climate Science, Icahn School of Medicine at Mount Sinai, New York, NY 10029, USA

* Correspondence: youssef.oulhote@mssm.edu

**Abstract:** Background: Folate is critical for many physiological processes, and low folate levels have been associated with a wide range of health outcomes, including chronic diseases and developmental outcomes. Many environmental chemicals are suspected to contribute to the etiology of health outcomes related to folate deficiency. However, little is known about how these pollutants influence folate levels as potential mechanistic pathways. Objective: To investigate the individual and joint associations between a mixture of 39 pollutants and red blood cell (RBC) folate concentrations in the U.S. population. Methods: We used available data on 27,938 participants, aged 18–80 from the U.S. National Health and Nutrition Examination survey (2007–2016), with available RBC folate concentrations and 39 environmental pollutants' concentrations. We estimated covariate-adjusted independent and joint associations between environmental pollutants and RBC folate, and compared evidence from two complimentary mixture approaches: exposome-wide association study (ExWAS) and quantile-based g computation (Q-gcomp). Results: In the ExWAS analysis, 12 environmental chemicals, including metals (cadmium, arsenic, lead, and mercury), perfluoroalkyl substances, phthalates, phenols and parabens, and polycyclic aromatic hydrocarbons, were inversely associated with RBC folate, whereas four environmental pollutants, including metals (manganese and selenium) and two phthalate metabolites, were positively associated with RBC folate. Q-gcomp showed convergent results with the ExWAS analysis; a quartile increase in the metal and PFAS mixtures was significantly associated with a decrease of −38.4 ng/mL (95%CI: −52.3, −24.4) and −48.9 ng/mL (95%CI: −57.6, −39.6) in RBC folate concentrations, respectively. Conclusion: The present study shows that higher exposure to PFASs, metals, and PAHs are associated with lower RBC folate concentrations. However, given the cross-sectional design, we cannot make inferences about the directionality of the observed associations.

**Keywords:** folate; pollutants; NHANES; mixtures; metals; PFAS; EDCs; PAHs

## 1. Introduction

Folate is the generic term for naturally occurring folate forms in foods, and folic acid, also known as vitamin $B_9$ or Vitamin M, is the synthetic form of folate used for dietary supplements and fortified foods. Folate is vital in humans for several metabolic reactions involved in the formation and transfer of methyl groups. These metabolic reactions in humans include the following: biosynthesis of purines and thymidine, amino acid homeostasis of glycine, serine, and methionine, epigenetic maintenance, homocysteine remethylation, hematopoiesis, and immune responses [1,2]. Folate deficiency has been linked to anemia [1,2] and hyperhomocystinemia [3], which has been associated with increased cardiovascular, cerebrovascular, and thromboembolic diseases. There is also epidemiologic evidence to sµggest folate is inversely associated with various cancers including lung, oropharynx, esophagus, stomach, colorectal, pancreas, cervix, ovary, prostate, and breast cancers, as well as leukemia [4–6]. Additionally, low folate levels have been associated with a range of developmental outcomes, including autism, neural tube defects, neurodevelopment, still birth, preterm birth, and recurrent pregnancy loss [7–16]. A recent NHANES biomonitoring study sµggested that, althoµgh blood folate concentrations in the US population have not decreased recently, the prevalence of folate insufficiency is about 20% in the US population [7].

There are both modifiable and non-modifiable factors associated with low folate levels. Established modifiable factors affecting folate levels include intake of certain medications, alcohol use, smoking, and dietary intake of folic acid supplements [17–20]. On the other hand, single nucleotide polymorphisms in certain genes are genetic, non-modifiable risk factors that affect folate levels. These include SNPs in 5,10-methylenetertahydrofolate, and other genes responsible for the metabolism of vitamins, as well as mutations in solute carrier family 46 member 1 (SLC46A1), a gene responsible for folate transport [21].

Recently, exposure to environmental chemicals has been sµggested as a potential modifiable risk factor for low folate levels. Environmental chemicals refer to chemicals that are present in air, water, food, soil, dust, or other environmental media such as consumer products [15]. These chemicals are often ubiquitous in the environment, and some may persist for several years. Many of these chemicals had limited testing for their effects on human health and even less is known about the combined exposure to many environmental chemicals [22].

The objective of this study is to investigate the associations between individual chemicals, chemical mixtures, and red blood cell (RBC) folate levels among the U.S. adult population using available data from the National Health and Nutrition Examination Survey (NHANES; 2007–2016). We compared evidence from two complimentary statistical approaches developed to examine chemical mixtures: exposome-wide association study (ExWAS) and a quantile-based g computation (Q-gcomp).

## 2. Methods

### 2.1. Population and Data Collection

The National Health and Nutrition Examination Survey (NHANES) is a cross-sectional, nationwide study designed for the assessment of the health and nutritional status of noninstitutionalized adults and children in the United States, conducted by the Centers for Disease Control and Prevention (CDC). Questionnaires were administered by study staff at an in-home visit and biological specimens were collected at mobile examination centers (MEC) [23].

This analysis included 27,938 NHANES participants aged 18 years and older. All measures of environmental chemicals and RBC folate concentrations were conducted as part of the NHANES program at the CDC, and laboratory methods for blood and urine samples have been described thoroughly at: https://wwwn.cdc.gov/nchs/nhanes/search/datapage.aspx?Component=Laboratory (accessed 1 December 2018). All the data used in this analysis are available at the CDC website and were extracted from the following link: https://wwwn.cdc.gov/nchs/nhanes/Default.aspx (accessed 1 December 2018).

### 2.2. RBC Folate Measurement

RBC folate was processed, stored, and shipped to the Division of Laboratory Sciences, National Center for Environmental Health, and Centers for Disease Control and Prevention for analysis. RBC folate concentrations were measured using a microbiological assay, which was described in detail elsewhere [24].

### 2.3. Assessment of Environmental Exposure Biomarkers

We included six environmental chemical families in this analysis: phthalates, heavy metals, per- and polyfluoroalkyl substances (PFASs), phenols and parabens, polyaromatic hydrocarbons (PAHs), and cotinine. These environmental chemical families included 39 environmental chemical biomarkers and metabolites. Phthalates, arsenic, phenols and parabens, and PAHs were measured in urine samples collected at mobile examination centers (MECs) [23]. PFASs and cotinine were measured in serum samples collected at MECs, whereas metals were measured in whole blood samples.

### 2.4. Phthalates (ng/mL)

Measures of urinary phthalate metabolites were performed in a subsample comprising one-third of the participants in all the included cycles. There were 11 phthalate metabolites included in this study: Mono (carboxyisoctyl) phthalate (MCOP), Mono-2-ethyl-5-carboxypentyl phthalate (MECPP), Mono-n-butyl phthalate (MBP), Mono-(3-carboxypropyl) phthalate (MCPP), Mono-ethyl phthalate (MEP), Mono-(2-ethyl-5-hydroxyhexyl) phthalate (MEHHP), Mono-(2-ethyl)-hexyl phthalate (MEHP), Mono-isobutyl phthalate (MiBP), Mono-isononyl phthalate (MNP), Mono-(2-ethyl-5-oxohexyl) phthalate (MEOHP), and Mono-benzyl phthalate (MBzP). Urine samples for the quantification of phthalate metabolites were stored at −20 °C until they arrived at the National Center for Environmental Health for testing. They were quantified using high performance liquid chromatography–electrospray ionization–tandem mass spectrometry (HPLC-ESI-MS/MS). The percentage coefficient of variation (CV) for phthalates ranged from 1.5% to 18.9%. There was a range in limits of detection (MCOP: 0.2–0.7 ng/mL; MECPP: 0.2–0.5 ng/mL; MBP: 0.4–0.6 ng/mL; MCPP: 0.2–0.4 ng/mL; MEP: 0.462–1.2 ng/mL; MEHHP: 0.2–0.7 ng/mL; MEHP: 0.5–1.1 ng/mL; MiBP: 0.2–0.8 ng/mL; MNP: 0.5–1.232 ng/mL; MEOHP: 0.2–0.6 ng/mL; MBzP: 0.2–0.3 ng/mL) based on the NHANES cycle.

### 2.5. Heavy Metals

Blood metals were measured in all participants in all cycles, whereas urine metals were determined only in subsamples of participants in all cycles. Heavy metals measured in blood included cadmium (µg/L), lead (µg/dL), manganese (µg/L), mercury (µg/L), and selenium (µg/L). Blood samples for the quantification of heavy metals were stored at −30 °C until they arrived at the National Center for Environmental Health for testing. Samples of total urinary arsenic samples (µg/L) were stored at −30 °C until they arrived at the National Center for Environmental Health for testing. They were quantified using inductively coupled plasma-mass spectrometry (ICP-MS). The percent CV for metals ranged from 1.2% to 11.3%. There was a range in the limits of detection (cadmium: 0.10–0.28 µg/L; lead: 0.07–0.37 µg/dL; manganese: 0.99–1.06 µg/dL; mercury: 0.16–0.325 µg/dL; selenium: 24.48–30.0 µg/dL; arsenic: 0.26–1.25 µg/dL) based on the NHANES cycle.

## 2.6. PFAS (ng/mL)

Measures of serum PFAS compounds were performed in a one third subsample of participants in all the included cycles. There were 7 PFAS compounds included in this study: Perfluorooctanoic acid (PFOA), Perfluorooctane sulfonic acid (PFOS), Perfluorononanoic acid (PFNA), Perfluoroundecanoic acid (PFUA), Perfluorohexane sulfonic acid (PFHxS), Perfluorodecanoic acid (PFDeA), and 2-(N-methylperfluorooctanesulfonamido)acetic acid (Me-PFOSA-AcOH). Serum samples for the quantification of PFASs were stored at −30 °C until they arrived at the National Center for Environmental Health for testing. They were quantified using solid phase extraction coupled with high performance liquid chromatography–turbo ion spray ionization–tandem mass spectrometry (on-line SPE-HPLC-TIS-MS/MS). The percent CV for PFASs ranged from 8.6% to 12.8%. There was a range of the limits of detection (PFDeA: 0.1–0.2 ng/mL; Me-PFOSA-AcOH: 0.09–0.2 ng/mL; PFNA: 0.08–0.1 ng/mL; PFUA: 0.1–0.2 ng/mL; PFOS: 0.1–0.2 ng/mL) based on NHANES cycle. The limit of detection for PFHxS and PFOA was 0.1 ng/mL for all NHANES cycles.

## 2.7. Phenols and Parabens (ng/mL)

Measures of urinary phenols and parabens were performed in a one third subsample of participants in all the included cycles. There were two phenols and 3 parabens measured in this study: bisphenol A (BPA), triclosan, methyl paraben (MBP), butyl paraben (BPB), and propyl paraben (PBP). Urine samples for the quantification of phenols and parabens were stored at −20 °C until they arrived at the National Center for Environmental Health for testing. They were quantified using on-line solid phase extraction coupled with high performance liquid chromatography and tandem mass spectrometry (on-line SPE-HPLC-MS/MS). The percent CV for phenols and parabens ranged from 2.3% to 13.5%. There was a range of the limits of detection (BPA: 0.2–0.4 ng/mL; Triclosan: 1.7–02.3 ng/mL; butyl paraben: 0.1–0.2 ng/mL; propyl paraben: 0.1–0.2 ng/mL) based on NHANES cycle. The limit of detection for methyl paraben was 1.0 ng/mL for all NHANES cycles.

## 2.8. PAH (ng/L)

Measures of urinary phthalate metabolites were performed in a subsample of one third of the participants in four cycles (2007–2014) and were not performed in the last cycle (2015–2016). There were 10 PAHs measured in this study: 1-hydroxynaphthalene, 2-hydroxynaphthalene, 3-hydroxyfluorene, 2-hydroxyfluorene, 3-hydroxyphenanthrene, 1-hydroxyphenanthrene, 2-hydroxyphenanthrene, 1-hydroxypyrene, 9-hydroxyfluorene, and 4-phenanthrene. Urine samples for the quantification of PAH were stored at −20 °C until they arrived at the National Center for Environmental Health for testing. They were quantified using on-line SPE-HPLC-MS/MS. The percent CV for PAHs ranged from 2.1% to 13%. There was a range of the limits of detection (1-hydroxynaphthalene: 44.0–60.0 ng/L; 2-hydroxynaphthalene: 42.0–90.0 ng/L; 3-hydroxyfluorene: 4.95–10.0 ng/L; 2-hydroxyfluorene: 8.0–10.041 ng/L; 3-hydroxyphenanthrene: 4.95–10.0 ng/L; 1-hydroxyphenanthrene: 7.778–10.0 ng/L; 2-hydroxyphenanthrene: 4.95–10.0 ng/L; 1-hydroxypyrene: 4.95–70.0 ng/L; 9-hydroxyfluorene: 10.0–18.243 ng/L) based on the NHANES cycle.

## 2.9. Cotinine (ng/mL)

Samples of serum cotinine were stored at −20 °C until they arrived at the National Center for Environmental Health for testing. Cotinine was measured by isotope-dilution high-performance liquid chromatography/atmospheric pressure chemical ionization tandem mass spectrometric (ID HPLC-ACPI MS/MS) method. The percent CV for cotinine ranged from 4% to 40.6%. The limit of detection for serum cotinine was 0.015 ng/mL for all NHANES cycles.

## 3. Covariates

All data on covariates was extracted from the CDC/NHANES website. We identified potential confounders that were associated with environmental chemicals and RBC folate from prior research. Questionnaire data were collected for participants' sex, age, race, education, and family poverty-to-income ratio (FPR: family's income divided by the poverty level threshold for the family size and the survey year; a FPR of 1 indicates a family income at 100% of the federal poverty level) at the in-home visit. Urinary creatinine (mg/dL) was assessed from laboratory data and $log_2$-transformed for analyses to address skewness and limit the influence of outliers. The healthy eating index (HEI) was also calculated from 24 h dietary recall interviews at the MECs, and was included as a proxy for dietary patterns that may influence both chemical concentrations and RBC folate. The HEI measures overall diet quality based on adherence to the Dietary Guidelines for Americans and is validated in the U.S. population. It consists of adequacy components (total fruits, whole fruits, vegetables, greens/beans, whole grains, dairy, protein foods, seafood/plant proteins, fatty acids) and moderation components (refined grains, sodium, added sμgars, saturated fats). The 100-point scale assigns a higher score for better quality of overall diet. Finally, NHANES cycle was also included in all models to account for secular trends in both RBC folate levels and environmental chemical concentrations. Final models therefore included the following confounders: age, sex, race, education, FPR, urinary creatinine, HEI, and NHANES cycle.

## 4. Statistical Methods

We described distributions of adult sociodemographic characteristics using frequencies and percentages for categorical variables and mean with an accompanying standard deviation for continuous variables. The sample size, percent below the limit of detection (LOD), geometric mean, geometric standard error, interquartile range, and maximum values for each chemical, as well as RBC folate were calculated and presented in descriptive analyses. Environmental chemical concentrations were $log_2$-transformed and the influence of outliers was limited. Additionally, values below the limit of detection were replaced by the limit of detection divided by the square root of 2.

We conducted descriptive analyses to compare RBC folate concentrations by adult sociodemographic characteristics using Student's *t* test or One-way Analysis of Variance (ANOVA) (with Tukey's test for each category) depending on the number of categories for each sociodemographic characteristic. We calculated the Pearson correlation coefficients for the correlations between different chemicals and between chemicals and RBC folate.

To investigate the individual and joint associations between chemicals and RBC folate, we used two complimentary methods that can consider multiple correlated exposures in the context of environmental health studies: exposome-wide association study (ExWAS) and quantile-based g computation (Q-gcomp).

ExWAS addresses potential issues with type 1 error rate due to multiple comparisons; this method corrects for multiplicity by performing traditional linear regression and applying a threshold for effective tests (TEF) for significance testing [25,26]. The TEF is calculated based on the number of exposures and applies a Bonferroni correction based on the number of exposures.

As a complementary analysis, we used Q-gcomp to investigate the joint associations of multiple chemicals with RBC folate. This method does not assume linearity or additivity, and it does not assume that all components of the mixture have the same direction of effect [27]. We ran Q-gcomp analyses separately for the different families of pollutants, metals, PFASs, phthalates, PAHs, and phenols and parabens.

Because each NHANES cycle contains different amounts of missing data for each chemical, and not all chemicals were measured for all NHANES cycles, our dataset contained missing values for chemicals during the NHANES cycles, as they were not collected or because some chemical families, such as phthalates, phenols and parabens, PFASs, and PAHs were only measured in a subset of participants. To assess the impact of missing values on our study, we conducted a sensitivity analysis using multivariable imputation by chained equations (MICE). MICE is an imputation method that creates multiple imputed datasets to generate more accurate standard error values when using simulated datasets [28]. Based on previous research and imputation guidelines, we generated 70 imputed datasets [28]. We used the Rubin's rule to combine the results from the 70 imputed datasets for the ExWAS and Q-gcomp analyses [29]. All statistical analyses were conducted using R version 3.5.2. (R Core Team, Vienna, Austria, 2018), and SAS version 9.4 (SAS Institute, Inc, Cary, NC, USA).

## 5. Results

NHANES participants in our sample were predominantly male (48.7%), non-Hispanic white (41.5%), had some college or an associate in arts degree (28.90%), and had not smoked in the past 30 days (79.5%), (Table 1). The geometric mean urinary creatinine concentration was 98.94 (GSD: 2.09) mg/dL, and the average FPR was 2.44 (SD: 1.63). The geometric mean RBC folate concentration was 515.7 ng/mL (geometric standard deviation (GSD) = 243.7 ng/mL). The mean age was 48 (SD: 18.48) years old. RBC folate concentrations were higher among females, participants aged 65 years and older, non-Hispanic whites, participants that had at least a college degree, those who have not smoked in the past 30 days, participants in the highest family income-to-poverty ratio, participants in the lowest quartile of urinary creatinine values, and in the highest quartile of the HEI (Table 1). Geometric mean concentrations and the distribution of phthalates, metals, PFASs, PAHs, and phenols and parabens, are displayed in Table 2.

**Table 1.** Mean concentrations of red blood cell (RBC) folate according to participants characteristics (NHANES; 2007–2016). Abbreviations: standard deviation (SD); family income-to-poverty ratio (FPR); healthy eating index (HEI). The *p*-Value calculation for Overall RBC Folate is not applicable (N/A).

| | N | Mean | SD | *p*-Value |
|---|---|---|---|---|
| Overall RBC Folate | 27,938 | 515.7 | 243.7 | N/A |
| Sex | | | | <0.001 |
| Male | 13,599 | 500.1 | 232.5 | - |
| Female | 14,339 | 530.6 | 252.9 | <0.001 |
| Age | | | | <0.001 |
| 18 to 34 | 8022 | 439.1 | 172.1 | - |
| 35 to 64 | 13,650 | 506.3 | 220.4 | <0.001 |
| 65 and Older | 6266 | 634.4 | 315.0 | <0.001 |
| Race | | | | <0.001 |
| Mexican American | 4441 | 478.4 | 199.2 | - |
| Other Hispanic | 3012 | 483.1 | 200.7 | 0.918 |
| Non-Hispanic White | 11,605 | 584.4 | 273.4 | <0.001 |
| Non-Hispanic Black | 5768 | 440.6 | 210.3 | <0.001 |
| Other | 3112 | 483.9 | 211.4 | 0.861 |
| Education | | | | <0.001 |
| Less than 9th Grade | 3107 | 489.8 | 236.0 | - |
| 9th to 11th Grade | 4094 | 495.5 | 242.6 | 0.921 |
| High School Graduate/GED | 6309 | 514.4 | 255.4 | <0.001 |
| Some College or AA | 8074 | 519.6 | 246.0 | <0.001 |
| College Graduate or Above | 6254 | 539.0 | 229.1 | <0.001 |
| Missing | 100 | 473.0 | 301.1 | 0.984 |
| Smoking Status | | | | <0.001 |
| Has not Smoked in Last 30 Days | 22,200 | 533.6 | 250.6 | - |
| Smoked in Last 30 Days | 5729 | 446.7 | 200.6 | 0.540 |
| Missing | 9 | 448.5 | 134.0 | 0.999 |

**Table 1.** *Cont.*

| | N | Mean | SD | *p*-Value |
|---|---|---|---|---|
| FPR | | | | <0.001 |
| Lowest Quartile | 6335 | 475.5 | 223.7 | - |
| 2nd Quartile | 6349 | 516.3 | 251.2 | <0.001 |
| 3rd Quartile | 6365 | 528.9 | 242.9 | <0.001 |
| Highest Quartile | 6401 | 547.5 | 244.1 | <0.001 |
| Missing | 2488 | 501.3 | 258.4 | <0.001 |
| Urinary Creatinine | | | | <0.001 |
| Lowest Quartile | 6376 | 548.9 | 258.1 | - |
| 2nd Quartile | 6372 | 531.8 | 253.3 | <0.001 |
| 3rd Quartile | 6473 | 500.0 | 225.0 | <0.001 |
| Highest Quartile | 6469 | 471.4 | 210.1 | <0.001 |
| Missing | 2248 | 549.4 | 288.3 | 0.999 |
| Cycle | | | | 0.251 |
| 2007–2008 | 5600 | 538.0 | 265.0 | - |
| 2009–2010 | 6019 | 496.2 | 232.8 | <0.001 |
| 2011–2012 | 5269 | 486.0 | 224.5 | <0.001 |
| 2013–2014 | 5636 | 533.7 | 247.4 | 0.88 |
| 2015–2016 | 5414 | 524.7 | 242.1 | 0.03 |
| HEI | | | | <0.001 |
| Lowest Quartile | 6534 | 474.7 | 229.2 | - |
| 2nd Quartile | 6533 | 498.7 | 237.6 | <0.001 |
| 3rd Quartile | 6534 | 528.8 | 251.1 | <0.001 |
| Highest Quartile | 6534 | 565.4 | 249.5 | <0.001 |
| Missing | 1803 | 499.0 | 232.5 | <0.001 |

**Table 2.** Concentrations of environmental chemicals among adult NHANES participants from 2007 to 2016. Abbreviations: geometric mean (GM); geometric standard deviation (GSD); interquartile range (IQR); limit of detection (LOD).

| Exposure | N | % < LOD | GM | GSD | IQR |
|---|---|---|---|---|---|
| Phthalates (ng/mL) | | | | | |
| Mono(carboxyisoctyl) phthalate (MCOP) | 9012 | 1.22% | 11.34 | 4.17 | 23.98 |
| Mono-2-ethyl-5-carboxypentyl phthalate (MECPP) | 9012 | 0.23% | 15.19 | 3.25 | 22.90 |
| Mono-n-butyl phthalate (MBP) | 9012 | 2.24% | 11.83 | 3.44 | 19.94 |
| Mono-(3-carboxypropyl) phthalate (MCPP) | 9012 | 9.55% | 2.10 | 3.67 | 3.70 |
| Mono-ethyl phthalate (MEP) (ng/mL) | 9012 | 0.13% | 61.78 | 4.94 | 153.48 |
| Mono-(2-ethyl-5-hydroxyhexyl) phthalate (MEHHP) | 9012 | 0.67% | 9.68 | 3.51 | 15.90 |
| Mono-(2-ethyl)-hexyl phthalate (MEHP) | 9012 | 33.60% | 1.61 | 3.10 | 2.63 |
| Mono-isobutyl phthalate (MiBP) | 9012 | 2.00% | 7.49 | 3.12 | 12.00 |
| Mono-isononyl phthalate (MNP) | 9012 | 67.63% | 1.05 | 2.74 | 0.61 |
| Mono-(2-ethyl-5-oxohexyl) phthalate (MEOHP) | 9012 | 0.95% | 5.96 | 3.40 | 9.45 |
| Mono-benzyl phthalate (MBzP) | 9012 | 2.66% | 4.88 | 3.72 | 9.80 |
| Metals (μg/L) | | | | | |
| Cadmium (μg/L) | 22,401 | 15.71% | 0.36 | 2.24 | 0.38 |
| Lead | 22,401 | 0.29% | 12.0 | 20.1 | 11.4 |
| Manganese | 10,787 | 0.00% | 9.38 | 1.43 | 4.31 |
| Mercury | 22,401 | 9.85% | 0.90 | 2.69 | 1.22 |
| Selenium | 10,787 | 0.00% | 192.83 | 1.14 | 29.97 |
| Total arsenic | 9170 | 0.87% | 8.35 | 3.17 | 12.40 |
| PFAS (ng/mL) | | | | | |
| Perfluorodecanoic acid (PFDeA) | 8963 | 16.82% | 0.23 | 2.25 | 0.26 |
| Perfluorohexane sulfonic acid (PFHxS) | 8963 | 1.91% | 1.39 | 2.61 | 1.79 |
| 2-(N-methylperfluoroctanesulfonamido)acetic acid (Me-PFOSA-AcOH) | 8963 | 53.33% | 0.16 | 2.52 | 0.23 |
| Perfluorononanoic acid (PFNA) | 8963 | 1.53% | 0.91 | 2.11 | 0.88 |

**Table 2.** *Cont.*

| Exposure | N | % < LOD | GM | GSD | IQR |
|---|---|---|---|---|---|
| Perfluoroundecanoic acid (PFUA) | 8963 | 59.88% | 0.15 | 2.27 | 0.13 |
| Perfluorooctanoic acid (PFOA) | 8961 | 0.22% | 2.34 | 2.14 | 2.40 |
| Perfluorooctane sulfonic acid (PFOS) | 8961 | 0.39% | 7.49 | 2.61 | 9.59 |
| Phenols and parabens (ng/mL) | | | | | |
| Bisphenol A (BPA) | 9013 | 0.65% | 1.53 | 3.03 | 2.40 |
| Triclosan | 9013 | 7.51% | 10.93 | 7.05 | 37.47 |
| Butyl paraben | 9013 | 0.18% | 0.25 | 5.14 | 0.33 |
| Methyl paraben | 9013 | 2.49% | 59.09 | 6.03 | 213.80 |
| Propyl paraben (ng/mL) | 9013 | 0.18% | 7.33 | 9.78 | 43.70 |
| PAHs (ng/L) | | | | | |
| One hydroxynaphthalene | 7194 | 0.06% | 2235.54 | 4.68 | 5480.00 |
| Two hydroxynaphthalene | 7221 | 0.00% | 4474.30 | 3.20 | 8318.10 |
| Three hydroxyfluorene | 7256 | 1.86% | 104.31 | 3.97 | 208.15 |
| Two hydroxyfluorene | 7267 | 0.00% | 261.61 | 3.43 | 470.50 |
| Three hydroxyphenanthrene | 5439 | 1.84% | 79.04 | 2.80 | 118.80 |
| One hydroxyphenanthrene | 7280 | 0.38% | 123.95 | 2.56 | 164.73 |
| Two hydroxyphenanthrene | 5417 | 1.14% | 68.29 | 2.55 | 90.00 |
| One hydroxypyrene | 7253 | 7.33% | 118.89 | 2.84 | 176.30 |
| Nine hydroxyfluorene | 5448 | 0.00% | 304.70 | 3.00 | 490.23 |
| Cotinine (ng/mL) | 27,646 | 27.41% | 0.31 | 47.50 | 8.72 |

Within and between family chemical correlations varied between 0.10 and 0.98 for phthalates, −0.07 and 0.56 for metals, −0.19 and 0.78 for PFASs, 0.28 and 0.96 for PAHs, and −0.11 and 0.82 for phenols and parabens (Figure 1).

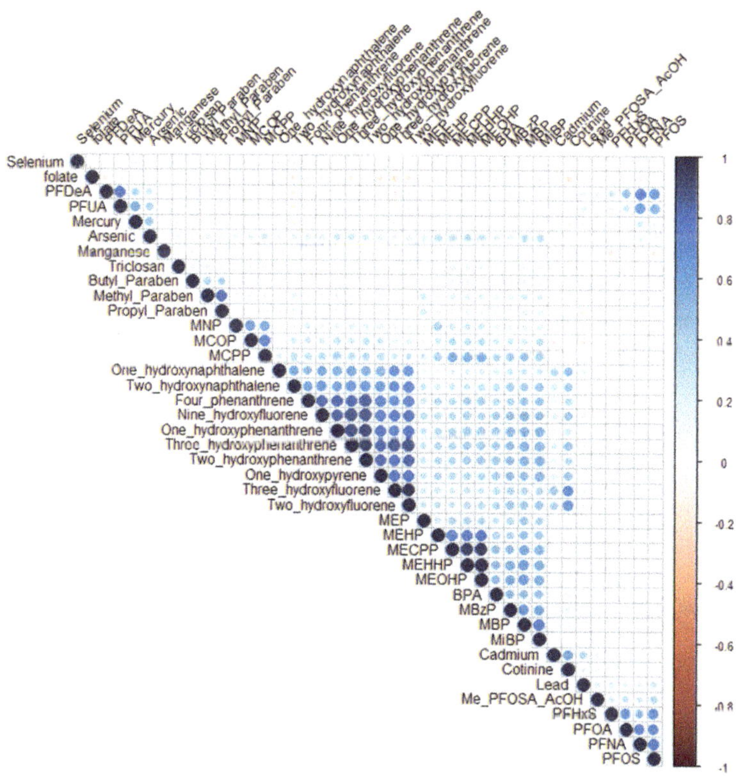


**Figure 1.** Pearson correlation heat map of included environmental pollutants and folate. Red circles indicate negative correlations and blue circles indicate positive correlations.

*5.1. ExWAS Analysis*

For the overall ExWAS analysis, the corrected *p* value was $2.01 \times 10^{-3}$. After adjusting for sex, age, race, education, smoking status, FPR, urinary creatinine, HEI, and NHANES cycle, 12 environmental chemicals, including metals, PFASs, and PAHs, were significantly inversely associated with RBC folate, and four environmental chemicals, including metals (manganese, selenium), and MBzP and MECPP phthalates, were significantly positively associated with RBC folate (Figure 2). For instance, a doubling of PFNA ($\beta = -48.3$; 95%CI: −57.4, −39.1), PFDeA ($\beta = -46.7$; 95%CI: −55.6, −37.8), PFOS ($\beta = -43.7$; 95%CI: −53.5, −33.9), PFUA ($\beta = -43.1$; 95%CI: −52.4, −33.9), lead ($\beta = -27.0$; 95%CI: −33.4, −20.7), cotinine ($\beta = -22.1$; 95%CI: −27.2, −17.1), mercury ($\beta = -21.6$; 95%CI: −27.2, −16.1), three hydroxyfluorene ($\beta = -17.4$; 95%CI: −32.7, −2.1), arsenic ($\beta = -16.3$; 95%CI: −24.4, −8.1), PFOA ($\beta = -14.6$; 95%CI: −24.4, −4.8), two hydroxy naphthalene ($\beta = -14.1$; 95%CI: −26.9, −1.2), and cadmium ($\beta = -7.3$; 95%CI: −14.1, −0.5) were associated with a statistically significant decrease in RBC folate after adjustment. A doubling of MBzP ($\beta = 14.8$; 95%CI: 3.9, 25.8), MECPP ($\beta = 13.2$; 95%CI: 2.2, 24.1), manganese ($\beta = 12.9$; 95%CI: 5.3, 20.4), and selenium ($\beta = 10.3$; 95%CI: 3.0, 17.6) were associated with a statistically significant increase in RBC folate after adjustment. No other chemicals were statistically significantly associated with a change in RBC folate after adjustment.

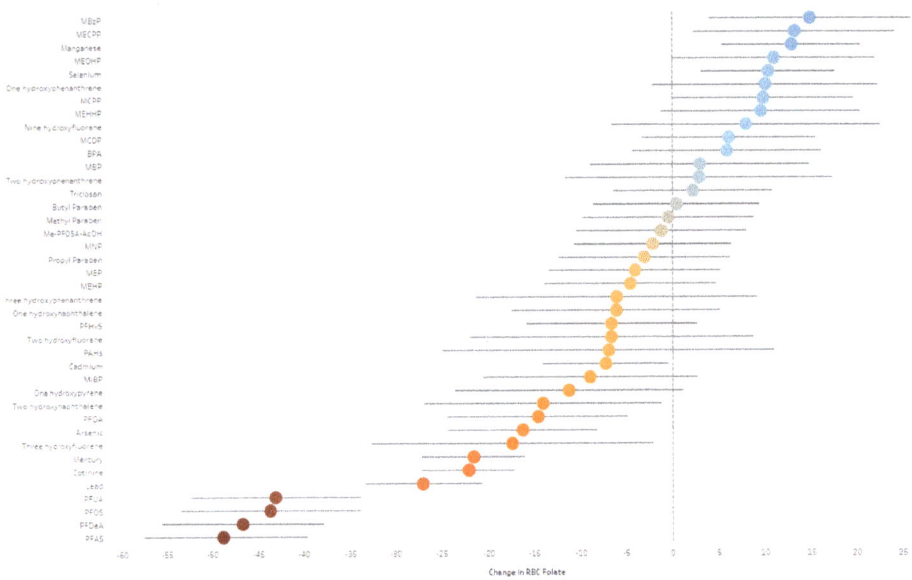


**Figure 2.** Estimates and 95% CIs for the associations between environmental chemical biomarkers and RBC folate using exposome-wide association study (ExWAS) analysis from the NHANES database from 2007 to 2016 (TEF = $2.01 \times 10^{-3}$). Models were adjusted for age, race, sex, family income-to-poverty ratio, education, NHANES cycle, and HEI. Additional adjustments for urinary creatinine were made for models with chemicals collected in urine. Estimates represent the change in RBC folate concentrations for each doubling in chemical concentrations. Blue illustrates a positive estimate and red illustrates a negative estimate.

*5.2. Q-Gcomp Analysis*

One quartile increases in the metal ($\beta = -38.36$; 95%CI −52.31, −24.42) and PFAS ($\beta = -48.86$; 95%CI: −57.56, −39.61) mixtures were significantly associated with a decrease in RBC folate after adjustment. No other chemical families were statistically significantly associated with a change in RBC folate after adjustment (Figure 3).

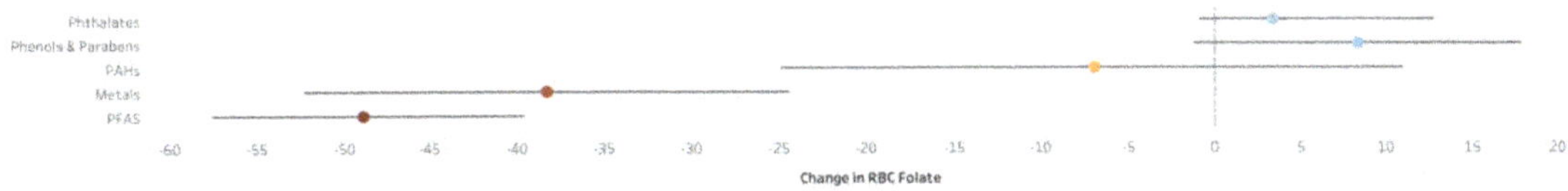


**Figure 3.** Estimates and 95% CIs for the associations between mixtures of environmental chemical biomarkers and RBC folate using quantile g computation (Q-gcomp) analysis from the NHANES database from 2007 to 2016. Models were adjusted for age, race, family income-to-poverty ratio, education, NHANES cycle, smoking status, and HEI. Additional adjustments for urinary creatinine were made for models with chemicals collected in urine. Estimates represent the associations between one quartile increases in an exposure family and changes in RBC folate concentrations.

The ExWAS sensitivity analysis using imputed datasets revealed 21 chemicals that were statistically significantly negatively associated with RBC folate and one chemical that was statistically significantly positively associated with RBC folate (Figure 4). For instance, a doubling of cotinine ($\beta$ = −31.1; 95%CI: −34.0, −28.2) was associated with a statistically significant decrease in RBC folate, and manganese ($\beta$ = 4.8; 95%CI: 1.2, 8.4) was associated with a statistically significant increase in RBC folate after adjustment. The Q-gcomp sensitivity analysis using imputed datasets revealed that one quartile increases in PFAS ($\beta$ = −29.9; 95%CI: −34.8, −24.9), metal ($\beta$ = −49.8; 95%CI: −56.2, −43.4), and PAH ($\beta$ = −10.4; 95%CI: −16.6, −4.3) mixtures were statistically significantly associated with decreases in RBC folate after adjustment (Figure 5). No other chemicals or chemical families were statistically significantly associated with changes in RBC folate after adjustment.

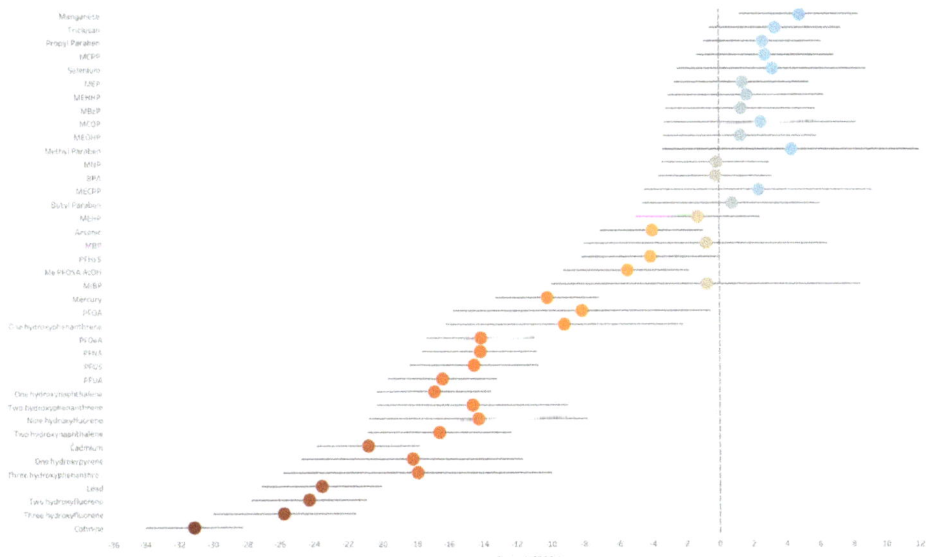


**Figure 4.** Pooled estimates and 95% CIs for the associations between environmental chemical biomarkers and RBC folate using exposome-wide association study (ExWAS) analysis from the NHANES database from 2007 to 2016 using 70 imputed datasets (TEF = 2.01 × $10^{-3}$). Models were adjusted for age, race, sex, family to income poverty ratio, education, NHANES cycle, and HEI. Additional adjustments for urinary creatinine were made for models with chemicals collected in urine. Estimates represent the change in RBC folate concentrations for each doubling in chemical concentrations. Blue illustrates a positive estimate and red illustrates a negative estimate.

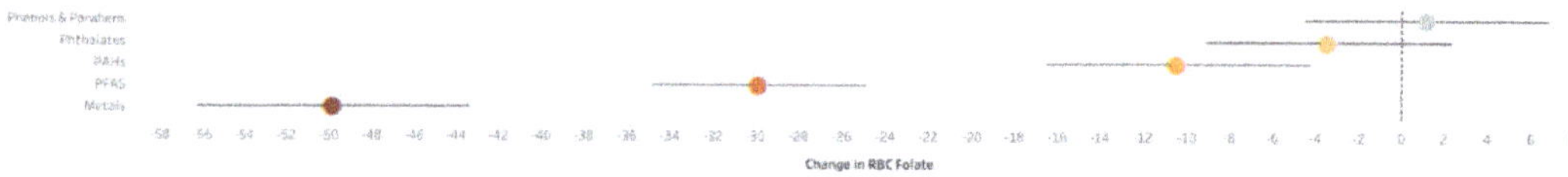


**Figure 5.** Pooled estimates and 95% CIs for the associations between environmental chemical mixtures and RBC folate using quantile g computation (Q-gcomp) analysis of adults from the NHANES database from 2007 to 2016 using 70 imputed datasets. Adjusted for age, race, family income-to-poverty ratio, education, NHANES cycle, smoking status, and diet. Additional adjustments for urinary creatinine were made for models with chemicals collected in urine. Estimates represent the association between a one quantile increase in the exposure family and a ng/mL change in RBC folate. Blue illustrates a positive estimate and red illustrates a negative estimate.

## 6. Discussion

In the present study, we used two statistical approaches, ExWAS and Q-gcomp, to evaluate the associations of 39 individual chemicals and 6 chemical mixtures with RBC folate concentrations in a sample of U.S. adults from NHANES (2007–2016). We found that several chemicals, including cadmium, lead, mercury, arsenic, PFDA, PFNA, PFUA, PFOA, PFOS, two hydroxynapthalene, three hydroxyfluorene, and cotinine were associated with lower RBC folate levels and MECPP, MBzP, manganese and selenium were associated with higher RBC folate levels. The ExWAS and complimentary Q-gcomp analysis yielded convergent results.

Although there are limited studies examining the associations between environmental chemicals and RBC folate concentrations, our findings are consistent with previous findings suggesting an inverse association between lead and folate among lead-exposed workers and smoking and folate among Inuit women of childbearing age [30,31]. Additionally, one cross-sectional study has examined the associations among PFASs, and a PFAS mixture and red blood cell folate using Bayesian kernel machine regression (BKMR) and Q-gcomp, and found comparable results using data from NHANES 2007–2010 [32].

The potential pathways by which chemicals may affect folate levels are unclear; however, a few experimental studies suggest possible biological mechanisms for the inverse associations between these environmental chemicals and RBC folate. For instance, PFASs have been shown to impact thyroid hormone levels [33,34] and thyroid stimulating hormones stimulate folate-dependent bioprocesses [35]. On the other hand, vitamin B complexes with folate have been shown to reduce cadmium and lead levels in rats, possibly by preventing absorption or facilitating increased excretion [36]. Also, mercury and PAHs are detoxified through the glutathione detoxification system which requires folate for the metabolic processing of cysteine, a precursor of glutathione [37–39]. Finally, PAHs, PFASs, lead, and cadmium, have all been associated with increased homocysteine (Hcy) concentrations [40–42]. Hcy is inversely associated with bioavailable folate due to folate's use in converting Hcy into either methionine or cysteine during one-carbon metabolism, and folate deficiency can cause Hcy buildup [43].

Regarding the observed positive associations, selenium has been shown to enhance concentrations of glutathione and would help to explain the positive associations between selenium and RBC folate observed in our study [39].

This study has several key limitations. First, the design of the study is cross-sectional with only one measurement representing exposure status available. This precludes making any causal claims, as the temporality of the relationship between environmental chemicals and folate is unclear. Given the use of biomarkers for measurements of environmental chemicals, we cannot exclude the potential for reverse causation, whereas folate levels impact measured biomarkers of exposure, and their metabolism. For instance, we cannot state whether these chemicals decrease the levels of folate or whether folate helps decrease the body's chemical burden, or impacts how folate is transported or metabolized in target tissues. The relationship may also be due to unmeasured confounders that may impact both exposure and RBC folate. For example, previous studies have shown that folate and PFASs share transport carriers [44]. Second, because there were NHANES cycles that did not include certain chemicals, there were periods where some chemicals were missing from the analysis, especially for PAHs in the last included NHANES cycle (2015–2016). These gap may introduce selection bias; however, results from analyses run with an imputed dataset were similar to the results in our main analysis. Also, the gaps in the data are largely due to the NHANES cycles and the subset of the participants that was representative of NHANES participants as a whole, and most likely were not related to the other variables in our analysis.

The strengths of this study include the breadth of environmental chemicals available through the NHANES dataset and the adoption of modern statistical approaches to analyze both mixtures and individual associations between environmental chemicals and RBC folate. Additionally, the large sample size and representativeness for the United States population provide increased generalization to non-institutionalized United States citizens, and adequate power for sensitivity analyses. Also, red blood cell folate is a long-term biomarker of folate status and is more resistant to acute changes in folate status and supplementation. Finally, we also adjusted for the HEI which is a good indicator of potential confounding by dietary patterns.

## 7. Conclusions

Our results suggest significant relationships between exposures to some environmental chemicals and RBC folate, and these findings may have implications for public health. First, a ubiquitous and continuous source of chemical exposures that has a modest inverse association with folate can have important implications for public health given the role of folate in many biological processes. Second, vulnerable populations with insufficient folate levels are further burdened by preventable modifiable environmental factors that reduce folate levels.

This study, to our knowledge, is the first to examine the associations between mixtures of metals, PAHs, phenols and parabens, and phthalates with RBC folate levels. Our study's results should be interpreted cautiously given the cross-sectional design. Future prospective studies can expand these preliminary findings by investigating temporally aligned exposures to environmental chemicals, folate levels, and potential health outcomes at later time points.

**Author Contributions:** M.M. and Y.O. conceived and designed the study, analyzed the data, and wrote the manuscript. K.R., R.B., Z.L. and N.L. supervised the methodological aspects, reviewed the manuscript, provided critical feedback, and edited for accuracy. All authors have read and agreed to the published version of the manuscript.

**Funding:** This work was funded by the National Institute of Environmental Health Sciences, grant N: R01ES032552.

**Institutional Review Board Statement:** This study is based on publicly available data from the National Health and Nutrition Examination Survey (NHANES). Since this manuscript is based on secondary analysis of data, the study was deemed exempt by the University of Massachusetts IRB.

**Informed Consent Statement:** Not applicable.

**Data Availability Statement:** All the data used in this manuscript are available at https://www.cdc.gov/nchs/nhanes/index.html. (accessed 1 December 2018).

**Conflicts of Interest:** The authors declare no conflicts of interest.

## References


1. Ducker, G.S.; Rabinowitz, J.D. One-Carbon Metabolism in Health and Disease. *Cell Metab.* **2017**, *25*, 27–42. [CrossRef] [PubMed]
2. Fowler, B. The folate cycle and disease in humans. *Kidney Int.* **2001**, *59*, 221–229. [CrossRef]
3. Son, P.; Lewis, L. Hyperhomocysteinemia. [Updated 2020 May 21]. In *StatPearls [Internet]*; StatPearls Publishing: Treasure Island, FL, USA, 2022. Available online: https://www.ncbi.nlm.nih.gov/books/NBK554408/ (accessed on 24 November 2024).
4. Keil, K.P.; Lein, P.J. DNA methylation: A mechanism linking environmental chemical exposures to risk of autism spectrum disorders? *Environ. Epigenetics* **2016**, *2*, dvv012. [CrossRef]
5. Kim, Y. Folate and carcinogenesis: Evidence, mechanisms, and implications. *J. Nutr. Biochem.* **1999**, *10*, 66–88. [CrossRef] [PubMed]
6. Kim, Y. Nutritional Epigenetics: Impact of Folate Deficiency on DNA Methylation and Colon Cancer Susceptibility. *J. Nutr.* **2005**, *135*, 2703–2709. [CrossRef]
7. Pfeiffer, C.M.; Sternberg, M.R.; Zhang, M.; Fazili, Z.; Storandt, R.J.; Crider, K.S.; Lavoie, D.J. Folate status in the US population 20 y after the introduction of folic acid fortification. *Am. J. Clin. Nutr.* **2019**, *110*, 1088–1097. [CrossRef]
8. Greenberg, J.A.; Bell, S.J.; Guan, Y.; Yu, Y.-H. Folic Acid Supplementation and Pregnancy: More Than Just Neural Tube Defect Prevention. *Rev. Obstet. Gynecol.* **2011**, *4*, 52–59. [PubMed] [PubMed Central]
9. Botto, L.D.; Moore, C.A.; Khoury, M.J.; Erickson, J.D. Neural-Tube Defects. *N. Engl. J. Med.* **1999**, *341*, 1509–1519. [CrossRef]
10. Czeizel, A.; Dudás, I.; Vereczkey, A.; Bánhidy, F. Folate Deficiency and Folic Acid Supplementation: The Prevention of Neural-Tube Defects and Congenital Heart Defects. *Nutrients* **2013**, *5*, 4760–4775. [CrossRef]
11. George, L.; Mills, J.L.; Johannson, A.L.V.; Nordmark, A.; Olander, B.; Granath, F.; Cnattingius, S. Plasma Folate Levels and Risk of Spontaneous Abortion. *JAMA* **2002**, *288*, 1867. [CrossRef]
12. Liu, X.; Lv, L.; Zhang, H.; Zhao, N.; Qiu, J.; He, X.; Zhang, Y. Folic acid supplementation, dietary folate intake and risk of preterm birth in China. *Eur. J. Nutr.* **2015**, *55*, 1411–1422. [CrossRef] [PubMed]
13. Naninck EF, G.; Stijger, P.C.; Brouwer-Brolsma, E.M. The Importance of Maternal Folate Status for Brain Development and Function of Offspring. *Adv. Nutr.* **2019**, *10*, 502–519. [CrossRef] [PubMed]
14. Watanabe, H.; Fukuoka, H.; Sμgiyama, T.; Nagai, Y.; Ogasawara, K.; Yoshiike, N. Dietary folate intake during pregnancy and birth weight in Japan. *Eur. J. Nutr.* **2008**, *47*, 341–347. [CrossRef] [PubMed]
15. Zhu, X.; Wei, L.; Cao, D.; Liu, C.; Tian, J.; Long, Y.; Mo, Z. Low serum folate status in the second trimester increase the risk of low birthweight in Chinese women. *J. Obstet. Gynaecol. Res.* **2018**, *44*, 2037–2044. [CrossRef]
16. Oulhote, Y.; Lanphear, B.; Braun, J.M.; Webster, G.M.; Arbuckle, T.E.; Etzel, T.; Forget-Dubois, N.; Seguin, J.R.; Bouchard, M.F.; MacFarlane, A.; et al. Gestational exposures to phthalates and folic acid, and autistic traits in Canadian children. *Environ. Health Perspect.* **2020**, *128*, 027004. [CrossRef]
17. Weggemans, R.M.; Groot, L.C.D.; Haller, J. Factors Related to Plasma Folate and Vitamin B12. The Seneca Study. *Int. J. Food Sci. Nutr.* **1997**, *48*, 141–150. [CrossRef]
18. Sanvisens, A.; Zuluaga, P.; Pineda, M.; Fuster, D.; Bolao, F.; Juncà, J.; Mμga, R. Folate deficiency in patients seeking treatment of alcohol use disorder. *Drug Alcohol Depend.* **2017**, *180*, 417–422. [CrossRef]
19. Zhou, Z.; Li, J.; Yu, Y.; Li, Y.; Zhang, Y.; Liu, L.; Huo, Y. Effect of Smoking and Folate Levels on the Efficacy of Folic Acid Therapy in Prevention of Stroke in Hypertensive Men. *Stroke* **2018**, *49*, 114–120. [CrossRef]
20. Stamm, R.; Hoμghton, L. Nutrient Intake Values for Folate during Pregnancy and Lactation Vary Widely around the World. *Nutrients* **2013**, *5*, 3920–3947. [CrossRef]
21. Zhao, R.; Aluri, S.; Goldman, I.D. The proton-coupled folate transporter (PCFT-SLC46A1) and the syndrome of systemic and cerebral folate deficiency of infancy: Hereditary folate malabsorption. *Mol. Asp. Med.* **2017**, *53*, 57–72. [CrossRef]
22. Kishi, R.; Grandjean, P. Health Impacts of Developmental Exposure to Environmental Chemicals. In *Health Impacts of Developmental Exposure to Environmental Chemicals*; Springer: Berlin/Heidelberg, Germany, 2020.
23. Centers for Disease Control and Prevention (CDC); National Center for Health Statistics (NCHS). *National Health and Nutrition Examination Survey Data [2007–2016]*; U.S. Department of Health and Human Services, Centers for Disease Control and Prevention: Hyattsville, MD, USA. Available online: https://www.cdc.gov/nchs/nhanes/index.html (accessed on 24 November 2024).
24. Centers for Disease Control and Prevention (CDC); National Center for Health Statistics (NCHS). *National Health and Nutrition Examination Survey Protocol 4000.04 [2015–2016]*; U.S. Department of Health and Human Services, Centers for Disease Control and Prevention: Hyattsville, MD, USA. Available online: https://wwwn.cdc.gov/nchs/data/nhanes/2015-2016/labmethods/FOLATE-I-MET-508.pdf (accessed on 24 November 2024).
25. Li, M.X.; Yeung, J.M.; Cherny, S.S.; Sham, P.C. Evaluating the effective numbers of independent tests and significant p-value thresholds in commercial genotyping arrays and public imputation reference datasets. *Hum. Genet.* **2012**, *131*, 747–756. [CrossRef] [PubMed]
26. Warembourg, C.; Maitre, L.; Tamayo-Uria, I.; Fossati, S.; Roumeliotaki, T.; Aasvang, G.M.; Basagaña, X. Early-Life Environmental Exposures and Blood Pressure in Children. *J. Am. Coll. Cardiol.* **2019**, *74*, 1317–1328. [CrossRef]

27. Keil, A.P.; Buckley, J.P.; O'Brien, K.M.; Ferguson, K.K.; Zhao, S.; White, A.J. A Quantile-Based g-Computation Approach to Addressing the Effects of Exposure Mixtures. *Environ. Health Perspect.* **2020**, *128*, 047004. [CrossRef] [PubMed]
28. Zhu, X. Comparison of four methods for handing missing data in longitudinal data analysis through a simulation study. *Open J. Stat.* **2014**, *4*, 933–944. [CrossRef]
29. Rubin, D.B. *Multiple Imputation for Nonresponse in Surveys*; John Wiley and Son: New York, NY, USA, 2004.
30. Duncan, K.; Erickson, A.C.; Egeland, G.M.; Weiler, H.; Arbour, L.T. Red blood cell folate levels in Canadian Inuit women of childbearing years: Influence of food security, body mass index, smoking, education, and vitamin use. *Can. J. Public Health* **2018**, *109*, 684–691. [CrossRef]
31. Bal, C.; Hocaoglu, A.; Büyükşekerci, M.; Alagüney, M.E.; Yılmaz, O.H.; Tutkun, E. Evaluation of folate and vitamin B12 status in lead exposed workers. *Toxicol. Lett.* **2015**, *42*, 294–298. [CrossRef]
32. Tian, Y.; Luan, M.; Zhang, J.; Yang, H.; Wang, Y.; Chen, H. Associations of single and multiple perfluoroalkyl substances exposure with folate among adolescents in Nhanes 2007–2010. *Chemosphere* **2022**, *307*, 135995. [CrossRef]
33. Lee, J.E.; Choi, K. Perfluoroalkyl substances exposure and thyroid hormones in humans: Epidemiological observations and implications. *Ann. Pediatr. Endocrinol. Metab.* **2017**, *22*, 6–14. [CrossRef]
34. Catargi, B.; Parrot-Roulaud, F.; Cochet, C.; Ducassou, D.; Roger, P.; Tabarin, A. Homocysteine, hypothyroidism, and effect of thyroid hormone replacement. *Thyroid. Off. J. Am. Thyroid. Assoc.* **1999**, *9*, 1163–1166. [CrossRef]
35. Barjaktarovic, M.; Steegers, E.A.P.; Jaddoe, V.W.V.; de Rijke, Y.B.; Visser, T.J.; Korevaar, T.I.M.; Peeters, R.P. The Association of Thyroid Function with Maternal and Neonatal Homocysteine Concentrations. *J. Clin. Endocrinol. Metab.* **2017**, *102*, 4548–4556. [CrossRef]
36. Tandon, S.K.; Flora, S.J.; Behari, J.R.; Ashquin, M. Vitamin B complex in treatment of cadmium intoxication. *Ann. Clin. Lab. Sci.* **1984**, *14*, 487–492. [PubMed]
37. Sobrino-Plata, J.; Meyssen, D.; Cuypers, A.; Escobar, C.; Hernández, L. Glutathione is a key antioxidant metabolite to cope with mercury and cadmium stress. *Plant Soil* **2014**, *377*, 369–381. Available online: https://doi-org.silk.library.umass.edu/10.1007/s11104-013-2006-4 (accessed on 24 November 2024). [CrossRef]
38. Branco, V.; Matos, B.; Mourato, C.; Diniz, M.; Carvalho, C.; Martins, M. Synthesis of glutathione as a central aspect of PAH toxicity in liver cells: A comparison between phenanthrene, benzo[b]fluoranthene and their mixtures. *Ecotoxicol. Environ. Saf.* **2021**, *208*, 111637. [CrossRef] [PubMed]
39. Richie, J.J.P.; Das, A.; Calcagnotto, A.M.; Aliaga, C.A.; El-Bayoumy, K. Age related changes in selenium and glutathione levels in different lobes of the rat prostate. *Exp. Gerontol.* **2012**, *47*, 223–228. Available online: https://doi-org.silk.library.umass.edu/10.1016/j.exger.2011.11.015 (accessed on 24 November 2024). [CrossRef]
40. Mallah, M.A.; Mallah, M.A.; Liu, Y.; Xi, H.; Wang, W.; Feng, F.; Zhang, Q. Relationship Between Polycyclic Aromatic Hydrocarbons and Cardiovascular Diseases: A Systematic Review. *Front. Public Health* **2021**, *9*, 763706. [CrossRef]
41. Min, J.-Y.; Lee, K.-J.; Park, J.-B.; Min, K.-B. Perfluorooctanoic acid exposure is associated with elevated homocysteine and hypertension in US adults. *Occup. Environ. Med.* **2012**, *69*, 658–662. Available online: http://www.jstor.org/stable/23567816 (accessed on 24 November 2024). [CrossRef]
42. Ledda, C.; Cannizzaro, E.; Lovreglio, P.; Vitale, E.; Stufano, A.; Montana, A.; Li Volti, G.; Rapisarda, V. Exposure to Toxic Heavy Metals Can Influence Homocysteine Metabolism? *Antioxidants* **2019**, *9*, 30. [CrossRef]
43. Blom, H.J.; Smulders, Y. Overview of homocysteine and folate metabolism. With special references to cardiovascular disease and neural tube defects. *J. Inherit. Metab. Dis.* **2011**, *34*, 75–81. [CrossRef]
44. Zhang, Y.; Mustieles, V.; Wang, Y.-X.; Sun, Y.; Agudelo, J.; Bibi, Z.; Torres, N.; Oulhote, Y.; Slitt, A., Messerlian, C. Folate concentrations and serum perfluoroalkyl and polyfluoroalkyl substance concentrations in adolescents and adults in the USA (National Health and Nutrition Examination Study 2003–2016): An observational study. *Lancet Planet. Health* **2023**, *7*, e449–e458. [CrossRef]

*toxics*

MDPI

*Article*

# Independent and Combined Associations of Urinary Heavy Metal Exposures with Serum α-Klotho in Middle-Aged and Older Adults

**Xinliang Zheng [1,†], Wenxin Zhou [1,†], Zhuoying Jiang [1], Chan Ding [1], Minqian Feng [1], Yongxin Li [1], Fitri Kurniasari [2], Shuanghua Xie [3,*] and Huadong Xu [1,*]**

1 School of Public Health, Zhejiang Provincial People's Hospital (Affiliated People's Hospital), Hangzhou Medical College, 182 Tianmushan Road, Xihu District, Hangzhou 310013, China; zxl2695291160@163.com (X.Z.); zzzhouwx@foxmail.com (W.Z.); jiangzhuoying0304@163.com (Z.J.); 130232023252@hmc.edu.cn (C.D.); 130232024250@hmc.edu.cn (M.F.); 21617018@zju.edu.cn (Y.L.)

2 Department of Environmental Health, Faculty of Public Health, University of Indonesia, Depok 16424, West Java, Indonesia; fitri.kurniasari04@ui.ac.id

3 Department of Central Laboratory, Beijing Obstetrics and Gynecology Hospital, Capital Medical University, Beijing Maternal and Child Health Care Hospital, Beijing 100026, China

* Correspondence: xiesh2021@mail.ccmu.edu.cn (S.X.); xuhuadong@hmc.edu.cn (H.X.)

† These authors contributed equally to this work.

**Abstract:** α-Klotho is an anti-aging protein linked to various age-related diseases. Environmental metal exposure has been associated with oxidative stress and aging, but its effect on α-Klotho levels remains unclear. This study investigated the relationship between urinary metal concentrations and serum α-Klotho levels using data from the National Health and Nutrition Examination Survey (NHANES) 2007–2016 cycles. A total of 4071 adults aged 40 to 79 years were included in the analysis. After adjusting for potential confounders, positive associations were found between serum α-Klotho levels and barium (Ba), cesium (Cs), and molybdenum (Mo), while tungsten (W) and uranium (U) were negatively correlated with α-Klotho levels. The combined effects of multiple metals were further analyzed using the qgcomp model, which demonstrated a negative correlation between increased metal mixtures and serum α-Klotho levels. Specifically, U, total arsenic (t-As), W, cadmium (Cd), antimony (Sb), and lead (Pb) contributed to the reduction of α-Klotho levels, while Ba, Cs, dimethylarsinic acid (DMA), Mo, thallium (Tl), and cobalt (Co) were positively associated with α-Klotho levels. These findings suggest that exposure to certain metals, particularly in combination, may reduce serum α-Klotho levels, potentially accelerating aging processes. Further studies should investigate the underlying mechanisms responsible for these associations.

**Keywords:** α-Klotho; urinary metals; NHANES; metal mixtures; aging biomarkers

## 1. Introduction

The Klotho protein family, including α-Klotho and β-Klotho, plays a central role in regulating aging and longevity. Of particular interest is α-Klotho, a soluble form of the protein that has been shown to exert protective effects on various organ systems, such as the cardiovascular, renal, and nervous systems [1,2]. Animal studies have demonstrated that α-Klotho contributes to an extended lifespan and delayed onset of age-related diseases, such as kidney disease and neurodegeneration [1,3–5]. In humans, higher α-Klotho levels have been linked to reduced all-cause mortality, highlighting its potential as a therapeutic target for age-related conditions [6]. Recent research has further linked α-Klotho to the pathophysiology of chronic diseases, such as cardiovascular disease [7], cancer [8], and diabetes [9], highlighting its potential as both a biomarker for aging and a therapeutic target for various age-related diseases.

Environmental exposure to heavy metals is a widespread global health concern. These metals can enter the human body through inhalation, ingestion, and dermal absorption, leading to various adverse health outcomes, including neurodevelopmental disorders, cardiovascular diseases, and cancer [10]. Arsenic (As), lead (Pb), and cadmium (Cd) are well-documented toxic metals [11,12], while antimony (Sb), tungsten (W), and molybdenum (Mo) also pose potential health risks. Sb exposure has been associated with oxidative stress and immunotoxicity [13], W has been implicated in carcinogenesis and systemic toxicity [14], and Mo can be toxic at high levels, impairing enzymatic functions and metabolism [15]. Environmental metal exposure has also been linked to accelerated aging processes, indicating that metals contribute to increased oxidative stress, DNA damage, and impaired cellular function, all of which are hallmarks of aging [16]. Therefore, examining the relationship between metal exposure and aging biomarkers, such as α-Klotho, is critical for understanding how environmental pollutants influence aging and contribute to age-related diseases.

A growing body of research has explored the relationship between α-Klotho levels and environmental pollutants, including organic contaminants such as polycyclic aromatic hydrocarbons [17], perchlorates, nitrates, thiocyanates [18], and dichlorobenzene [19]. Emerging studies have elucidated the impact of heavy metal exposure on α-Klotho levels. A study using NHANES data found that higher Pb levels are associated with lower serum α-Klotho, further supporting the link between heavy metal exposure and aging-related processes [20]. Additionally, exposure to Cd and Pb has been linked to oxidative stress, with evidence indicating that α-Klotho homeostasis may be disrupted in individuals with kidney dysfunction, especially at more severe stages [21]. Another investigation demonstrated that α-Klotho partially mediated the association between blood Pb levels and estimated glomerular filtration rate (eGFR), suggesting a potential role of α-Klotho in Pb-induced renal dysfunction [22]. Furthermore, studies on three essential elements identified a negative correlation between serum α-Klotho and blood copper (Cu) levels [23]. These findings underscore the importance of investigating the effects of heavy metal exposure on serum α-Klotho levels, especially the potential synergistic effects of multiple metal exposures on health. Given the ubiquity and persistence of metal pollutants, it is essential to explore how combined metal exposure influences α-Klotho levels, particularly in the general population.

The goal of this study was to investigate the association between urinary metal concentrations and serum α-Klotho levels using data from the National Health and Nutrition Examination Survey (NHANES), which is a nationally representative survey that provides comprehensive health data on the U.S. population, making it an invaluable resource for environmental health studies [24,25]. We used multiple linear regression and quantile g-computation (qgcomp) models to evaluate the independent and combined effects of urinary metals on serum α-Klotho levels. By examining a wide range of urinary metals and their mixtures, this study aims to provide new insights into the relationship between environmental metal exposure and aging biomarkers.

## 2. Materials and Methods

### *2.1. Study Design and Participants*

This study analyzed data from five cycles of the NHANES conducted between 2007 and 2016 (2007–2008, 2009–2010, 2011–2012, 2013–2014, 2015–2016). NHANES emphasizes environmental exposures and their impacts on health outcomes. Participants were selected based on the availability of data on urinary metals and serum α-Klotho levels, as shown in Figure 1. Initially, 17,389 adults aged 40–79 years were included in the analysis, as serum α-Klotho levels were only assessed in individuals within this age group. After excluding participants with incomplete data on serum α-Klotho ($n$ = 3625), urinary metals ($n$ = 9420), or covariates ($n$ = 273), the final study population consisted of 4071 participants. The NHANES study protocol was reviewed and approved by the Institutional Review Board of the National Center for Health Statistics (NCHS), and informed consent was obtained from all participants. No additional ethical approval was required for this secondary data analysis.

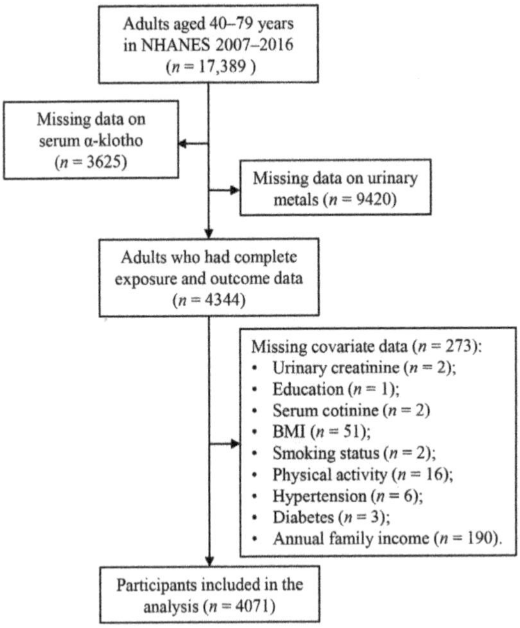


**Figure 1.** Flow diagram of selection of study participants from NHANES 2007–2016.

### 2.2. Measurement of Urinary Metal Levels

Urine samples were collected, stored at −30 °C, and subsequently shipped to the National Center for Environmental Health (NCEH) for analysis. Urinary concentrations of total arsenic (t-As), barium (Ba), cobalt (Co), Mo, cesium (Cs), Cd, Pb, Sb, thallium (Tl), W, and uranium (U) were quantified using inductively coupled plasma mass spectrometry (ICP-MS). For As species, including dimethylarsinic acid (DMA), arsenobetaine, monomethylarsonic acid, arsenocholine, arsenous (III) acid, and arsenic (V) acid, high-performance liquid chromatography (HPLC) was used. However, only DMA had a detection rate exceeding 70%, while other arsenic species exhibited lower detection rates. For elements measured by ICP-MS and other techniques, values below the limit of detection (LOD) were imputed as LOD divided by the square root of two, following NHANES protocols. Detailed information on laboratory procedures for measuring urinary metals and arsenic species can be found on the NHANES website.

### 2.3. Measurement of Serum α-Klotho Levels

Serum samples were stored at −80 °C until further analysis. α-Klotho levels were measured using an ELISA kit from IBL International (Gunma, Japan). The assay was validated prior to the study, demonstrating excellent sensitivity (4.33 pg/mL, compared to the manufacturer's claim of 6.15 pg/mL) and linearity ($R^2$ = 0.998 and 0.997 for high and low α-Klotho concentrations). Intra-assay precision was 3.2–3.9% for recombinant samples and 2.3–3.3% for human samples, while inter-assay precision was 2.8–3.5% for recombinant samples and 3.4–3.8% for human samples. All samples were analyzed in duplicate, and results met the laboratory's acceptance criteria. Additional methodological details can be found on the NHANES website (https://wwwn.cdc.gov/Nchs/Data/Nhanes/Public/2015/DataFiles/SSKL_I.htm) (accessed on 5 December 2024).

### 2.4. Covariates

Several covariates were selected based on their known associations with α-Klotho levels, as reported in previous literature [19,20,26,27], including age, sex, smoking status, physical activity, body mass index (BMI), diabetes mellitus, hypertension, race/ethnicity, education level, annual family income, marital status, serum cotinine, and NHANES cycle. Urinary creatinine levels were included to adjust for variability in urine concentration.

### 2.5. Statistical Analysis

Statistical analyses were performed using R software (version 4.2.1). Group differences in α-Klotho levels were evaluated using the Mann–Whitney U test for two-group comparisons and the Kruskal–Wallis test for multiple-group analyses. Urinary metal concentrations were analyzed both as continuous variables (after natural logarithmic transformation) and in quartiles. Multiple linear regression models were used to evaluate the association between serum α-Klotho levels and urinary metal concentrations, with results presented as the estimated percent changes in serum α-Klotho levels and their corresponding 95% confidence intervals (CIs) according to previous studies [28]. The $p$-value for trend was calculated by fitting urinary metal quartiles into linear models to assess dose–response relationships. All regression models were adjusted for age, sex, race/ethnicity, BMI, annual family income, smoking, education, marital status, hypertension, diabetes, NHANES cycle, physical activity, serum cotinine, and urinary creatinine.

In addition to analyzing single metal effects, the combined effects of multiple urinary metals on serum α-Klotho levels were assessed by adjusting for other metals. Finally, to investigate the impact of metal mixtures, the qgcomp model was implemented in the "qgcomp" R package. This model assigns positive or negative weights to urinary metals, estimating their combined exposure effect. The "qgcomp boot" function was used to assess the linearity of the exposure–response relationship and estimate the overall marginal effect.

## 3. Results

### 3.1. Characteristics of Study Participants and Serum α-Klotho Levels

A total of 4071 adults aged 40 to 79 years were included (Table 1), comprising 1999 males (49.1%) and 2072 females (50.9%). Serum α-Klotho levels varied significantly by age, sex, and race/ethnicity. Participants aged 40–49 years had the highest α-Klotho levels (883.5 ± 338.5 pg/mL), while those aged ≥ 70 years had the lowest levels (796.8 ± 264.3 pg/mL) ($p < 0.001$). Females had higher α-Klotho levels (882.4 ± 340.6 pg/mL) compared to males (819.5 ± 269.5 pg/mL) ($p < 0.001$), and non-Hispanic Black participants had the highest levels (905.5 ± 358.3 pg/mL) ($p < 0.001$). Serum α-Klotho levels were significantly higher in participants with hypertension (861.9 ± 309.9 pg/mL) compared to those without hypertension (839.3 ± 308.3 pg/mL) ($p = 0.002$). Underweight participants also had significantly higher α-Klotho (919.7 ± 331.3 pg/mL) than those in other BMI categories ($p = 0.002$). Significant variations in α-Klotho levels were also observed across NHANES cycles ($p < 0.001$), with the highest levels in the 2011–2012 cycle (897.5 ± 330.9 pg/mL) and the lowest in the

2015–2016 cycle (817.7 ± 329.3 pg/mL). Regarding marital status, participants who were never married had significantly higher serum α-Klotho levels (890.6 ± 405.3 pg/mL) compared to those who were married/cohabiting (849.1 ± 288.1 pg/mL) ($p$ = 0.040). However, no significant differences were observed across education levels, family income, serum cotinine levels, physical activity, smoking status, or diabetes status.

**Table 1.** Distribution of serum α-Klotho levels based on the characteristics of study participants in the NHANES 2007–2016.

| Characteristic | N | (%) | Serum α-Klotho Levels (Mean ± SD in pg/mL) | $p$ Value |
|---|---|---|---|---|
| Age, years | | | | <0.001 |
| 40–49 | 1144 | 28.10 | 883.5 ± 338.5 | |
| 50–59 | 1059 | 26.01 | 870.1 ± 306.9 | |
| 60–69 | 1142 | 28.05 | 837.0 ± 302.2 | |
| ≥70 | 726 | 17.83 | 796.8 ± 264.3 | |
| Sex | | | | <0.001 |
| Male | 1999 | 49.10 | 819.5 ± 269.5 | |
| Female | 2072 | 50.90 | 882.4 ± 340.6 | |
| Race/ethnicity | | | | <0.001 |
| Mexican American | 632 | 15.52 | 857.8 ± 297.9 | |
| Non-Hispanic White | 1775 | 43.60 | 817.0 ± 282.6 | |
| Non-Hispanic Black | 788 | 19.36 | 905.5 ± 358.3 | |
| Others | 876 | 21.52 | 868.2 ± 313.4 | |
| Education | | | | 0.088 |
| <High school | 1119 | 27.49 | 854.3 ± 337.6 | |
| High school | 871 | 21.40 | 829.7 ± 275.1 | |
| >High school | 2081 | 51.12 | 859.1 ± 306.7 | |
| Annual family income | | | | 0.970 |
| <USD 25,000 | 1279 | 31.42 | 855.0 ± 323.2 | |
| USD 25,000–64,999 | 1406 | 34.54 | 845.6 ± 293.9 | |
| ≥USD 65,000 | 1386 | 34.05 | 854.2 ± 311.6 | |
| Marital status | | | | 0.040 |
| Married/cohabiting | 2645 | 64.97 | 849.1 ± 288.1 | |
| Widowed/divorced/separated | 1083 | 26.60 | 844.9 ± 323.4 | |
| Never married | 343 | 8.43 | 890.6 ± 405.3 | |
| Smoking status | | | | <0.001 |
| Never | 2081 | 51.12 | 872.9 ± 304.6 | |
| Current | 768 | 18.87 | 833.6 ± 314.8 | |
| Former | 1222 | 30.02 | 826.4 ± 311.3 | |
| BMI, kg/m$^2$ | | | | 0.002 |
| Underweight (<18.5) | 40 | 0.98 | 919.7 ± 331.3 | |
| Normal weight (18.5–24.9) | 953 | 23.41 | 875.9 ± 315.3 | |
| Overweight (25–29.9) | 1415 | 34.76 | 836.9 ± 294.2 | |
| Obese (≥30) | 1663 | 40.85 | 848.3 ± 317.0 | |

Table 1. *Cont.*

| Characteristic | N | (%) | Serum α-Klotho Levels (Mean ± SD in pg/mL) | *p* Value |
|---|---|---|---|---|
| Physical activity | | | | 0.879 |
| Sedentary | 1197 | 29.40 | 860.5 ± 331.0 | |
| Insufficient | 596 | 14.64 | 846.3 ± 300.6 | |
| Moderate | 556 | 13.66 | 839.9 ± 285.4 | |
| High | 1722 | 42.30 | 850.8 ± 304.1 | |
| Diabetes | | | | 0.123 |
| No | 3356 | 82.44 | 839.6 ± 326.9 | |
| Yes | 715 | 17.56 | 854.0 ± 305.4 | |
| Hypertension | | | | 0.002 |
| No | 2189 | 53.77 | 839.3 ± 308.3 | |
| Yes | 1882 | 46.23 | 861.9 ± 309.9 | |
| Serum cotinine | | | | 0.421 |
| <LOD | 1184 | 29.08 | 854.3 ± 294.3 | |
| ≥LOD | 2887 | 70.92 | 850.4 ± 315.3 | |
| NHANES cycle | | | | <0.001 |
| 2007–2008 | 910 | 22.35 | 851.4 ± 330.0 | |
| 2009–2010 | 835 | 20.51 | 845.4 ± 290.7 | |
| 2011–2012 | 733 | 18.01 | 897.5 ± 330.9 | |
| 2013–2014 | 807 | 19.82 | 849.1 ± 254.3 | |
| 2015–2016 | 786 | 19.31 | 817.7 ± 329.3 | |

### *3.2. Distribution of Urinary Metal Concentrations*

The distribution of urinary metal concentrations among the study participants is presented in Table 2. The detection rates for the 12 urinary metals ranged from 70.4% (for Sb) to 100% (for Cs and Mo). The highest mean urinary concentrations were observed for Mo at 51.28 μg/L, followed by t-As at 19.86 μg/L and DMA at 5.72 μg/L. The lowest mean concentrations were found for uranium (U) at 0.0121 μg/L and Sb at 0.074 μg/L. The 95th percentile concentrations ranged from 0.0351 μg/L for U to 139.40 μg/L for Mo, indicating considerable variability in exposure levels across participants. Additionally, positive correlations were observed among the urinary metal concentrations, as shown in Figure S1, suggesting that participants with higher levels of one metal often had elevated levels of others. These inter-metal correlations highlighted the complexity of metal exposures in this population

Table 2. The distributions of urinary metals among study participants in the NHANES 2007–2016.

| Elements | Detection Rates (%) | Mean (μg/L) | Percentile (μg/L) | | | | |
|---|---|---|---|---|---|---|---|
| | | | 5th | 25th | Median | 75th | 95th |
| t-As | 99.2 | 19.86 | 1.56 | 3.76 | 7.66 | 16.60 | 63.87 |
| DMA | 78.5 | 5.72 | 1.20 | 2.00 | 3.59 | 6.38 | 17.20 |
| Ba | 99.2 | 1.85 | 0.21 | 0.53 | 1.07 | 2.15 | 5.40 |
| Cd | 96.5 | 0.441 | 0.049 | 0.145 | 0.281 | 0.547 | 1.368 |
| Co | 99.7 | 0.499 | 0.090 | 0.202 | 0.336 | 0.535 | 1.271 |

**Table 2.** *Cont.*

| Elements | Detection Rates (%) | Mean (μg/L) | Percentile (μg/L) | | | | |
|---|---|---|---|---|---|---|---|
| | | | 5th | 25th | Median | 75th | 95th |
| Cs | 100 | 5.11 | 1.23 | 2.70 | 4.39 | 6.58 | 11.11 |
| Mo | 100 | 51.28 | 7.42 | 20.10 | 38.10 | 66.04 | 139.40 |
| Pb | 98.7 | 0.71 | 0.10 | 0.27 | 0.48 | 0.83 | 1.89 |
| Sb | 70.4 | 0.074 | 0.016 | 0.028 | 0.046 | 0.078 | 0.192 |
| Tl | 99.5 | 0.178 | 0.038 | 0.087 | 0.149 | 0.233 | 0.407 |
| W | 82.9 | 0.110 | 0.013 | 0.027 | 0.060 | 0.121 | 0.336 |
| U | 84.1 | 0.0121 | 0.0014 | 0.0028 | 0.0055 | 0.0113 | 0.0351 |

### 3.3. Relationships Between Urinary Metals and Serum α-Klotho Levels

The relationships between individual urinary metal concentrations and serum α-Klotho levels were assessed after adjusting for potential confounders (Table S1). After adjusting for age, sex, race/ethnicity, BMI, annual family income, education, marital status, hypertension, diabetes, NHANES cycle, physical activity, serum cotinine, and urinary creatinine, significant positive associations were observed for Ba (percent change = 1.96, 95% CI: 1.19–2.74), Cs (percent change = 2.67, 95% CI: 1.21–4.14), and Mo (percent change = 1.05, 95% CI: 0.05–2.05). Quartile-based analyses revealed that participants in higher quartiles (Q2–Q4) of urinary Ba, Q3–Q4 of Cs, and Q4 of Mo exhibited significantly elevated serum α-Klotho levels compared to the reference quartile (Q1). Conversely, inverse associations were identified for W (percent change = −0.90, 95% CI: −1.69 to −0.10) and U (percent change = −1.65, 95% CI: −2.43 to −0.86). Participants in Q4 of W and Q3–Q4 of U demonstrated significantly lower serum α-Klotho levels relative to Q1.

Subsequently, using mutually adjusted models, the combined effects of multiple urinary metals on serum α-Klotho levels were examined (Table 3). After adjusting for other covariates and metals, Ba, Cs, and Mo remained positively associated with serum α-Klotho levels, with percent change values of 2.10 (95% CI: 1.24, 2.96), 2.81 (95% CI: 0.86, 4.80), and 1.40 (95% CI: 0.22, 2.59), respectively. In contrast, W and U were negatively associated with serum α-Klotho levels (W: percent change = −0.97, 95% CI: −1.88, −0.05; U: percent change = −1.58, 95% CI: −2.42, −0.74). Participants with higher urinary levels of Ba and Cs (Q2, Q3, Q4) had significantly higher serum α-Klotho levels, while those with elevated levels of Sb and U (Q2, Q3, Q4) exhibited significantly lower serum α-Klotho levels.

**Table 3.** Associations of multiple urinary metals with serum α-Klotho levels in the NHANES 2007–2016.

| Metals | Percent Change of Serum α-Klotho (95% CI) [a] | | | | | *p* for Trend |
|---|---|---|---|---|---|---|
| | Continuous | Q1 | Q2 | Q3 | Q4 | |
| tAs | −0.62 (−1.66, 0.42) | Ref. | −0.83 (−3.28, 1.68) | −2.40 (−5.14, 0.43) | −2.06 (−5.10, 1.08) | 0.159 |
| DMA | −0.35 (−1.92, 1.25) | Ref. | −1.17 (−3.61, 1.33) | 0.70 (−2.28, 3.76) | 0.21 (−3.20, 3.74) | 0.646 |
| Ba | 2.10 (1.24, 2.96) *** | Ref. | 4.46 (2.36, 6.61) *** | 4.32 (2.05, 6.64) *** | 5.12 (2.65, 7.65) *** | <0.001 |
| Cd | −0.69 (−1.75, 0.38) | Ref. | −0.55 (−3.22, 2.19) | −0.62 (−2.89, 1.70) | −0.14 (−2.23, 2.00) | 0.586 |
| Co | −0.28 (−1.49, 0.95) | Ref. | −0.42 (−2.61, 1.83) | 0.28 (−2.26, 2.89) | 1.12 (−1.68, 3.99) | 0.290 |
| Cs | 2.81 (0.86, 4.80) ** | Ref. | 1.75 (−0.66, 4.21) | 4.46 (1.54, 7.47) ** | 4.32 (1.03, 7.72) * | 0.005 |
| Mo | 1.40 (0.22, 2.59) * | Ref. | −0.39 (−2.54, 1.82) | 0.70 (−1.78, 3.23) | 0.35 (−2.42, 3.20) | 0.641 |
| Pb | −0.48 (−1.65, 0.70) | Ref. | 0.35 (−1.81, 2.55) | −0.48 (−2.90, 1.99) | −0.35 (−3.10, 2.48) | 0.206 |

**Table 3.** *Cont.*

| Metals | Percent Change of Serum α-Klotho (95% CI) [a] | | | | | p for Trend |
|---|---|---|---|---|---|---|
| | Continuous | Q1 | Q2 | Q3 | Q4 | |
| Sb | −0.69 (−1.86, 0.49) | Ref. | −2.33 (−4.47, −0.14) * | −2.53 (−4.81, −0.20) * | −1.99 (−4.53, 0.61) | 0.206 |
| Tl | −0.62 (−2.18, 0.96) | Ref. | −0.83(−3.07, 1.46) | 0.63 (−2.01, 3.33) | −0.55 (−3.47, 2.45) | 0.794 |
| W | −0.97 (−1.88, −0.05) * | Ref. | −0.69 (−2.75, 1.41) | 0.91 (−1.39, 3.25) | −1.72 (−4.20, 0.82) | 0.342 |
| U | −1.58 (−2.42, −0.74) ** | Ref. | −2.19 (−4.19, −0.15) * | −2.46 (−4.61, −0.27) * | −3.74 (−6.03, −1.40) ** | 0.002 |

[a] Adjusted for age, sex, race/ethnicity, BMI, annual family income, smoking, education, marital status, hypertension, diabetes, NHANES cycle, physical activity, serum cotinine, and urinary creatinine as well as other metals. * $p < 0.05$; ** $p < 0.01$; *** $p < 0.001$.

### *3.4. Association Between Metal Mixtures and Serum α-Klotho by the Qgcomp Model*

To investigate the combined effects of multiple urinary metals on serum α-Klotho levels, the qgcomp model was employed (Figure 2). The regression index weights revealed that U, t-As, W, Cd, Sb, and Pb contributed negatively to serum α-Klotho levels, with U being the primary contributor to the overall negative association. In contrast, Ba, Cs, DMA, Mo, Tl, and Co showed positive associations with serum α-Klotho levels, with Ba having the greatest positive effect. Furthermore, the combined effect of the metal mixture was analyzed based on the quantile range (Figure 2B). The results demonstrated a negative correlation between the mixture of twelve urinary metals and serum α-Klotho levels. A linear decrease in serum α-Klotho levels was observed across increasing quartiles of the metal mixture, with a percent change of −0.61 (95% CI: −1.07, −0.14) ($p = 0.002$), suggesting that higher exposure to multiple metals is associated with reduced serum α-Klotho levels.

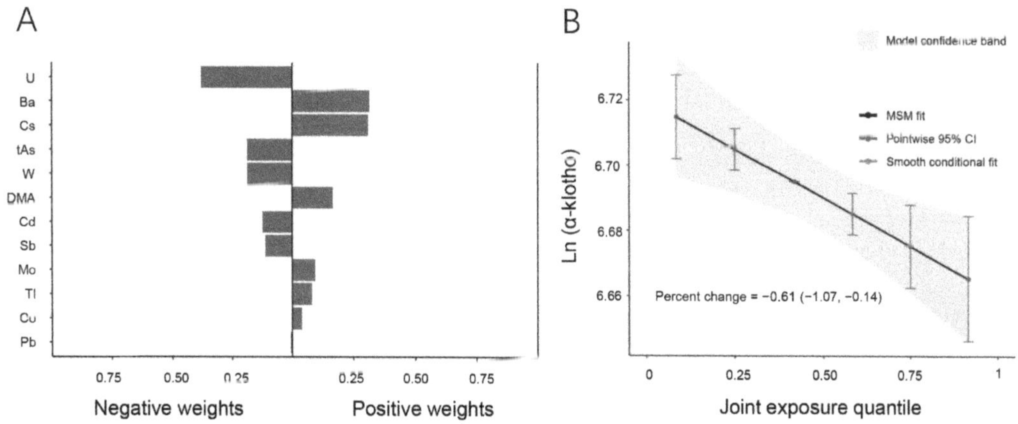


**Figure 2.** Associations between metal mixtures and serum α-Klotho by the qgcomp model. (**A**) Direction and magnitude of the assigned weights for each metal in association with serum α-Klotho. (**B**) Combined effects of twelve urinary metals levels on serum α-Klotho (95% CI). The model was adjusted for age, sex, race/ethnicity, BMI, annual family income, smoking, education, marital status, hypertension, diabetes, NHANES cycle, physical activity, serum cotinine, and urinary creatinine.

## 4. Discussion

This study comprehensively analyzed the relationship between urinary metal exposures and serum α-Klotho levels using data from the NHANES 2007–2016 cycles [20,29]. While previous studies have explored the associations between α-Klotho and environmental pollutants, especially organic chemicals, the effects of mixed metal exposure on α-Klotho levels remain largely unexplored. Our study is the first to systematically examine both individual and combined metal exposures and their effects on α-Klotho levels in a large, nationally representative sample. This research filled a critical gap in the literature by addressing the previously unexplored relationship between mixed metal exposure and α-Klotho levels.

Although the relationship between metal exposure and α-Klotho remains under investigation, prior studies have demonstrated that heavy metals could impact α-Klotho levels, primarily through oxidative stress and kidney function impairment [10,30]. Previous research has shown that Pb exposure negatively correlates with α-Klotho levels and mediates its effect on kidney function, while Cd and Pb have been linked to oxidative-stress-related Klotho dysregulation, particularly in individuals with renal impairment [21,22]. Additionally, studies on trace elements found that a combined effect of selenium (Se), Cu, and zinc (Zn) decreased α-Klotho concentrations [23]. Our study extends these findings by assessing the effects of multiple metals on α-Klotho simultaneously, rather than focusing on single-metal exposures. We observed that urinary W and U were negatively associated with α-Klotho levels, and our quantile g-computation model revealed a dose-dependent decrease in α-Klotho with increasing metal mixture exposure. These findings suggest that exposure to multiple metals may have a cumulative or synergistic effect, amplifying their negative impact on aging biomarkers. Unlike previous studies that reported significant associations between Cd and Pb with α-Klotho [20], we did not observe statistically significant effects for these metals. This discrepancy may be attributed to differences in study design, population characteristics, or the influence of co-exposures in our multi-metal analysis, which could obscure individual metal effects.

Given the central role of α-Klotho in aging and disease prevention, it is important to consider what constitutes a normal reference range for this biomarker. Currently, there is no universally established reference range for serum α-Klotho protein levels. Most studies on α-Klotho concentrations are based on data from the NHANES [19,20,31–34]. In our study, the quartile-based analysis of α-Klotho levels provides insight into how varying degrees of metal exposure may affect this anti-aging protein. While the specific health effects of small fluctuations in α-Klotho levels remain unclear, previous research suggests that reduced α-Klotho levels are associated with aging-related diseases. In this context, the observed associations between metal exposure and α-Klotho variations may have long-term implications for health and aging processes.

Our study also compared metal-associated effects on α-Klotho between different demographic groups. Notably, our analysis revealed that individuals who were never married exhibited higher serum α-Klotho levels than those who were married or cohabiting. This observation might reflect differences in psychosocial stress or lifestyle behaviors, which can influence oxidative stress [35] and, in turn, α-Klotho expression. Similarly, individuals with hypertension had significantly higher α-Klotho levels than those without hypertension. Previous studies have suggested that lower α-Klotho levels are associated with an increased risk of hypertension, identifying it as a potential risk factor for elevated blood pressure [4,36]. This discrepancy between our findings and prior research may be due to differences in study populations, measurement methods, or unmeasured confounders. The higher α-Klotho levels observed in hypertensive individuals in our study could represent a compensatory response to vascular stress or endothelial dysfunction. Additionally, potential residual confounding from factors such as medication use, kidney function, or inflammatory status may have influenced the observed association [6,37]. Moreover, α-Klotho levels varied significantly across NHANES cycles. This variation might reflect underlying population-level differences in environmental exposures, dietary patterns, or methodological factors related to sample collection and processing. Future studies should explore whether these variations are linked to temporal trends in metal exposure or other environmental stressors that may impact aging and disease susceptibility.

Interestingly, while most non-essential metals were associated with lower α-Klotho levels, we found that Ba and Mo were positively correlated with α-Klotho. Both metals are considered essential trace elements with antioxidative properties that may counteract oxidative-stress-induced α-Klotho depletion [15,38]. These metals may support the maintenance of α-Klotho levels, counteracting the oxidative damage caused by other environmental stressors. Furthermore, the potential therapeutic implications of these metals in maintaining α-Klotho levels could warrant further investigation into their possible use in anti-aging interventions. This contrasts with the negative effects observed for heavy metals, underscoring the complexity of metal interactions in biological systems. In addition to these compounding effects, it is plausible that antagonistic interactions may also occur between certain metals, either through functional interference or competition at receptor sites [39], which could modify the overall impact on α-Klotho levels. Further research is needed to determine the specific biological roles of different metals in modulating aging processes.

Moreover, our study emphasized the significance of considering metal mixtures rather than focusing solely on individual metal exposures. Using the quantile qgcomp model, we observed a clear dose–response relationship between increasing quartiles of metal mixtures and decreasing serum α-Klotho levels. This suggested that exposure to multiple metals in combination might have compounded or synergistic effects, amplifying their negative impact on aging biomarkers. This finding highlighted the necessity of studying metal mixtures, as they more accurately reflected real-world environmental exposures [40]. Previous research had predominantly focused on individual metal exposures [20,34], but our study demonstrated that the combined effect of multiple metals was likely stronger and more significant in influencing health outcomes, particularly in the context of aging.

The biological mechanisms through which metals influenced α-Klotho levels remain to be fully understood. However, oxidative stress appeared to be a central pathway. α-Klotho is a potent antioxidant and anti-inflammatory protein, and its deficiency is associated with increased ROS production and exacerbated oxidative stress [32]. Previous studies suggested that metals like Cd and Pb, known for their ability to induce oxidative damage, might reduce α-Klotho production, thereby promoting aging [20]. On the other hand, metals like Ba and Mo, which possess antioxidative properties [41,42], might mitigate oxidative damage and protected against age-related cellular dysfunction. These findings underscore the complexity of metal toxicity, as certain metals might have dual effects depending on exposure levels, the presence of other metals, and individual susceptibility.

Despite the valuable insights provided by our study, several limitations must be acknowledged. First, while urinary metals are widely used as biomarkers of exposure, they do not fully capture the total body burden of metals. Additionally, urinary metal concentrations might not reflect long-term accumulation, particularly for metals that accumulate in tissues over time [43]. Second, due to the nature of our cross-sectional study, establishing cause-and-effect relationships was not feasible. Longitudinal studies are needed to validate these associations and better understand the long-term effects of metal exposure on α-Klotho levels and aging. Furthermore, while we adjusted for several confounders, unmeasured factors, such as genetic predisposition, diet, and lifestyle, might also affect the relationship between metal exposure and α-Klotho levels. Moreover, we primarily examined the effects of individual metals and overall metal mixtures but did not explore specific interactions between chemically similar metals, such as Sb + As or Cd + Pb, which may exert unique combined effects. Future research should employ interaction models or machine learning algorithms to investigate whether certain metal pairs have synergistic or antagonistic effects on α-Klotho levels. Lastly, the potential impact of repeated freezing and thawing cycles on serum α-Klotho measurements cannot be ruled out, which might have introduced some variability in the results.

## 5. Conclusions

This study was the first to investigate the effects of twelve urinary metals on serum α-Klotho levels using the NHANES database. Our findings indicated that exposure to metals, especially in combination, was associated with decreased serum α-Klotho levels, potentially influencing aging processes. The identification of both positive and negative correlations underscored the complex biological effects of metals on aging. Further research is needed to clarify the mechanisms through which metals, individually and in mixtures, regulate α-Klotho and impact health. Longitudinal studies should explore causal relationships, while mechanistic investigations can elucidate metal-induced effects on α-Klotho regulation. Additionally, assessing the combined toxicity or protective effects of metal mixtures and the therapeutic potential of metals positively linked to α-Klotho may provide valuable insights into aging-related interventions. Despite its limitations, this study provided a foundation for future research on environmental metal exposure and its impact on aging biomarkers.

**Supplementary Materials:** The following supporting information can be downloaded at: https://www.mdpi.com/article/10.3390/toxics13040237/s1, Figure S1: Pairwise Pearson correlation matrix among ln-transformed urinary metals among study population in the NHANES 2007–2016; Table S1: Associations of single urinary metals with serum α-Klotho levels in the NHANES 2007–2016.

**Author Contributions:** Conceptualization, S.X., F.K. and H.X.; methodology, X.Z. and H.X.; validation, W.Z. and Z.J.; formal analysis, X.Z., C.D., Y.L. and M.F.; data curation, X.Z. and W.Z.; writing—original draft preparation, X.Z. and W.Z.; writing—review and editing, Z.J., M.F., F.K., S.X. and H.X.; visualization, X.Z.; supervision, H.X.; project administration, H.X.; funding acquisition, X.Z. and H.X. All authors have read and agreed to the published version of the manuscript.

**Funding:** This research was funded by the Innovation and Entrepreneurship Training Program for College Students of Zhejiang Province (S202413023126), the National Natural Science Foundation of China (82404231), and the Key Discipline of Zhejiang Province in Public Health and Preventive Medicine (First Class, Category A).

**Institutional Review Board Statement:** The NHANES was conducted following the Declaration of Helsinki and approved by the National Center for Health Statistics Institutional Review Board. NCHS IRB/ERB Protocol Number or Description: Continuation of Protocol #2005-06, Continuation of Protocol #2005-06, Protocol #2011-17, Continuation of Protocol #2011-17, and Continuation of Protocol #2011-17. Information regarding the specific approval codes and dates is available at: https://www.cdc.gov/nchs/nhanes/about/erb.html?CDC_AAref_Val=https://www.cdc.gov/nchs/nhanes/irba98.htm (accessed on 10 February 2025).

**Informed Consent Statement:** Not applicable.

**Data Availability Statement:** The raw data utilized in this study are publicly accessible through the National Health and Nutrition Examination Survey at: https://www.cdc.gov/nchs/nhanes/index.htm (accessed on 10 November 2024).

**Acknowledgments:** The authors would like to thank the NHANES project for providing the publicly available data.

**Conflicts of Interest:** The authors declare no conflicts of interest.

## References

1. Prud'homme, G.J.; Wang, Q. Anti-Inflammatory Role of the Klotho Protein and Relevance to Aging. *Cells* **2024**, *13*, 1413. [CrossRef] [PubMed]

2. Abraham, C.R.; Mullen, P.C.; Tucker-Zhou, T.; Chen, C.D.; Zeldich, E. Klotho Is a Neuroprotective and Cognition-Enhancing Protein. *Vitam. Horm.* **2016**, *101*, 215–238. [CrossRef]
3. Charrin, E.; Dabaghie, D.; Sen, I.; Unnersjö-Jess, D.; Möller-Hackbarth, K.; Burmakin, M.; Mencke, R.; Zambrano, S.; Patrakka, J.; Olauson, H. Soluble Klotho Protects against Glomerular Injury through Regulation of ER Stress Response. *Commun. Biol.* **2023**, *6*, 208. [CrossRef]
4. Prud'homme, G.J.; Kurt, M.; Wang, Q. Pathobiology of the Klotho Antiaging Protein and Therapeutic Considerations. *Front. Aging* **2022**, *3*, 931331. [CrossRef]
5. Gupta, S.; Moreno, A.J.; Wang, D.; Leon, J.; Chen, C.; Hahn, O.; Poon, Y.; Greenberg, K.; David, N.; Wyss-Coray, T.; et al. KL1 Domain of Longevity Factor Klotho Mimics the Metabolome of Cognitive Stimulation and Enhances Cognition in Young and Aging Mice. *J. Neurosci.* **2022**, *42*, 4016–4025. [CrossRef]
6. Yan, Y.; Chen, J. Association between Serum Klotho Concentration and All-Cause and Cardiovascular Mortality among American Individuals with Hypertension. *Front. Cardiovasc. Med.* **2022**, *9*, 1013747. [CrossRef]
7. Akhiyat, N.; Ozcan, I.; Gulati, R.; Prasad, A.; Tchkonia, T.; Kirkland, J.L.; Lewis, B.; Lerman, L.O.; Lerman, A. Patients With Coronary Microvascular Dysfunction Have Less Circulating α-Klotho. *J. Am. Heart Assoc.* **2024**, *13*, e031972. [CrossRef]
8. Ligumsky, H.; Merenbakh-Lamin, K.; Keren-Khadmy, N.; Wolf, I.; Rubinek, T. The Role of α-Klotho in Human Cancer: Molecular and Clinical Aspects. *Oncogene* **2022**, *41*, 4487–4497. [CrossRef]
9. Qiu, S.; Li, C.; Zhu, J.; Guo, Z. Associations between the TyG Index and the α-Klotho Protein in Middle-Aged and Older Population Relevant to Diabetes Mellitus in NHANES 2007–2016. *Lipids Health Dis.* **2024**, *23*, 188. [CrossRef]
10. Balali-Mood, M.; Naseri, K.; Tahergorabi, Z.; Khazdair, M.R.; Sadeghi, M. Toxic Mechanisms of Five Heavy Metals: Mercury, Lead, Chromium, Cadmium, and Arsenic. *Front. Pharmacol.* **2021**, *12*, 643972. [CrossRef]
11. Rehman, K.; Fatima, F.; Waheed, I.; Akash, M.S.H. Prevalence of Exposure of Heavy Metals and Their Impact on Health Consequences. *J. Cell. Biochem.* **2018**, *119*, 157–184. [CrossRef]
12. Zhong, Q.; Zhou, W.; Lin, J.; Sun, W.; Qin, Y.; Li, X.; Xu, H. Independent and Combined Associations of Blood Manganese, Cadmium and Lead Exposures with the Systemic Immune-Inflammation Index in Adults. *Toxics* **2023**, *11*, 659. [CrossRef] [PubMed]
13. Periferakis, A.; Caruntu, A.; Periferakis, A.-T.; Scheau, A.-E.; Badarau, I.A.; Caruntu, C.; Scheau, C. Availability, Toxicology and Medical Significance of Antimony. *Int. J. Environ. Res. Public Health* **2022**, *19*, 4669. [CrossRef]
14. Bolt, A.M.; Mann, K.K. Tungsten: An Emerging Toxicant, Alone or in Combination. *Curr. Environ. Health Rep.* **2016**, *3*, 405–415. [CrossRef]
15. Schwarz, G.; Belaidi, A.A. Molybdenum in Human Health and Disease. *Met. Ions Life Sci.* **2013**, *13*, 415–450. [CrossRef] [PubMed]
16. Maldonado, E.; Morales-Pison, S.; Urbina, F.; Solari, A. Aging Hallmarks and the Role of Oxidative Stress. *Antioxidants* **2023**, *12*, 651. [CrossRef] [PubMed]
17. Chen, Y.-Y.; Chen, W.-L. The Relationship between Polycyclic Aromatic Hydrocarbons Exposure and Serum Klotho among Adult Population. *BMC Geriatr.* **2022**, *22*, 198. [CrossRef]
18. Guo, X.; Wu, B.; Hu, W.; Wang, X.; Su, W.; Meng, J.; Lowe, S.; Zhao, D.; Huang, C.; Liang, M.; et al. Associations of Perchlorate, Nitrate, and Thiocyanate with Metabolic Syndrome and Its Components among US Adults: A Cross-Sectional Study from NHANES. *Sci. Total Environ.* **2023**, *879*, 163083. [CrossRef]
19. Zhu, J.; Wei, Y. Exposure to P-Dichlorobenzene and Serum α-Klotho Levels among US Participants in Their Middle and Late Adulthood. *Sci. Total Environ.* **2023**, *858*, 159768. [CrossRef]
20. Kim, D.; Lee, S.; Choi, J.-Y.; Lee, J.; Lee, H.-J.; Min, J.-Y.; Min, K.-B. Association of α-Klotho and Lead and Cadmium: A Cross-Sectional Study. *Sci. Total Environ.* **2022**, *843*, 156938. [CrossRef]
21. Jain, R.B. Serum Klotho and Its Associations with Blood and Urine Cadmium and Lead across Various Stages of Glomerular Function: Data for US Adults Aged 40–79 Years. *Environ. Sci. Pollut. Res.* **2022**, *29*, 57412–57420. [CrossRef]
22. Jiang, L.; Guo, T.; Zhong, X.; Cai, Y.; Yang, W.; Zhang, J. Serum Protein α-Klotho Mediates the Association between Lead, Mercury, and Kidney Function in Middle-Aged and Elderly Populations. *Environ. Health Prev. Med.* **2025**, *30*, 24–00296. [CrossRef] [PubMed]
23. Zhang, Y.; Li, T.; Ding, X.; Liu, L.; Xu, P.; Ma, Y.; Xing, H.; Keerman, M.; Niu, Q. Elevated Serum Copper, Zinc, Selenium, and Lowered α-Klotho Associations: Findings from NHANES 2011–2016 Dataset. *Biol. Trace Elem. Res.* **2025**, *203*, 1395–1404. [CrossRef]
24. Briefel, R.R. Assessment of the US Diet in National Nutrition Surveys: National Collaborative Efforts and NHANES. *Am. J. Clin. Nutr.* **1994**, *59*, 164S–167S. [CrossRef]
25. Ahluwalia, N.; Dwyer, J.; Terry, A.; Moshfegh, A.; Johnson, C. Update on NHANES Dietary Data: Focus on Collection, Release, Analytical Considerations, and Uses to Inform Public Policy. *Adv. Nutr.* **2016**, *7*, 121–134. [CrossRef] [PubMed]

26. Chen, Y.; Pan, Z.; Shen, J.; Wu, Y.; Fang, L.; Xu, S.; Ma, Y.; Zhao, H.; Pan, F. Associations of Exposure to Blood and Urinary Heavy Metal Mixtures with Psoriasis Risk among U.S. Adults: A Cross-Sectional Study. *Sci. Total Environ.* **2023**, *887*, 164133. [CrossRef] [PubMed]
27. Kamizono, Y.; Shiga, Y.; Suematsu, Y.; Imaizumi, S.; Tsukahara, H.; Noda, K.; Kuwano, T.; Fujimi, K.; Saku, K.; Miura, S. Impact of Cigarette Smoking Cessation on Plasma α-Klotho Levels. *Medicine* **2018**, *97*, e11947. [CrossRef] [PubMed]
28. Xu, H.; Mao, Y.; Hu, Y.; Xu, B. Association between Exposure to Polyfluoroalkyl Chemicals and Increased Fractional Exhaled Nitric Oxide in Adults. *Environ. Res.* **2021**, *198*, 110450. [CrossRef]
29. Liang, M.; Guo, X.; Ding, X.; Song, Q.; Wang, H.; Li, N.; Su, W.; Liang, Q.; Sun, Y. Combined Effects of Multiple Metals on Hearing Loss: A Bayesian Kernel Machine Regression Approach. *Ecotoxicol. Environ. Saf.* **2022**, *247*, 114279. [CrossRef]
30. Chen, R.; Yin, H.; Cole, I.S.; Shen, S.; Zhou, X.; Wang, Y.; Tang, S. Exposure, Assessment and Health Hazards of Particulate Matter in Metal Additive Manufacturing: A Review. *Chemosphere* **2020**, *259*, 127452. [CrossRef]
31. Zhu, X.; Lu, X.; Yin, T.; Zhu, Q.; Shi, S.; Cheang, I.; Yue, X.; Tang, Y.; Liao, S.; Zhou, Y.; et al. Renal Function Mediates the Association Between Klotho and Congestive Heart Failure Among Middle-Aged and Older Individuals. *Front. Cardiovasc. Med.* **2022**, *9*, 1–10. [CrossRef]
32. Jena, S.; Sarangi, P.; Das, U.K.; Lamare, A.A.; Rattan, R. Serum α-Klotho Protein Can Be an Independent Predictive Marker of Oxidative Stress (OS) and Declining Glomerular Function Rate in Chronic Kidney Disease (CKD) Patients. *Cureus* **2022**, *14*, e25759. [CrossRef] [PubMed]
33. Guan, Z.; Ma, L.; Wu, C. Association between Serum Klotho and Physical Frailty in Middle-Aged and Older Adults: Finding From the National Health and Nutrition Examination Survey. *J. Am. Med. Dir. Assoc.* **2023**, *24*, 1173–1178.e2. [CrossRef]
34. Guan, G.; Cai, J.; Zheng, S.; Xiang, Y.; Xia, S.; Zhang, Y.; Shi, J.; Wang, J. Association between Serum Manganese and Serum Klotho in a 40–80-Year-Old American Population from NHANES 2011–2016. *Front. Aging* **2023**, *4*, 1–8. [CrossRef]
35. Picard, M. Pathways to Aging: The Mitochondrion at the Intersection of Biological and Psychosocial Sciences. *J. Aging Res.* **2011**, *2011*, 814096. [CrossRef]
36. Yu, L.; Kang, L.; Ren, X.Z.; Diao, Z.L.; Liu, W.H. Circulating α-Klotho Levels in Hemodialysis Patients and Their Relationship to Atherosclerosis. *Kidney Blood Press. Res.* **2018**, *43*, 1174–1182.
37. Chung, C.-P.; Chang, Y.-C.; Ding, Y.; Lim, K.; Liu, Q.; Zhu, L.; Zhang, W.; Lu, T.-S.; Molostvov, G.; Zehnder, D.; et al. α-Klotho Expression Determines Nitric Oxide Synthesis in Response to FGF-23 in Human Aortic Endothelial Cells. *PLoS ONE* **2017**, *12*, e0176817. [CrossRef]
38. Cannas, D.; Loi, E.; Serra, M.; Firinu, D.; Valera, P.; Zavattari, P. Relevance of Essential Trace Elements in Nutrition and Drinking Water for Human Health and Autoimmune Disease Risk. *Nutrients* **2020**, *12*, 2074. [CrossRef]
39. Yu, X.; Tian, X.; Wang, Y.; Zhu, C. Metal-Metal Interaction and Metal Toxicity: A Comparison between Mammalian and D. Melanogaster. *Xenobiotica* **2021**, *51*, 842–851. [CrossRef]
40. Renaud, M.; El Morabet, H.; Reis, F.; da Silva, P.M.; Siciliano, S.D.; Sousa, J.P.; Natal-da-Luz, T. Are Structural and Functional Endpoints of Soil Communities Similarly Affected by Metal Mixtures?—A Terrestrial Model Ecosystem Approach. *Sci. Total Environ.* **2021**, *795*, 148909. [CrossRef]
41. Heesterbeek, T.J.; Rouhi-Parkouhi, M.; Church, S.J.; Lechanteur, Y.T.; Lorés-Motta, L.; Kouvatsos, N.; Clark, S.J.; Bishop, P.N.; Hoyng, C.B.; den Hollander, A.I.; et al. Association of Plasma Trace Element Levels with Neovascular Age-Related Macular Degeneration. *Exp. Eye Res.* **2020**, *201*, 108324. [CrossRef] [PubMed]
42. Adamus, J.P.; Ruszczyńska, A.; Wyczałkowska-Tomasik, A. Molybdenum's Role as an Essential Element in Enzymes Catabolizing Redox Reactions: A Review. *Biomolecules* **2024**, *14*, 869. [CrossRef] [PubMed]
43. Martinez-Morata, I.; Sobel, M.; Tellez-Plaza, M.; Navas-Acien, A.; Howe, C.G.; Sanchez, T.R. A State-of-the-Science Review on Metal Biomarkers. *Curr. Environ. Health Rep.* **2023**, *10*, 215–249. [CrossRef] [PubMed]

toxics

MDPI

*Article*

# Effects of Co-Exposure to Benzene, Toluene, and Xylene, Polymorphisms of microRNA Genes, and Their Interactions on Genetic Damage in Chinese Petrochemical Workers

**Shuangqi Li [1,†], Xiaojing Liao [2,†], Rui Ma [1,3,†], Na Deng [1], Haimei Wu [1], Zhaorui Zhang [2], Liping Chen [1], Qing Wang [1], Qilong Liao [1], Qianxi Li [2], Xinyi Ouyang [2], Yongmei Xiao [1,*,‡] and Qifei Deng [2,*,‡]**

1 Department of Occupational and Environmental Health, School of Public Health, Sun Yat-Sen University, 74 Zhongshan 2nd Road, Yuexiu District, Guangzhou 510080, China; shuangqi0717@163.com (S.L.)
2 School of Public Health, Guangzhou Medical University, Xinzao Road, Panyu District, Guangzhou 511436, China
3 Huadu Center for Disease Control and Prevention, Guangzhou 510801, China
* Correspondence: xiaoym@mail.sysu.edu.cn (Y.X.); dengqifei@126.com (Q.D.); Tel./Fax: +86-20-87332851 (Y.X.); +86-20-37103529 (Q.D.)
† These authors contributed equally to this work.
‡ These authors jointly supervised this work.

**Abstract:** Benzene, toluene, and xylene (BTX) co-exist in human environments, yet their individual and combined effects on genetic damage at low exposure levels are not fully understood. Additionally, single nucleotide polymorphisms in microRNAs (mirSNPs) might be involved in cancer etiology by affecting the related early health damage. To investigate the influence of BTX exposure, mirSNPs, and their interactions on genetic damage, we conducted a cross-sectional study in 1083 Chinese petrochemical workers, quantifying the BTX cumulative exposure levels and multiple genetic damage biomarkers. Additionally, we genotyped multiple common mirSNPs. Benzene and a BTX mixture were positive associated with the olive tail moment (OTM) and tail DNA% ($p < 0.05$). Higher levels of toluene and xylene enhanced the association of benzene with genetic damage levels. Genotypes and/or mutant allele counts of miR-4482-related rs11191980, miR-4433-related rs136547, miR-27a-related rs2594716, miR-3130-related rs725980, and miR-3928-related rs878718 might significantly influence genetic damage levels. Stronger effect estimates of benzene/BTX exposure were found in carriers of miR-196a-2-related rs11614913 heterozygotes and of wild homozygotes of miR-1269b-related rs12451747, miR-612-related rs12803915, and miR-4804-related rs266437. Our findings provide further support of the involvement of BTX co-exposure, mirSNPs, and their gene–environment interactions in determining the severity of DNA strand break in a complex manner.

**Keywords:** BTX co-exposure; microRNA; genetic polymorphisms; genetic damage; gene–environment interaction; petrochemical workers

## 1. Introduction

Benzene, toluene, and xylene (BTX), characterized by a single benzene ring, are vital petrochemical materials which are commonly used in the production of a large number of petrochemicals, ranging from various solvents to drugs. Due to their growing significance in producing everyday products, BTX have a vast and steadily growing market. According to "BTX Market Size & Share Analysis-Growth Trends & Forecasts (2024–2029)" [1], the global annual demand for BTX is nearly 108 million metric tons, with a demand growth rate of approximately 5%, and the global BTX market is estimated to register a compound annual growth rate (CAGR) of more than 3.5% by 2028. Owing to the dramatic increase in the production and usage of BTX and their related downstream products, volatile BTX that are consequently released are ubiquitously distributed in various human living and working environments. As a major player in the Asia-Pacific region's BTX market, China's growing petrochemical industry has led to rising BTX pollution levels, posing significant health risks to populations exposed to these chemicals both at work and in the environment [2].

After entering into the body, mainly through inhalation, BTX compounds can be metabolized by cytochrome P450 (CYP) and other enzymes to generate reactive metabolites to cause multiple adverse health effects, ranging from neurological impairment to cancers [3–5]. Thus, BTX are one of the focuses of great concern in view of their deleterious health effects associated with chronic or acute exposure [3–5]. Benzene has received more attention than the other BTX components, as there is conclusive evidence to support the assertion that it has strong genotoxicity and can cause cancers such as leukemia and lymphohematopoietic malignancies in chronically exposed humans, even at relatively low levels of exposure [5]. Thus, benzene has been classified as a known human carcinogen (Group 1) by the International Agency for Research on Cancer (IARC) [6,7]. Toluene and xylene, on the other hand, have been the subject of relatively limited and not fully conclusive research [3,4]. Even so, their effects on genetic damage, the most critical early biologic event for cancer development, have attracted more and more attention in recent years. Furthermore, since toluene and xylene frequently co-exist with benzene in various human environments and share similar enzyme-mediated biotransformation, their simultaneous exposure might alter benzene metabolism and then affect its toxic effects [8]. Previous research in humans and mice suggests that simultaneous exposure to high levels of benzene and toluene ($\geq$50 ppm) can impact benzene metabolism and increase benzene-related genetic damage [9]. However, different co-exposure dose ranges demonstrate disparate effects, which might be caused by the dose-dependency of benzene metabolism [9]. With more effective control actions having been implemented to reduce airborne BTX (especially benzene) levels to close to or below the occupational and community air standards, their health effects and underlying mechanisms at lower co-exposure levels have attracted significant attention [10–12]. We previously evaluated the effects of BTX co-exposure on pulmonary function [13] and declines in hematologic parameters [10] in Chinese petrochemical workers with long-term low-dose exposure. Research on genetic damages utilizing low co-exposure levels would further characterize the benzene/toluene/xylene dose–response relations and their interactions and provide more important data for risk assessment and management in relation to the public [12].

In addition to environmental hazards, genetic damage levels are also determined by individual genetic predisposition [14]. Studying genetic determinants of environmental health effects can provide a scientific basis for identifying high-risk groups within exposed populations. However, data on genetic factors conferring susceptibility or resistance to BTX-related genotoxicity is relatively limited, with most research focused on polymorphisms in metabolic enzyme genes and DNA damage repair genes [15]. Thus, exploring additional genetic factors linked to BTX-related genotoxicity is essential. MicroRNAs (miRNAs) are highly conserved endogenous noncoding RNAs that post-transcriptionally regulate gene expressions through translational inhibition or mRNA degradation [16]. MiRNA-mediated gene expression regulations are important for the cellular response to environmental stress and genetic damage, and therefore are extensively implicated in various human diseases like cancers [17]. The miRNA biogenesis process begins with pri-miRNA transcripts, which are cut to form pre-miRNAs and then mature into miRNA duplexes after cytoplasmic export. The mature miRNA duplex's 5p or 3p strands pair with argonaute proteins to create an RNA-induced silencing complex that targets mRNA for expression suppression, with targeting specificity determined by the miRNA seed sequence's complementarity to the mRNA's 'seed-match' region [16]. It has been demonstrated that any sequence alteration in miRNA genes (including pri-miRNAs, pre-miRNAs, mature miRNAs, and seed regions), especially single nucleotide polymorphisms (SNPs, i.e., mirSNPs), can alter the biogenesis, activity, or bioavailability of the corresponding miRNAs, and eventually exert significant impacts on the expression and/or functions of numerous targets [18]. Thus, mirSNPs are important genetic determinants for individual variations in the cellular response to environmental hazards, phenotypes, and disease susceptibility [19]. A large number of epidemiological studies have demonstrated that mirSNPs are associated with cancer risk [20]. Our previous study in Chinese coke oven workers elucidated that rs11614913, located in the mature sequence of miR-196a2, and its interactions with environmental factors might affect oxidative damage levels, a type of cancer-related early health damage [21]. This preliminarily suggested that mirSNPs might be involved in cancer etiology by affecting the related early health damage. However, most genetic variations known to be located within miRNA genes according to the databases for miRNA-related SNPs (i.e., miRNASNP) have yet to be tested for their links to cancer-related early health damage, especially genetic damage, in the contexts of BTX exposure.

Given that understanding the effects of low-dose BTX co-exposure, mirSNPs, and their interactions on genetic damage levels is important for the development of early prevention strategies for exposed populations, we conducted a preliminary cross-sectional study in Chinese petrochemical workers with long-term occupational exposure primarily to low-dose BTX components. We previously conducted a follow-up study in these workers to evaluate the hematological effects of low-dose BTX co-exposure [10]. In the present study, we quantified their occupational BTX exposure levels by calculating cumulative exposure (CE), measured many genetic damage indices, and genotyped multiple common mirSNPs which were screened out from the miRNASNP database in the baseline stage. We separately evaluated the individual effects of BTX components and SNPs on genetic damage levels, as well as the BTX interactions and the gene–environment interactions. The present study may further enhance our knowledge about the environmental and genetic determinants of the severity of genetic damage and provide further theoretical underpinning for the health surveillance and early screening of BTX-exposed populations.

## 2. Materials and Methods

### 2.1. Study Subjects

As described previously [10], we recruited a total of 1443 BTX-exposed workers from two large state-owned petrochemical plants located in Guangzhou and Maoming, respectively, in southern China. Participants were selected based on the following criteria: (1) workers who had been employed in workplaces where BTX were the primary occupational hazards for at least one year; (2) workers without a history of serious diseases, such as tumors, cardiopulmonary diseases, or chronic immune diseases; (3) workers who had not taken medicine or undergone X-ray examinations in the week before the survey; and (4) workers who had completed the occupational questionnaire and physical examinations and had provided some biological sample materials.

In the present study, we further excluded non-Han subjects and those without sufficient heparin-anticoagulated peripheral venous blood samples for the measurement of genetic damage biomarkers. Finally, a total of 1083 workers were selected in this study. All participants understood the purpose and significance of this study and signed written informed consent forms. They were then interviewed by trained personnel using a pre-tested occupational questionnaire and provided information including their demographic characteristics, lifestyle habits (such as smoking and alcohol consumption), personal and family history of serious diseases, and occupational experience (such as workplaces, type of work, and duration of exposure). Individuals who smoked ≥1 cigarette/day for ≥1 year were defined as smokers, and those who consumed alcohol at least once a week for ≥1 year were defined as alcohol drinkers. After the interview, we collected from each subject ~5 mL of heparin sodium-anticoagulated fasting elbow venous blood for single-cell gel electrophoresis (SCGE) and the cytokinesis-block micronucleus (CBMN) assay. We also collected ~2 mL of ethylenediaminetetraacetic acid (EDTA)-anticoagulated venous blood from each subject. However, after the detection of hematologic parameters [10] and other indicators (such as blood biochemical parameters), only 667 subjects had sufficient EDTA-anticoagulated blood samples for DNA extraction. Thus, there were only 667 subjects in the mirSNP analysis.

### 2.2. Individual BTX Exposure Assessment

To assess long-term occupational BTX exposure, we calculated BTX CE levels for all participants in the present study as mentioned in our previous study [10]. In brief, we monitored ambient BTX concentrations in the workplaces over the three years preceding the study. BTX concentrations were measured using thermal desorption and capillary gas chromatography coupled with hydrogen flame ionization detector following the protocols and quality control methods recommended by the National Institute for Occupational Safety and Health (NIOSH) method 1501. The concentrations below the limits of detection (LOD) were replaced by LOD/2. We calculated 8 h-TWA concentrations for BTX components and then calculated CE levels (mg/m$^3$ $\times$ year) by multiplying the three-year mean 8 h-TWA concentrations in workplaces by work years.

### 2.3. CBMN Cytometry Assay

We performed the CBMN cytometry assay to evaluate chromosome damage levels using the standard method described by Fenech [22] with minor modifications. We added 0.5 mL of heparin sodium-anticoagulated blood to the prepared 1640 culture medium which contained bovine serum and phytohemagglutinin, and incubated the cultures at 37 °C with a carbon dioxide concentration of 5% for 44 h. Then, we added cytochalasin B (6 μg/L) into the cell culture medium and continued to incubate for another 28 h. Cell cultures were centrifuged at 1500 rpm for 10 min in a low-temperature centrifuge at 4 °C to remove the supernatant culture medium. We treated cells with 5 mL of 0.075 mol/L KCl to lyse red blood cells, and then removed the supernatant. We repeatedly added 5 mL of fixative consisting of methanol/acetic acid (3:1) into the culture tube, centrifuged the mixture at 1200 rpm for 10 min, and then discarded the supernatant. After the last centrifugation, we retained about 150 μL of liquid and resuspended the cell pellet. The suspension was dropped onto a clean glass slide, stained with a 10% Giemsa staining solution, and finally observed under a microscope. The frequency of micronuclei (MN), nucleoplasmic bridges (NPBs), and nuclear buds (NBUDs) were evaluated according to Fenech's criteria [23].

### 2.4. SCGE Assay

We performed the SCGE assay to evaluate DNA strand breakage levels using the standard method described by Singh [24] with some modifications. We centrifugated 3 mL of heparin sodium-anticoagulated blood to separate white blood cells, and then used a lymphocyte separation solution to separate lymphocytes, which were washed with phosphate-buffered saline (PBS) to adjust the cell concentrations to 106–107 cells/mL. The slides were immersed in 75% alcohol for a whole night. After being air-dried, the frosted glass slides were washed twice with double distilled water (ddH$_2$O). When the glass slides were dry, the first layer was covered with melted typical-melting-point agarose (NMPA) and kept at 4 °C to be solidified. Then, 100 μL of the lymphocyte suspension was mixed thoroughly with 100 μL of 0.5% low-melting-point agarose (LMPA) at 37 °C, which was then used to quickly cover the first agarose layer. The slides were then immersed in a lysing solution (2.5 M NaCl, 100 mM Na2-EDTA, 10 mM Tris-base, 5 g sodium sarcosinate, pH 10, and 1% TritonX-100, 10% DMSO added fresh) at 4 °C for overnight to lyse the cells and permit DNA unfolding. Afterward, the slides were washed twice with PBS and put in a 0.3 mol/L NaOH buffer at 4 °C for 20 min to allow DNA unwinding. Electrophoresis was conducted for the next 20 min at 300 mA and 25 V using a horizontal electrophoresis tank at 4 °C. After electrophoresis, the slides were immersed in the Tris-HCL neutralization buffer for 10 min and washed gently. Then, the slides were stained by 50 μL of 2 μg/mL PI staining solution for 25 min in the dark. After staining, slides were rinsed in distilled water and observed (within 24 h) under a fluorescence microscope equipped with an emission wavelength of 590 nm and an excitation wavelength of 549 nm. We used the comet assay software project 1.2.3beta1(CASP), (https://casp-uk.net/, accessed on 1 December 2013) to analyze randomly photographed pictures and calculated the olive tail moment (OTM), the percentage of tail DNA (Tail DNA%), and tail moment of the comet after observing 50 cells in each slide. All of these steps were performed in the dark to avoid additional DNA damage [24].

*2.5. Selection and Genotyping of mirSNPs*

Based on the miRNASNP v2.0 (https://ngdc.cncb.ac.cn/databasecommons/database/id/1681, accessed on 1 December 2013) a solid public database providing miRNA-related SNPs, we performed an integrative bioinformatic analysis to screen out SNPs on the seed sequences, mature sequences, and precursor sequences for all human miRNAs in the miRBase19.0 database (http://www.mirbase.org/, accessed on 1 December 2013). We selected the most promisingly functional SNPs based on a series of criteria: (1) common SNPs with a minor allele frequency (MAF) $\geq$ 0.05 in the Chinese Han population (CHB) were chosen; (2) SNPs located on the miRNA seed sequences or mature miRNA sequences were prioritized; and (3) for SNPs located on miRNA precursor sequences, we performed an extensive literature review and only selected the SNPs who or whose corresponding miRNAs were reported to be associated with leukemia pathogenesis, toxic metabolism, genetic damage, and/or related mechanisms. Finally, a total of 61 mirSNPs were selected.

We used the iPLEX system (Sequenom) (https://www.cd-genomics.com/sequenom-massarray-iplex-gold.html, accessed on 1 December 2013) for SNP genotyping. Before the Sequenom experiments, we used Sequenom's primer design software Assay design 3.1 (Laboratory Corporation of America Holdings, Burlington, NC, USA) to design the PCR reaction and single-base extension primers for the selected mirSNPs according to their sequence information. The primers for 46 mirSNPs were successfully designed (success rate was 75.41%) (Table S1), while the primer design for the other 15 mirSNPs failed (Table S2). Then, we replaced the 15 mirSNPs (called original mirSNPs) with other SNPs (Table S2) according to the following criteria: (a) the SNPs were located in the regions from 1000 kb upstream to 1000 kb downstream of the original mirSNPs; (b) the SNPs were in high linkage disequilibrium (LD) (i.e., r2 $\geq$ 0.8) with the original mirSNPs; (c) the primers for SNPs can be successfully designed; and (d) when multiple SNPs met the above three criteria, the strongest LD SNP was prioritized.

A total of 667 subjects with sufficient EDTA-anticoagulated blood samples were included in the mirSNP analysis. Genomic DNA was extracted from 400 µL of EDTA-anticoagulated blood samples using DNA extraction kit (Tiangen, Beijing, China) according to the manufacturer's protocol. The selected 61 SNPs were genotyped using Sequenom MassArray system (Beijing Bomiao Biological Co., Ltd., Beijing, China). For each selected SNP, 10% of samples were further randomly selected for repeated genotyping, and the results were 100% concordant.

*2.6. Statistical Analyses*

BTX CE levels, OTM, tail DNA%, and tail moments were natural logarithm (ln)-transformed to obtain a normal distribution. All these ln-transformed biomarkers were standardized before statistical analyses to improve the comparability of the effect estimates. Unless otherwise stated, we adjusted for several primary variables in the statistical analyses, including age (continuous), gender (male/female), smoking status (smokers/non-smokers), pack-years of smoking (continuous), drinking status (drinkers/non-drinkers), factory location (Guangzhou/Maoming), and body mass index (BMI, calculated as weight in kilograms divided by height in meters squared) (continuous).

We divided the participants according to their general characteristics, including age ($\leq$40 vs. >40, which was the median age), gender (female vs. male), smoking status (non-smokers vs. smokers), drinking status (non-drinkers vs. drinkers), and BMI (<24 kg/m$^2$ vs. $\geq$24 kg/m$^2$). We evaluated the between-characteristic differences in genetic damage levels via multivariable covariance analysis. In addition, we used covariate-adjusted generalized linear models to evaluate the associations of individual BTX (as independent variables) with genetic damage indicators (as dependent variables) in the total population.

For benzene, which was observed to be associated with genetic damage biomarkers, we further assessed the between-characteristic differences in its association by adding an interaction term of benzene CE levels (continuous) and general characteristics (categorical) into covariate-adjusted generalized linear models.

Then, we used generalized weighted quantile sum (gWQS) models and interaction analysis to assess the impact of BTX co-exposure on genetic damage indices. The weighted quartile sum (wqs) index for the three BTX components was divided into four quartiles, and the dataset was randomly split into training (40%) and validation sets (60%), with significance testing for β based on independent data, and we used 10,000 bootstrap iterations to enhance prediction sensitivity and stability. The contribution of each BTX component was evaluated by its weight in the models. For components that were not found to be associated with genetic damage, we further evaluate their modifying effects on benzene's genetic damage effects. We divided the subjects into three exposure groups according to the tertile CE levels of toluene and xylene, respectively. Then, we assessed their modifying effects on the associations of benzene with genetic damage by adding an interaction term of benzene CE levels (continuous) and exposure groups (continuous and categorical) into covariate-adjusted generalized linear models.

All SNPs were tested for the Hardy–Weinberg equilibrium (HWE) in the total population by a goodness-of-fit Chi-square test. The between-genotype differences in genetic damage levels were examined by means of multivariate analysis of covariance. We assessed the associations of the number of variant alleles of SNPs (as the independent variable) and genetic damage levels (as the dependent variable) in the total population using covariate-adjusted multivariate linear regression models. To explore the gene–environment interactions of benzene and the BTX mixture with SNPs, we evaluated their mutual effect modification on each other's associations with genetic damage by adding their interaction terms (including those of environment factors (continuous) and genotypes (categorical) and those of the number of SNP variant alleles (continuous) and exposure groups (categorical)) into covariate-adjusted generalized linear models.

All data analyses were carried out in RStudio software (version 4.1.2) and SPSS 26.0 (SPSS, Chicago, IL, USA). Two-sided $p < 0.05$ was considered statistically significant.

## 3. Results

### 3.1. Subject Characteristics

Table 1 shows the general characteristics, BTX CE levels, and genetic damage indices in the 1083 participants in the present study. Subjects had a mean age of 40.01 years, the majority of them were male (73.68%), and most workers were non-smokers (68.79%). About half of the subjects consumed alcohol (45.43%). More than half of the subjects were working in Maoming (65. 28%) and had a relatively long occupational BTX exposure history (mean work years: 19.21). Their average BMI was 23.20 $kg/m^2$. Their median CE levels of benzene, toluene, and xylene were 0.66, 0.78, and 1.46 $mg/m^3 \times$ year, respectively. The median frequencies of MN, NPB, and NBUD were 9, 1, and 2 per 1000 cells, respectively. The median levels of OTM, tail DNA%, and tail moments were 0.35, 1.50, and 0.13, respectively. We then compared the genetic damage levels between subjects with different general characteristics, and found that females had higher MN frequency, OTM, and tail moments after adjusting for other primary covariates ($p < 0.05$) (Table S3).

Since 416 subjects in the total population were not tested for SNPs due to their limited EDTA-anticoagulated blood samples, we also compared their general characteristics, BTX CE levels, and genetic damage indices with those who were included in subsequent mirSNP analysis (Table S4). We found that there were significant differences in terms of most of the general characteristics between these two populations ($p < 0.05$). However, BTX CE levels and genetic damage levels were not significantly different after adjusting for these primary covariables (all $p > 0.05$) (Table S4).

**Table 1.** General characteristics, BTX exposure levels, and genetic damage levels in petrochemical workers (n = 1083).

| Variables | Mean ± SD, n (%), or Median (25th Percentile, 75th Percentile) |
|---|---|
| General characteristics | |
| Age (years) | 40.0 ± 7.0 |
| Gender [male/female (%male)] | 798/285 (73.68) |
| Smoking status [smoker/nonsmoker (%smoker)] | 338/745 (31.21) |
| Pack-years of smoking | 2.8 ± 6.2 |
| Drinking status [drinker/nondrinker (%drinker)] | 492/591 (45.43) |
| Factory location [Maoming/Guangzhou (%Maoming)] | 707/376 (65.28) |
| Working years (years) | 19.2 ± 7.8 |
| BMI (kg/m$^2$) | 23.2 ± 3.0 |
| BTX CE levels (mg/m$^3$ × year) | |
| Benzene | 0.66 (0.37, 1.00) |
| Toluene | 0.78 (0.50, 1.21) |
| Xylene | 1.46 (0.61, 2.50) |
| Genetic damage indices | |
| MN frequency (per 1000 cells) | 9 (6, 13) |
| NPB frequency (per 1000 cells) | 1 (0, 2) |
| NBUD frequency (per 1000 cells) | 2 (1, 3) |
| OTM | 0.35 (0.20, 1.18) |
| Tail DNA% | 1. 50 (0.86, 4.83) |
| Tail moment | 0.13 (0.05, 0.69) |

Abbreviations: BTX, benzene, toluene, and xylene; BMI, body mass index; CE, cumulative exposure; MN, micronucleus; NPB, nucleoplasmic bridge; NBUD, nuclear bud; OTM, olive tail moment; Tail DNA%, percentage of DNA in the comet tail.

### 3.2. Individual and Combined Effects of BTX Components with Genetic Damage

We first divided BTX into two groups based on the mean values and compared the levels of genetic damage between the high-exposure and low-exposure groups (Table 2). In the high-benzene and high-xylene groups, tail DNA% was significantly higher than in the low exposure groups ($p < 0.05$). We further estimated the associations of single BTX components with genetic damage indices. We found that a 1-SD increase in ln-transformed benzene CE levels was associated with a 0.048-SD increase in ln-transformed OTM (95% CI: 0.007, 0.090) and a 0.073-SD increase in ln-transformed tail DNA% (95% CI: 0.027, 0.119) in the total population (Table 2). These associations of ln-transformed benzene with genetic damage indices were more pronounced in subjects older than 40 years (all $P_{\text{interaction}} < 0.05$) (Table S5). Consistently, benzene was also significantly positively correlated with OTM and tail DNA% ($p < 0.05$) in subjects included in the mirSNP analysis (Figure S1). However, we did not find any significant associations of BTX components with tail moments and the indicators of chromosomal damage (all $p > 0.05$) (Table 2), thus we did not consider these indicators in the subsequent analyses.

The combined effects of BTX components with OTM and tail DNA% in gWQS models are shown in Figure 1. A quartile increase in the wqs index of ln-transformed BTX was associated with a 0.054 increase in OTM (95% CI: 0.005, 0.103) and a 0.075 increase in tail DNA% (95% CI: 0.020, 0.130), respectively. The main contributor with the highest weight was benzene, with its weighted percentage being 0.809 in OTM and 0.766 in tail DNA%. Although the individual effects of toluene and xylene on genetic damage levels and their contributions to BTX's combined effects were limited, we further investigated their modifying effects on the associations of benzene. As shown in Figure 2, we observed that in comparison to the low-exposure groups, the associations of benzene CE levels with OTM and tail DNA% were significantly stronger in subjects with medium toluene exposure levels and in workers with medium and higher xylene exposure levels ($P_{\text{interaction}} < 0.05$).

Interestingly, the magnitude of these associations was significantly increased with the increase in xylene exposure levels ($P_{trend} < 0.05$) (Figure 2).

**Table 2.** Associations of single BTX CE levels with genetic damage indices.

| BTX Components | MN Frequency | NPB Frequency | NBUD Frequency | OTM | Tail DNA% | Tail Moment |
|---|---|---|---|---|---|---|
| Benzene | | | | | | |
| High group [a] | 10.26 ± 5.87 | 1.39 ± 1.76 | 2.63 ± 2.87 | 1.31 ± 1.00 | 4.98 ± 3.42 | 0.91 ± 1.12 |
| Low group [a] | 9.20 ± 5.29 | 1.38 ± 1.48 | 1.85 ± 1.77 | 0.50 ± 0.76 | 2.02 ± 2.57 * | 0.29 ± 0.83 |
| $\beta_{std}$ (95% CI) [b] | −0.057 (−0.142, 0.029) | −0.032 (−0.122, 0.057) | −0.015 (−0.102, 0.073) | 0.048 (0.007, 0.090) | 0.073 (0.027, 0.119) | 0.041 (−0.001, 0.084) |
| $P_{trend}$ [b] | 0.193 | 0.480 | 0.742 | 0.022 | 0.002 | 0.057 |
| Toluene | | | | | | |
| High group [a] | 9.71 ± 5.66 | 1.38 ± 1.60 | 1.39 ± 1.66 | 0.79 ± 0.97 | 3.07 ± 3.29 | 0.52 ± 1.07 |
| Low group [a] | 9.71 ± 5.55 | 1.39 ± 1.66 | 2.31 ± 2.71 | 0.75 ± 0.89 | 2.96 ± 3.12 * | 0.47 ± 0.89 |
| $\beta_{std}$ (95% CI) [b] | 0.051 (−0.132, 0.030) | −0.053 (−0.136, 0.030) | 0.020 (−0.062, 0.102) | 0.023 (−0.019, 0.066) | 0.034 (−0.012, 0.081) | 0.014 (−0.029, 0.057) |
| $P_{trend}$ [b] | 0.219 | 0.211 | 0.634 | 0.276 | 0.150 | 0.533 |
| Xylene | | | | | | |
| High group [a] | 9.22 ± 5.68 | 1.33 ± 1.40 | 1.63 ± 1.75 | 0.42 ± 0.69 | 1.72 ± 2.25 | 0.23 ± 0.79 |
| Low group [a] | 10.06 ± 5.53 | 1.42 ± 1.76 | 2.64 ± 2.70 | 1.22 ± 1.00 | 4.68 ± 3.47 | 0.84 ± 1.09 |
| $\beta_{std}$ (95% CI) [b] | −0.072 (−0.170, 0.025) | −0.050 (−0.152, 0.051) | −0.019 (−0.118, 0.080) | −0.004 (−0.054, 0.045) | 0.001 (−0.054, 0.056) | −0.020 (−0.071, 0.031) |
| $P_{trend}$ [b] | 0.144 | 0.331 | 0.704 | 0.864 | 0.962 | 0.435 |

Abbreviations: BTX, benzene, toluene, and xylene; CE, cumulative exposure; MN, micronucleus; NPB, nucleoplasmic bridge; NBUD, nuclear bud; OTM, olive tail moment; Tail DNA%, percentage of DNA in the comet tail. [a]: The mean ± SD for each genetic damage indicator. [b]: Generalized linear models (GLM) with adjustment for age, gender, smoking status, pack-years of smoking, drinking status, factory location, and BMI. BTX CE were included as a continuous variable in the GLM. *: $p < 0.05$ for the between-group differences which were determined by multivariable covariance analysis with adjustment for age, gender, smoking status, pack-years of smoking, drinking status, factory location, and BMI.

### 3.3. Influences of SNPs on Genetic Damage Levels

The basic information for 46 mirSNPs and 15 replaced SNPs are presented in Tables S1 and S2, respectively. The genotype distributions for 11 SNPs did not conform to the Hardy–Weinberg equilibrium (all $P_{HWE} < 0.05$), and thus were excluded from the following analysis. Rs73112689 were also excluded because all the subjects were of the same genotype (CC). The other 49 SNPs were distributed as expected under the Hardy–Weinberg equilibrium (all $P_{HWE} > 0.05$) (Tables S1 and S2), and were included in the following analysis.

We first compared the levels of OTM and tail DNA% in workers carrying different genotypes, and then investigated the associations of the number of variant alleles with OTM and tail DNA% (Table S6 and Figure 3). We found that after adjusting for multiple confounding factors, the genotypes and/or the numbers of mutant alleles of rs11191980, rs1365477, rs2594716, rs725980, and rs878718 significantly influenced OTM and/or tail DNA% (Table S6 and Figure 3). Specifically, for rs11191980, when compared with carriers of wild homozygotes (TT) and heterozygotes (TC), workers with mutant homozygotes (CC) had significantly lower mean OTM (TT: −0.82; TC: −0.65; CC: −1.40; $p < 0.015$) and tail DNA% (TT: 0.58; TC: 0.73; CC: −0.07; $p = 0.004$). For rs1365477, carriers of wild homozygotes (CC) had significant higher OTM (CC: −0.77; CT: −1.05; CT + TT: −1.02; $p < 0.045$) and tail DNA% (CC: 0.63; CT: 0.31; CT + TT: 0.34; $p < 0.025$) when compared with the carriers of CT or T alleles (i.e., CT + TT), and the number of mutant T alleles was negatively associated with both OTM ($\beta = -0.185$, $P_{trend} = 0.019$) and tail DNA% ($\beta = -0.227$, $P_{trend} = 0.009$). For rs2594716, when compared with carriers of wild homozygotes (CC) and/or C allele (i.e., CT + CC), subjects with mutant homozygotes (TT) had significantly lower mean OTM (CC: −0.80; CT + CC: −0.78; TT: −0.99; $p < 0.025$) and tail DNA% (CT + CC: 0.62; TT: 0.42; $p = 0.026$), and the number of mutant T alleles was significantly negatively associated with OTM ($\beta = -0.084$, $P_{trend} = 0.029$). For rs725980, when compared with carriers of wild homozygotes (GG), workers with GC or mutant C alleles (i.e., GC + CC) had significant higher OTM (GG: −0.87; GC: −0.70; GC + CC: −0.71; $p < 0.020$) and tail DNA% (GG: 0.53; GC: 0.70; GC + CC: 0.69; $p < 0.035$). Furthermore, the number of rs725980 C alleles was positively associated with OTM ($\beta = 0.085$, $P_{trend} = 0.034$) and tail DNA% ($\beta = 0.092$, $P_{trend} = 0.038$). For rs878718, when compared with the carriers of wild homozygotes (AA), workers with an AG genotype and mutant G alleles (i.e., AG + GG) had significant higher tail DNA% (AA: 0.55; AG: 0.63; AG + GG: 0.62; $p < 0.045$). However, we did not observe any statistically significant between-genotype differences (all $p > 0.05$) or associations (all $P_{trend} > 0.05$) in the two genetic damage indicators for other SNPs (Table S6).

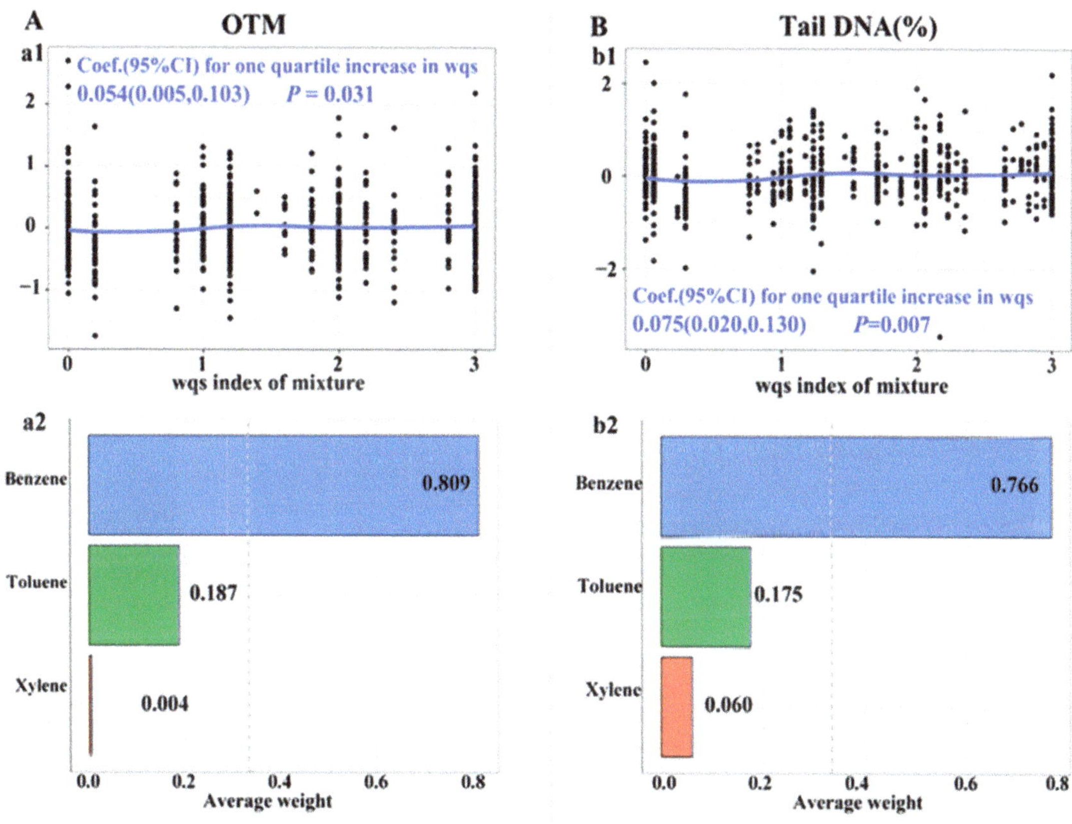


**Figure 1.** The dose–effect relationship of co-exposure to the BTX mixture (**a1**,**b1**) with (**A**) OTM and (**B**) tail DNA%, as well as the contribution of individual BTX components (**a2**,**b2**). Abbreviations: wqs, weighted quartile sum index for BTX mixture; Coef. (95% CIs), coefficients and 95% confidence intervals; OTM, olive tail moment; Tail DNA%, percentage of DNA in the comet tail. The gWQS models were adjusted by age, gender, smoking status, pack-years of smoking, drinking status, factory location, and BMI.

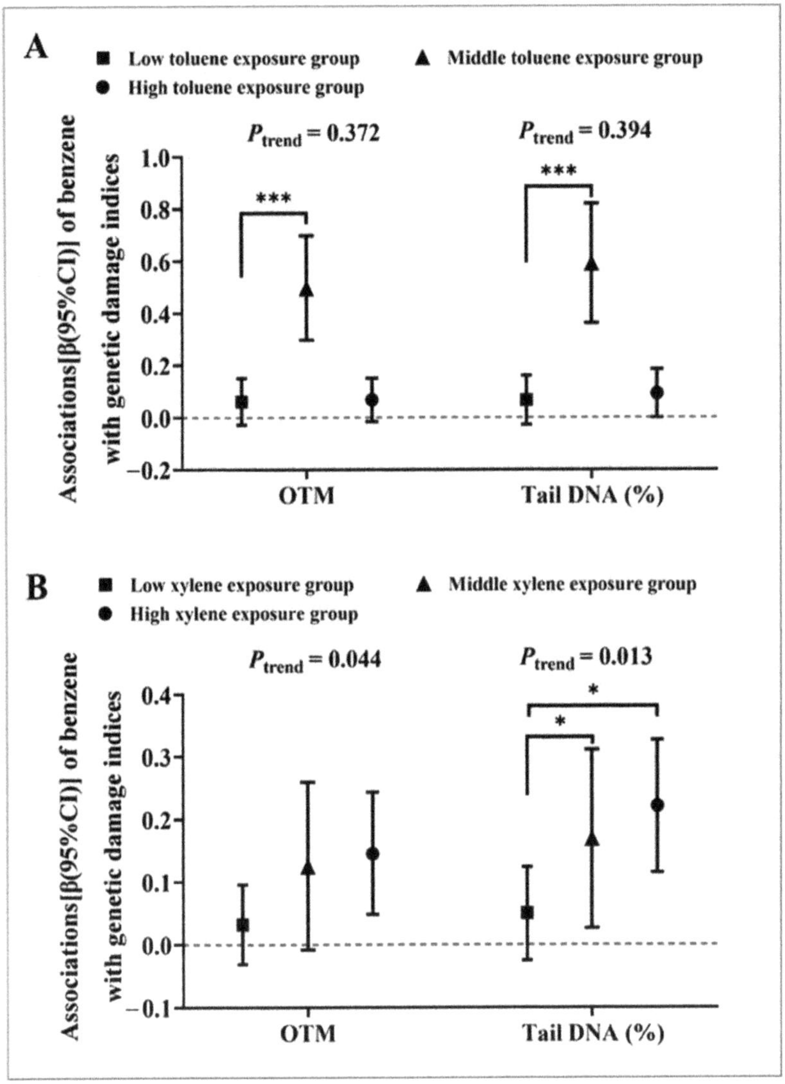


**Figure 2.** Modifying effects of (**A**) toluene and (**B**) xylene on the associations [β (95% CI)] of benzene with OTM and tail DNA%. Abbreviations: OTM, olive tail moment; Tail DNA%, percentage of DNA in the comet tail. The lines represent the associations of benzene CE levels with genetic damage indices which were analyzed by generalized linear models adjusted for age, gender, smoking status, pack-years of smoking, drinking status, factory location, and BMI. The red dashed line represents the baseline (no association, β = 0). Significant levels are annotated as *** $P_{interaction} < 0.001$ in comparison to the low-exposure group and * $P_{interaction} < 0.05$ in comparison to the low-exposure group.

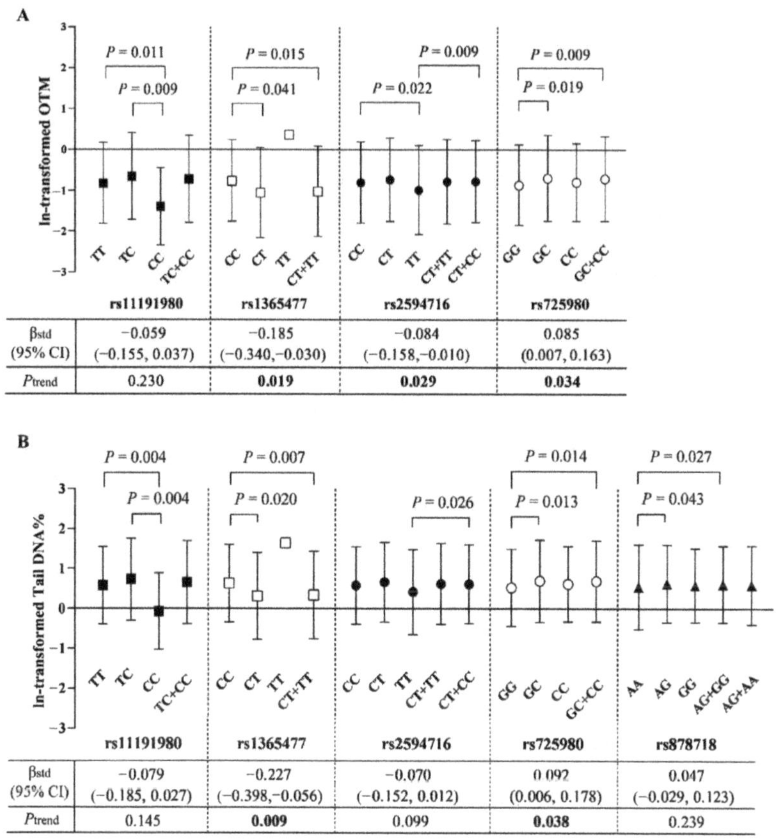


**Figure 3.** Significant effects of SNPs and/or their genotypes on (**A**) OTM and (**B**) tail DNA%. Abbreviations: OTM, olive tail moment; tail DNA%, percentage of DNA in the comet tail. The lines represent the levels of ln-transformed OTM or tail DNA% (error bars absent for condition where only two available samples). The between-genotype differences were evaluated by means of multivariate analysis of covariance, and the associations of the number of variant alleles with OTM and tail DNA% were evaluated by means of multivariate linear regression models with adjustment for age, gender, smoking status, pack-years of smoking, drinking status, factory location, and BMI. Bolded $p$-values indicate statistical significance.

### 3.4. Effect of Gene–Environment Interactions on Genetic Damage Levels

To explore the effect of gene–environment interactions of exposure to benzene and the BTX mixture with SNPs on genetic damage biomarkers, we evaluated their mutual effect modification on each other's associations with OTM and tail DNA%. We observed that the positive associations of benzene and/or the BTX mixture with OTM and tail DNA% were significantly different among different genotypes of rs11614913, rs12451747, rs12803915, and/or rs266437, with more pronounced effect estimates ($\beta_{std} \geq 0.080$, $P_{trend} < 0.05$) in carriers of rs11614913 TC heterozygotes and of wild homozygotes of rs12451747 (i.e., CC), rs12803915 (i.e., GG), and rs266437 (i.e., CC) ($P_{interaction} \leq 0.05$) (Figure 4 and Table S7). However, SNPs which were found to be associated with genetic damage levels (including rs11191980, rs1365477, rs2594716, rs725980, and rs878718) had no modifying effects on the effect estimates of exposure to benzene and the BTX mixture (Table S7).

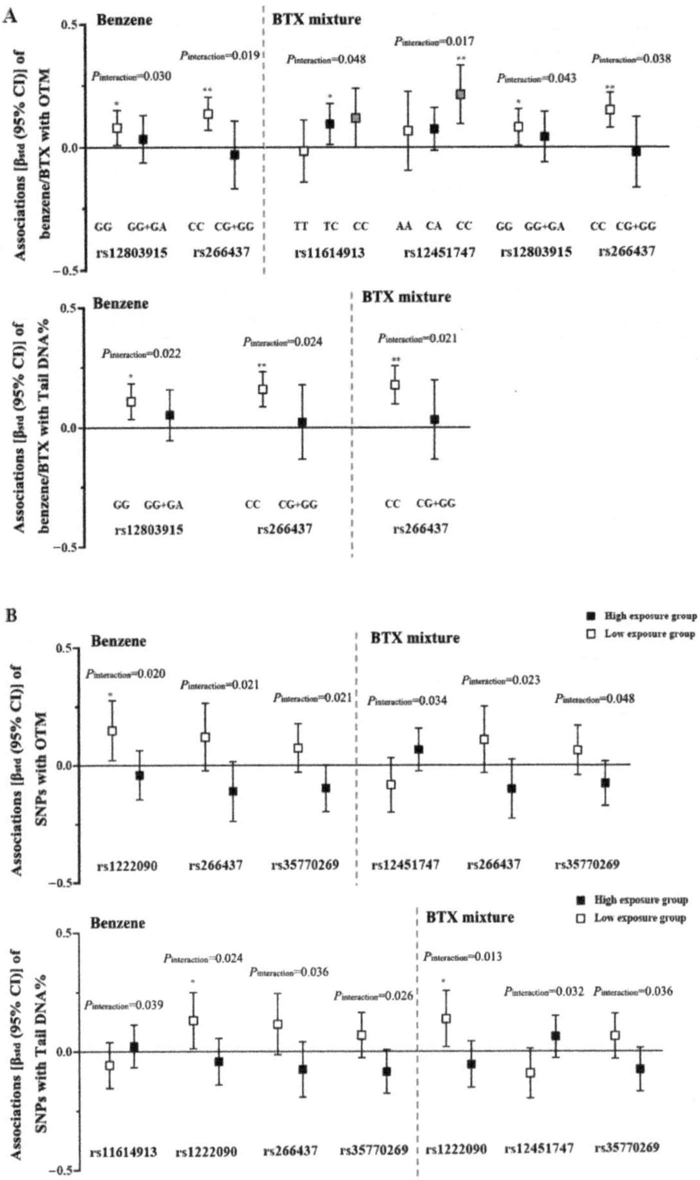


**Figure 4.** Significant modifying effects of (**A**) SNPs and (**B**) benzene/BTX exposure on each other's associations with OTM and tail DNA%, with $P_{\text{interaction}} < 0.05$. Abbreviations: OTM, olive tail moment; Tail DNA%, percentage of DNA in the comet tail. The lines represent the associations [$\beta_{\text{std}}$ (95% CI)] evaluated by multivariate linear regression models with adjustment for age, gender, smoking status, pack-years of smoking, drinking status, factory location, and BMI. * $P_{\text{trend}} < 0.05$, and ** $P_{\text{trend}} < 0.01$.

We then investigated the modifying effects of benzene and the BTX mixture on the associations of SNPs with genetic damage levels. We stratified the subjects included in mirSNP analysis into two exposure groups based on the median benzene CE levels and BTX wqs index. We observed that the effect estimates of rs11614913, rs12220909, rs12451747, rs266437, and/or rs35770269 on OTM and/or tail DNA% were significantly different in workers with different exposure levels of benzene and/or the BTX mixture ($P_{interaction} < 0.05$) (Figure 4 and Table S8). Interestingly, the positive associations of rs12220909 with OTM and/or tail DNA% were more pronounced ($\beta_{std} > 0.130$, $P_{trend} \leq 0.030$) in workers with lower exposure levels of benzene and BTX mixture, while they were weaker in workers with higher exposure levels ($\beta_{std} < -0.040$, $P_{trend} > 0.05$). However, exposure to benzene and the BTX mixture had no modifying effects on the effect estimates of SNPs that were associated with genetic damage levels (Table S8).

## 4. Discussion

To the best of our knowledge, the present study was the first exploration into the effects of BTX exposure, along with polymorphisms in miRNA genes, and the gene–environment interactions on genetic damage in Chinese petrochemical workers. We found that exposure to benzene and the BTX mixture might induce a significant increase in DNA strand break levels. Interestingly, the effects of benzene were significantly enhanced by higher exposure levels of toluene and xylene. Furthermore, these effects of benzene and BTX mixture were more pronounced in carriers of rs11614913 heterozygotes and of wild homozygotes of rs12451747, rs12803915, and rs26643. In addition, there were significant negative associations of rs1365477 and rs2594716, and positive associations of rs725980, with DNA strand break levels in the total population. Furthermore, the positive associations of rs12220909 with DNA strand break levels were more pronounced in workers with lower exposure levels to benzene and the BTX mixture. Our findings provide further support for the involvement of BTX co-exposure, mirSNPs, and their gene–environment interactions in determining the severity of genetic damage in a complex manner.

In epidemiological studies of BTX components, especially at low exposure levels, quality of exposure assessment is closely related to the ability to detect their health risks. Internal exposure biomarkers have a short biological resident time and are very susceptible to confounding factors such as smoking and diet [25], making them less suitable for long-term low-dose exposure assessment. Given that inhalation is the most common exposure route for volatile BTX components, and that the TWA concentrations of BTX components in our participants' workplaces were relatively stable and considerably lower than their commonly recommended occupational exposure limit [10], we used long-term environment monitoring data and work years to derive individual cumulative exposure estimates.

Our findings are consistent with previous studies showing that low-dose benzene exposure is associated with genetic damage. Several recent comprehensive meta-studies have indicated that compared to the control group, benzene exposure, even lower than 3.25 mg/m$^3$, might induce significant increases in various genetic damage indictors in blood lymphocytes [12,15]. A study involving workers with benzene cumulative doses ranging from 1.19 to 20.87 mg/m$^3$ $\times$ year showed a significant association between benzene exposure dose and PIG-A mutant frequencies and MN frequencies [26]. Li et al. suggested that low occupational benzene exposure ranging from 0.33 mg/m$^3$ to 1.08 mg/m$^3$ could induce a significantly increased MN frequency in lymphocytes [27]. The median CE levels and 8 h-TWA concentrations of benzene for our subjects were 0.66 mg/m$^3$ $\times$ year and 0.036 mg/m$^3$, respectively, which were lower than the levels in the above-mentioned studies. Even at such low exposure levels, the present study still observed significant associations of benzene CE levels with OTM and tail DNA%, further proving that long-term exposure to even lower benzene levels could still induce a significant increase in DNA strand break levels. We further found that the effect of a low dose of benzene on DNA strand break was more pronounced in subjects older than 40 years. Age is an important biological factor influencing susceptibility to the toxic effects of environmental hazards by affecting the efficiency of the pathways involved in metabolism and cytotoxic outcomes [28]. Gaikwad et al. [29] found that compared to younger subjects, older ones were more susceptible to oxidative DNA damage caused by exposure to genotoxic substances.

Furthermore, older workers were exposed to BTX for extended periods, which may lead to the accumulation of more genetic damage.

BTX components frequently co-exist in various human environments. Recent studies suggest caution in interpreting the health effects of mixed environmental exposures due to complex interactions among multiple components [30]. To address the complexities of mixed BTX exposures in real-world settings, we employed both single-pollutant models and combined exposure models to better understand each compound's toxicological role. We adopted both gWQS models and interaction analysis in the present study to explore the combined effects of three BTX components on genetic damage indices. Although the individual effects of toluene and xylene were not significant and their contributions to the combined BTX effects were limited, interaction analysis revealed that benzene's genotoxicity was more pronounced in individuals with moderate to high toluene and xylene exposure levels and was significantly increased with higher xylene exposure. Simultaneous exposure to BTX compounds may alter the metabolism mechanisms and further influence the toxicity of each component [8]. Earlier studies addressing co-exposure to benzene and toluene at high concentrations demonstrated a reduction in benzene-induced genotoxicity, which may be related to the dose-dependent competitive inhibition of metabolism [31]. Conversely, another study indicated that at lower exposure levels (benzene at 50 ppm and toluene at 100 ppm), the induction of CYP2E1 by toluene could lead to the increased metabolism of benzene into its genotoxic metabolite hydroquinone, potentially causing greater genetic damage [9]. In the context of the frequent low-dose co-existence of BTX compounds in human environments, our findings, along with those of previous studies, suggest that the genetic damage induced by benzene at low doses may be influenced by concurrent exposure to toluene and xylene. However, it is important to note that these interactions at low doses may involve distinct metabolic pathways compared to those at higher doses. Therefore, our study highlights the need for comprehensive management strategies that consider not only the levels of individual compounds like benzene but also the potential interactions at low doses of toluene and xylene.

In addition to the influence of BTX components, individually and in various combinations, on genetic damage, we also evaluated the involvement of genetic polymorphisms on miRNA genes. We observed the significant effects of the genotypes and/or the numbers of mutant alleles of rs11191980, rs1365477, rs2594716, rs725980, and rs878718 on DNA strand break levels. Rs11191980 is in high linkage disequilibrium with rs45596840 situated within the seed sequence of miR-4482. Mumtaz et al. found that the expression of mir-4482 was decreased in prostate cancer tissues when compared with the adjacent normal tissues and could inhibit the progression of prostate cancer cells by suppressing the expression of ETS-related gene [32]. Rs7259810 is in high linkage disequilibrium with rs2241347 in the mature miR-3130 sequence. Mir-3130 has been found to inhibit the expression of NDUFS1 to promote the invasiveness of lung adenocarcinoma in vivo and in vitro [33] and could also regulate the miR-3130-3p/NFYA/SATB1 axis to promote the occurrence and development of endometrial cancer cells [34]. Rs1365477 is in high linkage disequilibrium with rs12473206 located in the mature region of miR-4433. Wu et al. identified that mir-4433 could induce apoptosis through targeting Bcr-Abl genes and suppress the growth of leukemia cells [35]. Rs2594716 is closely linked to rs895819, which is positioned within the loop of the pre-miR-27a sequence. Previous studies have indicated a significant association between rs895819 and tumor susceptibility, with carriers of the mutant allele demonstrating a notably reduced risk of diffuse large B-cell lymphoma compared with individuals possessing the wild-type genotype [36]. Our findings also suggest that the population carrying the mutant allele at this specific locus exhibited lower genetic damage levels, suggesting that the mutant allele of rs2594716 (or rs895819) might exhibit a protective effect against cancer risk by reducing genetic damage. Rs878718 is tightly linked to rs5997893 located in the pre-miR-3928 sequence. Mir-3928 has been identified as a tumor-suppressive miRNA in both in vivo and in vitro, and is capable of downregulating oncogenes and upregulating p53, thereby inhibiting the progression of glioblastoma [37].

Collectively, our findings suggest potential roles for these SNPs in genetic damage, which could lead to differential cancer susceptibility. However, the mechanisms by which these SNPs influence miRNA biogenesis, activity, and/or bioavailability remain to be elucidated by further investigations.

In order to explore the gene–environment interactions, we further assessed the mutual modifying influence of SNPs and environment factors (including benzene and the BTX mixture) on each other's associations with genetic damage. The effects of benzene and the BTX mixture were found to be more pronounced among carriers of rs11614913 heterozygotes and wild-type homozygotes of rs12451747, rs12803915, and rs266437. Rs11614913 is a well-studied SNP located within the mature miRNA-196a2 sequence. Its mutant allele has been implicated in elevating the miRNA expression levels and enhancing the regulatory capacity of multiple target genes [38], eventually increasing the risk of cancers like acute lymphoblastic leukemia (ALL) in Chinese children [39]. The present study also found that individuals with the rs11614913 mutant allele might experience more severe DNA strand breaks as a result of exposure to benzene and the BTX mixture. However, our previous research observed that the rs11614913 mutant allele might attenuate the effects of lead, naphthalene, and benzo[a]pyrene on increased oxidative DNA damage among coke oven workers [21]. These seemingly contradictory results might be explained by the different balance of the functions of miR-196a2-targeting genes (including oncogenes or tumor suppression genes) in specific exposure conditions [40]. However, the regulation mechanisms of rs11614913 warrant further investigation. Rs12803915 is located in the mir-612 precursor coding region and has been shown to be significantly associated with ALL risk in a case–control study, with the mutant allele being protective [41]. It has been shown that rs12803915 could significantly influence the expression levels of mature miR-612 [42], which may further regulate the downstream targets and thereby affect the susceptibility to toxic effects of environmental hazards like benzene. Rs12451747 is located in the mature sequence of miR-1296b, which has been documented to be highly expressed in various cancers [43] and may be involved in the activation of the PI3K/AKT signaling pathway [44]. Rs266437 is linked to rs266435 in the hsa-mir-4804 precursor coding region, yet reports on the links of these loci and the associated miRNA with cancers are scarce. Overall, the present study might extend these findings by revealing the interactive effects of these SNPs with benzene/BTX exposure and suggesting that individuals with specific alleles at these loci may experience increased genetic damage subsequent to benzene/BTX exposure, potentially heightening the cancer risk. Furthermore, our study also observed a significant association of rs12220909 with higher genetic damage levels in the low-exposure group of benzene and/or the BTX mixture, which became weaker and insignificant in the high-exposure group. Rs12220909, situated in the seed sequence of mir-4293, has been implicated in tumorigenesis, with its heterozygotes often being regarded as a protective factor against cancers [45]. Our findings further suggest that the protective capacity of rs12220909 against tumorigenesis may be dose-dependent: the mutant allele might confer a protective advantage at higher exposures to benzene and BTX mixture, and may not provide the same levels of protection at lower exposures, potentially leading to increased genetic damage susceptibility.

The present study has several strengths. Firstly, we calculated individual BTX CE levels based on long-term average TWA concentrations and working years, thus providing a representation of environmental exposure profiles of petrochemical workers subjected to low BTX concentrations. Additionally, we performed an integrative bioinformatics analysis based on a solid public database and an extensive literature review to screen out multiple functional miRNA-related SNPs, which might help to systematically evaluate the effects of miRNA-related SNPs. However, there also existed some limitations in our study. First, our study is an exploratory cross-sectional study, and thus the findings could not demonstrate the causal associations. Additionally, although we selected petrochemical workers from workshops where BTX were the primary occupational hazards, they may still be exposed to other genotoxic hazards in their working and living environment, causing challenges in describing the genotoxicity of BTX in environments exposed to complex contaminants. Although we adjusted for general characteristics and factory location in our statistical analysis to minimize their confounding effects, further studies are needed to evaluate their influences on our results. Furthermore, the present study was limited to an ethnic Chinese occupational population, and it is uncertain whether our findings can be extrapolated to other populations. Additionally, in the subsequent studies, some research subjects were not included in the mir-SNP analysis due to limited biological samples, necessitating further examination of the representativeness of the results.

## 5. Conclusions

Conclusively, our study reveals that low-dose benzene exposure, particularly within BTX mixtures, significantly contributes to DNA strand breaks. The genotoxic effects of benzene are amplified by higher levels of toluene and xylene co-exposure. Furthermore, individuals harboring rs11614913 heterozygotes and wild homozygotes of rs12451747, rs12803915, and rs266437 appeared to be more vulnerable to the genotoxic effects of benzene and the BTX mixture. Moreover, the genotypes and/or the number of mutant alleles of rs11191980, rs1365477, rs2594716, rs725980, and rs878718 might influence DNA strand break levels. We also observed more pronounced positive associations of rs12220909 with DNA strand break levels only in workers with lower exposure levels of benzene and BTX mixture. These findings highlight the complex interactions between benzene exposure, mirSNPs, and genetic damage, emphasizing the need for further research to inform targeted interventions and refine risk assessment strategies for BTX-exposed workers. The present study contributes some novel insights into the individual and interactive effects of BTX and miRNA-related SNP on genetic damage, further shedding light on the risk assessment of genetic damage in BTX-exposed occupational populations.

**Supplementary Materials:** The following supporting information can be downloaded at: https://www.mdpi.com/article/10.3390/toxics12110821/s1, Table S1: Basic information of the mirSNPs included in the present study. Table S2: Basic information on the replaced SNPs for mirSNPs which failed in primer design in the present study. Table S3: Comparisons of genetic damage levels in subjects with different general characteristics. Table S4: General characteristics, BTX exposure levels, and genetic damage levels in workers that were or were not included in mirSNP study. Table S5: Associations of benzene CE levels with OTM and Tail DNA% in workers with different general characteristics. Table S6: Effects of SNPs and their genotypes on the levels of OTM and Tail DNA%. Table S7: Modifying effects of SNPs on the associations [βstd (95% CI)] of benzene and BTX mixture with OTM and Tail DNA%. Table S8: Modifying effects of benzene exposure on the associations [βstd (95% CI)] of SNPs (continuous) with OTM and Tail DNA%. Figure S1: Associations of BTX CE levels with OTM and Tail DNA% in subjects included in mirSNP analysis (n = 667).

**Author Contributions:** Conceptualization, Y.X. and Q.D.; Data curation, X.L., N.D. and H.W.; Formal analysis, S.L., X.L., R.M. and N.D.; Funding acquisition, Y.X. and Q.D.; Investigation, N.D., L.C. and Q.W.; Methodology, Q.L. (Qilong Liao); Project administration, Y.X. and Q.D.; Resources, Y.X.; Supervision, Y.X. and Q.D.; Validation, R.M., H.W. and Z.Z.; Visualization, Q.L. (Qianxi Li) and X.O.; Writing—original draft, S.L., X.L. and R.M.; Writing—review and editing, S.L. and Q.D. All authors have read and agreed to the published version of the manuscript.

**Funding:** The study was funded by the National Natural Scientific Foundation of China (Grant numbers: 81973006, 81973076, and 81402658), Guangdong Basic and Applied Basic Research Foundation (Grant numbers: 2020A1515010753; 2024A1515012072; 2024A1515030225), Science and Technology Planning Project of Guangzhou (Grant number: 202002030281), and the Young Teachers Training Program of Sun Yat-sen University (Grant number: 18ykpy14).

**Institutional Review Board Statement:** The study was conducted in accordance with the Declaration of Helsinki and was approved by the Ethical Review Committee of School of Public Health, Sun Yat-sen University (ethical approval code: [2011]-37). Written informed consent was obtained from all participants prior to their enrollment in this study.

**Informed Consent Statement:** Written informed consent was obtained from the participants for the publication of this study.

**Data Availability Statement:** The data presented in this study are available upon request from the corresponding author.

**Acknowledgments:** We thank all study participants, research staff, and students who participated in this work.

**Conflicts of Interest:** The authors declare no conflicts of interest.

## References

1. *Mordor Intelligence: BTX Market Size & Share Analysis-Growth Trends & Forecasts (2024–2029)*; Mordor Intelligence: Gachibowli Hyderabad, India, 2024; Available online: https://www.mordorintelligence.com/industry-reports/benzene-toluene-xylene-btx-market (accessed on 1 May 2024).
2. Ji, Y.; Gao, F.; Wu, Z.; Li, L.; Li, D.; Zhang, H.; Zhang, Y.; Gao, J.; Bai, Y.; Li, H. A review of atmospheric benzene homologues in China: Characterization, health risk assessment, source identification and countermeasures. *J. Environ. Sci.* **2020**, *95*, 225–239. [CrossRef] [PubMed]
3. *ATSDR: Toxicological Profile for Toluene*; U.S. Department of Health and Human Services, Public Health Service: Atlanta, GA, USA, 2017.
4. *ATSDR: Toxicological Profile for Xylenes*; U.S. Department of Health and Human Services, Public Health Service: Atlanta, GA, USA, 2007.
5. *ATSDR: Toxicological Profile for Benzene*; U.S. Department of Health and Human Services, Public Health Service: Atlanta, GA, USA, 2007.
6. Exposure to Benzene: A Major Public Health Concern. Available online: https://www.who.int/publications/i/item/WHO-CED-PHE-EPE-19.4.2 (accessed on 1 May 2024).
7. *IARC Monographs: On the Evaluation of Carcinogenic Risks to Humans*; IARC: Lyon, France, 2004; Volume 120.
8. *ATSDR: Interaction Profile for Benzene, Toluene, Ethylbenzene, and Xylenes (BTEX)*; U.S. Department of Health and Human Services, Public Health Service: Atlanta, GA, USA, 2004.
9. Bird, M.G.; Wetmore, B.A.; Letinski, D.J.; Nicolich, M.; Chen, M.; Schnatter, A.R.; Whitman, F.T. Influence of toluene co-exposure on the metabolism and genotoxicity of benzene in mice using continuous and intermittent exposures. *Chem. Biol. Interact.* **2010**, *184*, 233–239. [CrossRef] [PubMed]
10. Zhang, Z.; Liu, X.; Guo, C.; Zhang, X.; Zhang, Y.; Deng, N.; Lai, G.; Yang, A.; Huang, Y.; Dang, S.; et al. Hematological Effects and Benchmark Doses of Long-Term Co-Exposure to Benzene, Toluene, and Xylenes in a Follow-Up Study on Petrochemical Workers. *Toxics* **2022**, *10*, 502. [CrossRef]
11. Niu, Z.; Wen, X.; Wang, M.; Tian, L.; Mu, L. Personal exposure to benzene, toluene, ethylbenzene, and xylenes (BTEXs) mixture and telomere length: A cross-sectional study of the general US adult population. *Environ. Res.* **2022**, *209*, 112810. [CrossRef] [PubMed]
12. Zhou, Y.; Wang, K.; Wang, B.; Pu, Y.; Zhang, J. Occupational benzene exposure and the risk of genetic damage: A systematic review and meta-analysis. *BMC Public Health* **2020**, *20*, 1113. [CrossRef]
13. Liao, Q.; Du, R.; Ma, R.; Liu, X.; Zhang, Y.; Zhang, Z.; Ji, P.; Xiao, M.; Cui, Y.; Xing, X.; et al. Association between exposure to a mixture of benzene, toluene, ethylbenzene, xylene, and styrene (BTEXS) and small airways function: A cross-sectional study. *Environ. Res.* **2022**, *212*, 113488. [CrossRef]
14. León-Mejía, G.; Quintana-Sosa, M.; de Moya Hernandez, Y.; Rodríguez, I.L.; Trindade, C.; Romero, M.A.; Luna-Carrascal, J.; Ortiz, L.O.; Acosta-Hoyos, A.; Ruiz-Benitez, M.; et al. DNA repair and metabolic gene polymorphisms affect genetic damage due to diesel engine exhaust exposure. *Environ. Sci. Pollut. Res. Int.* **2020**, *27*, 20516–20526. [CrossRef]
15. Wang, T.; Cao, Y.; Xia, Z.; Christiani, D.C.; Au, W.W. Review on novel toxicological effects and personalized health hazard in workers exposed to low doses of benzene. *Arch. Toxicol.* **2024**, *98*, 365–374. [CrossRef]
16. Lujambio, A.; Lowe, S.W. The microcosmos of cancer. *Nature* **2012**, *482*, 347–355. [CrossRef]
17. Ali Syeda, Z.; Langden, S.S.S.; Munkhzul, C.; Lee, M.; Song, S.J. Regulatory Mechanism of MicroRNA Expression in Cancer. *Int. J. Mol. Sci.* **2020**, *21*, 1723. [CrossRef]
18. Króliczewski, J.; Sobolewska, A.; Lejnowski, D.; Collawn, J.F.; Bartoszewski, R. microRNA single polynucleotide polymorphism influences on microRNA biogenesis and mRNA target specificity. *Gene* **2018**, *640*, 66–72. [CrossRef] [PubMed]
19. Gong, J.; Tong, Y.; Zhang, H.M.; Wang, K.; Hu, T.; Shan, G.; Sun, J.; Guo, A.Y. Genome-wide identification of SNPs in microRNA genes and the SNP effects on microRNA target binding and biogenesis. *Hum. Mutat.* **2012**, *33*, 254–263. [CrossRef] [PubMed]
20. Pipan, V.; Zorc, M.; Kunej, T. MicroRNA Polymorphisms in Cancer: A Literature Analysis. *Cancers* **2015**, *7*, 1806–1814. [CrossRef]
21. Xie, Y.; Lin, T.; Yang, M.; Zhang, Z.; Deng, N.; Tang, M.; Xiao, Y.; Guo, H.; Deng, Q. Co-exposure to polycyclic aromatic hydrocarbons and metals, four common polymorphisms in microRNA genes, and their gene-environment interactions: Influences on oxidative damage levels in Chinese coke oven workers. *Environ. Int.* **2019**, *132*, 105055. [CrossRef] [PubMed]
22. Fenech, M. Cytokinesis-block micronucleus cytome assay. *Nat. Protoc.* **2007**, *2*, 1084–1104. [CrossRef]

23. Fenech, M. The cytokinesis-block micronucleus technique: A detailed description of the method and its application to genotoxicity studies in human populations. *Mutat. Res.* **1993**, *285*, 35–44. [CrossRef]
24. Singh, N.P.; McCoy, M.T.; Tice, R.R.; Schneider, E.L. A simple technique for quantitation of low levels of DNA damage in individual cells. *Exp. Cell Res.* **1988**, *175*, 184–191. [CrossRef]
25. Carrieri, M.; Bonfiglio, E.; Scapellato, M.L.; Maccà, I.; Tranfo, G.; Faranda, P.; Paci, E.; Bartolucci, G.B. Comparison of exposure assessment methods in occupational exposure to benzene in gasoline filling-station attendants. *Toxicol. Lett.* **2006**, *162*, 146–152 [CrossRef]
26. Cao, Y.; Wang, T.; Xi, J.; Tian, W.; Liu, W.; Sun, Y.; Liu, W.; You, X.; Li, A.; Zhang, G.; et al. Benchmark dose estimation for benzene-exposed workers in China: Based on quantitative and multi-endpoint genotoxicity assessments. *Environ. Pollut.* **2023**, *330*, 121765. [CrossRef]
27. Li, A.; Sun, Y.; Wang, T.; Wang, K.; Wang, T.; Liu, W.; Li, K.; Au, W.W.; Wang, Z.; Xia, Z.L. Effects of Micronucleus Frequencies and Mitochondrial DNA Copy Numbers among Benzene-Exposed Workers in China. *Environ. Mol. Mutagen.* **2020**, *61*, 355–360. [CrossRef]
28. Minatel, B.C.; Sage, A.P.; Anderson, C.; Hubaux, R.; Marshall, E.A.; Lam, W.L.; Martinez, V.D. Environmental arsenic exposure: From genetic susceptibility to pathogenesis. *Environ. Int.* **2018**, *112*, 183–197. [CrossRef] [PubMed]
29. Gaikwad, A.S.; Mahmood, R.; Ravichandran, B.; Kondhalkar, S. Evaluation of telomere length and genotoxicity among asphalt associated workers. *Mutat. Res. Genet. Toxicol. Environ. Mutagen.* **2020**, *858*, 503255. [CrossRef] [PubMed]
30. Yang, T.; Wang, J.; Huang, J.; Kelly, F.J.; Li, G. Long-term Exposure to Multiple Ambient Air Pollutants and Association with Incident Depression and Anxiety. *JAMA Psychiatry* **2023**, *80*, 305–313. [CrossRef] [PubMed]
31. Inoue, O.; Seiji, K.; Watanabe, T.; Kasahara, M.; Nakatsuka, H.; Yin, S.N.; Li, G.L.; Cai, S.X.; Jin, C.; Ikeda, M. Mutual metabolic suppression between benzene and toluene in man. *Int. Arch. Occup. Environ. Health* **1988**, *60*, 15–20. [CrossRef] [PubMed]
32. Mumtaz, S.; Usman Rashid, M.; Khan, R.U.; Malkani, N. miR-4482 and miR-3912 aim for 3′UTR of ERG mRNA in prostate cancer. *PLoS ONE* **2023**, *18*, e0286996. [CrossRef]
33. Zhan, J.; Sun, S.; Chen, Y.; Xu, C.; Chen, Q.; Li, M.; Pei, Y.; Li, Q. MiR-3130-5p is an intermediate modulator of 2q33 and influences the invasiveness of lung adenocarcinoma by targeting NDUFS1. *Cancer Med.* **2021**, *10*, 3700–3714. [CrossRef]
34. Pan, X.; Li, D.; Huo, J.; Kong, F.; Yang, H.; Ma, X. LINC01016 promotes the malignant phenotype of endometrial cancer cells by regulating the miR-302a-3p/miR-3130-3p/NFYA/SATB1 axis. *Cell Death Dis.* **2018**, *9*, 303. [CrossRef]
35. Wu, H.; Yin, J.; Ai, Z.; Li, G.; Li, Y.; Chen, L. Overexpression of miR-4433 by suberoylanilide hydroxamic acid suppresses growth of CML cells and induces apoptosis through targeting Bcr-Abl. *J. Cancer* **2019**, *10*, 5671–5680. [CrossRef]
36. Tang, W.; Xu, H.; Ma, D.; Ma, R.; Wu, J.; Yu, X.; Feng, J.; Liu, Q. Pre-miR-27a rs895819 polymorphism and risk of diffuse large B-cell lymphoma. *J. Clin. Lab. Anal.* **2020**, *34*, e23088. [CrossRef]
37. Mulcahy, E.Q.X.; Zhang, Y.; Colón, R.R.; Cain, S.R.; Gibert, M.K.; Dube, C.J.J.; Hafner, M.; Abounader, R. MicroRNA 3928 Suppresses Glioblastoma through Downregulation of Several Oncogenes and Upregulation of p53. *Int. J. Mol. Sci.* **2022**, *23*, 3930. [CrossRef]
38. Hoffman, A.E.; Zheng, T.; Yi, C.; Leaderer, D.; Weidhaas, J.; Slack, F.; Zhang, Y.; Paranjape, T.; Zhu, Y. microRNA miR-196a-2 and breast cancer: A genetic and epigenetic association study and functional analysis. *Cancer Res.* **2009**, *69*, 5970–5977. [CrossRef] [PubMed]
39. Tong, N.; Xu, B.; Shi, D.; Du, M.; Li, X.; Sheng, X.; Wang, M.; Chu, H.; Fang, Y.; Li, J.; et al. Hsa-miR-196a2 polymorphism increases the risk of acute lymphoblastic leukemia in Chinese children. *Mutat. Res.* **2014**, *759*, 16–21. [CrossRef] [PubMed]
40. Chen, C.; Zhang, Y.; Zhang, L.; Weakley, S.M.; Yao, Q. MicroRNA-196: Critical roles and clinical applications in development and cancer. *J. Cell. Mol. Med.* **2011**, *15*, 14–23. [CrossRef]
41. Gutierrez-Camino, A.; Lopez-Lopez, E.; Martin-Guerrero, I.; Piñan, M.A.; Garcia-Miguel, P.; Sanchez-Toledo, J.; Carbone Bañeres, A.; Uriz, J.; Navajas, A.; Garcia-Orad, A. Noncoding RNA-related polymorphisms in pediatric acute lymphoblastic leukemia susceptibility. *Pediatr. Res.* **2014**, *75*, 767–773. [CrossRef] [PubMed]
42. Kim, H.K.; Prokunina-Olsson, L.; Chanock, S.J. Common genetic variants in miR-1206 (8q24.2) and miR-612 (11q13.3) affect biogenesis of mature miRNA forms. *PLoS ONE* **2012**, *7*, e47454. [CrossRef]
43. Xie, Z.; Zhong, C.; Duan, S. miR-1269a and miR-1269b: Emerging Carcinogenic Genes of the miR-1269 Family. *Front. Cell Dev. Biol.* **2022**, *10*, 809132. [CrossRef] [PubMed]
44. Chen, L.; Liu, D.; Yi, X.; Qi, L.; Tian, X.; Sun, B.; Dong, Q.; Han, Z.; Li, Q.; Song, T.; et al. The novel miR-1269b-regulated protein SVEP1 induces hepatocellular carcinoma proliferation and metastasis likely through the PI3K/Akt pathway. *Cell Death Dis.* **2020**, *11*, 320. [CrossRef]
45. Ji, D.; An, M.; Fang, Q. Whether miR-4293 rs12220909 variant affects cancer susceptibility: Evidence from 11255 subjects. *Artif. Cells Nanomed. Biotechnol.* **2020**, *48*, 933–938. [CrossRef]

*toxics*

MDPI

*Article*

# Circ_0000284 Is Involved in Arsenite-Induced Hepatic Insulin Resistance Through Blocking the Plasma Membrane Translocation of GLUT4 in Hepatocytes via IGF2BP2/PPAR-γ

**Shiqing Xu, Zhida Hu, Yujie Wang, Qiyao Zhang, Zhi Wang, Teng Ma, Suhua Wang, Xiaohui Wang * and Li Wang ***

School of Public Health, Baotou Medical College, Inner Mongolia University of Science & Technology, Baotou 014040, China; 2022200097@stu.btmc.edu.cn (S.X.); 2021400116@stu.btmc.edu.cn (Z.H.); 2021400065@stu.btmc.edu.cn (Y.W.); 2020400068@stu.btmc.edu.cn (Q.Z.); 2022200104@stu.btmc.edu.cn (Z.W.); 102018924@btmc.edu.cn (T.M.); bt_wangsuhua@163.com (S.W.)

* Correspondence: 102018909@btmc.edu.cn (X.W.); 101995002@btmc.edu.cn (L.W.)

**Abstract:** Arsenic exposure can induce liver insulin resistance (IR) and diabetes (DM), but the underlying mechanisms are not yet clear. Circular RNAs (circRNAs) are involved in the regulation of the onset of diabetes, especially in the progression of IR. This study aimed to investigate the role of circRNAs in arsenic-induced hepatic IR and its underlying mechanism. Male C57BL/6J mice were given drinking water containing sodium arsenite (0, 0.5, 5, or 50 ppm) for 12 months. The results show that sodium arsenite increased circ_0000284 expression, decreased insulin-like growth factor 2 mRNA binding protein 2 (IGF2BP2) and peroxisome proliferator-activated receptor-γ (PPAR-γ), and inhibited cell membrane protein levels of insulin-responsive glucose transporter protein 4 (GLUT4) in the mouse livers, indicating that arsenic exposure causes liver damage and disruptions to glucose metabolism. Furthermore, sodium arsenite reduced glucose consumption and glycogen levels, increased the expression of circ_0000284, reduced the protein levels of IGF2BP2 and PPAR-γ, and inhibited GLUT4 protein levels in the cell membranes of insulin-treated HepG2 cells. However, a circ_0000284 inhibitor reversed arsenic exposure induced reductions in IGF2BP2, PPAR-γ, and GLUT4 levels in the plasma membrane. These results indicate that circ_0000284 is involved in arsenite-induced hepatic insulin resistance through blocking the plasma membrane translocation of GLUT4 in hepatocytes via IGF2BP2/PPAR-γ. This study provides a scientific basis for finding early biomarkers for the control of arsenic exposure and type 2 diabetes mellitus (T2DM), and discovering new prevention and control measures.

**Keywords:** arsenic exposure; diabetes mellitus; insulin resistance; circ_0000284; hepatotoxicity

## 1. Introduction

Diabetes mellitus (DM) can be influenced by genetic or environmental factors and is often characterised by hyperglycaemia and insulin abnormalities. The increasing prevalence of DM, particularly type 2 diabetes mellitus (T2DM), has put enormous pressure on healthcare resources, leading to a significant global public health problem [1,2]. Insulin resistance (IR) is the main aetiology and pathogenesis of T2DM. IR occurs due to the reduced sensitivity of the liver, fat, and other tissues to insulin. Notably, the liver is crucial for the maintenance of normal glucose homeostasis [3].

Arsenic is a toxic element found extensively in the environment, with an average concentration of about 5 mg/kg [4]. Although the World Health Organization (WHO) recommends a maximum arsenic concentration of 10 μg/L in drinking water, the recommendations for the maximum arsenic concentration in drinking water in over 40 countries exceed 10 μg/L [5]. About 200 million individuals globally are potentially exposed to elevated levels of arsenic in their drinking water [6]. Arsenic exposure is strongly associated with many human diseases, such as metabolic diseases, neurological diseases, skin diseases, and various cancers. In addition, arsenic exposure can lead to the occurrence of risk factors for cerebrovascular diseases, such as hypertension and T2DM [7].

Chronic arsenic exposure in humans can cause arsenic accumulation in the liver, affecting glucose metabolism, thus leading to IR and increasing the risk of T2DM [8]. A study showed that arsenic impairs glucose tolerance in mice after eight weeks of exposure to 50 mg/L inorganic arsenite in drinking water [9]. Another study showed that mice exposed to 20 ppm arsenite in drinking water for 12 months could develop IR [10]. Furthermore, the internal levels of arsenic in mice exposed to 50 ppm arsenite are comparable to the levels in highly exposed populations. Moreover, glucose tolerance is impaired in mice exposed to 50 ppm arsenite [9,11]. Therefore, a minimum of three doses should be selected to assess the dose–response correlation, adhering to established protocols for hazard identification and risk assessment [12]. In this study, 50 ppm, 5 ppm, and 0.5 ppm were selected as the maximum dose, medium dose, and low dose of sodium arsenite, respectively, to assess the effects of chronic sodium arsenite exposure on hepatic insulin resistance and its mechanism of action in mice.

Circular RNAs (circRNAs) are single-stranded non-coding RNAs with a covalent closed-loop structure. CircRNAs are involved in insulin resistance as microRNAs sponges or RNA-binding protein (RBP) sponges [13]. Circ_0000284 originates from the HIPK3 gene and has a length of 1099 nucleotides [14]. Circ_0000284 can cause hyperglycaemia and hepatic IR by sponging miR-192-5p [15]. Therefore, circ_0000284 may be involved in hepatic IR related to arsenic exposure.

The insulin-like growth factor 2 mRNA binding protein 2 (IGF2BP2) is an RBP involved in RNA localisation, stabilisation, and translation [16]. IGF2BP2 can participate in the development of liver cancer by binding to circRNAs [17]. Furthermore, IGF2BP2 was recognised as a T2DM-related gene as early as 2007, consistent with the findings of a meta-analysis of populations [18]. The liver-specific deletion of IGF2BP2 increases hepatic triglyceride accumulation and the risk of obesity, which are associated with IR-mediated T2DM [19,20]. However, it is unclear whether circ_0000284 promotes arsenic-induced hepatic IR by binding to IGF2BP2 and its downstream pathways.

Triglycerides accumulate in the liver when the transport rate of triglycerides from the liver to extrahepatic tissues is slowed down. This transport process may be related to the peroxisome proliferator-activated receptor-γ (PPAR-γ) [21]. In addition, hepatic PPAR-γ-deficient mice have a reduced glucose tolerance and insulin sensitivity [22]. The PPAR-γ activator ameliorates hepatic IR in arsenic-treated mice and HepG2 cells [23]. Glucose transporters (GLUTs) play a key role in insulin-stimulated glucose utilisation [24]. Although the insulin-responsive glucose transporter protein 2 (GLUT2) is the major GLUT isoform in the liver and is expressed at higher levels than insulin-responsive glucose transporter protein 4 (GLUT4), GLUT4 is a key regulator of systemic glucose homeostasis. GLUT4 is mainly expressed in adipose tissue, skeletal, and cardiac muscle cells [25]. However, it has been shown that GLUT4 is also involved in glucose metabolism in the liver, with IR significantly upregulating the expression of GLUT4 mRNA and protein in the liver, rather than GLUT2 expression [26]. The upregulating of GLUT4 can alleviate insulin resistance in the liver of mice [27]. In their study on the effects of metformin on hepatic glucose metabolism, Zhu et al. showed that the expression of GLUT4 in the liver is also significantly affected by metformin [28]. Furthermore, the downregulation of GLUT4 is the main pathological mechanism of hyperglycaemia induced by insulin resistance [29]. Therefore, we mainly investigated the expression of GLUT4 in hepatic IR induced by sodium arsenite. PPAR-γ and GLUT4 are elevated in diabetic rats. Notably, PPAR-γ regulates GLUT4 expression [30]. Although a specific GLUT4 knockdown leads to systemic glucose intolerance and IR in mouse muscle and liver tissues [31], the specific mechanism of action is unclear.

Herein, the role of circ_0000284 in arsenic exposure-induced hepatic IR is evaluated. The results reveal a novel molecular mechanism underlying hepatic IR and arsenic-induced T2DM. Therefore, this study provides a scientific basis for identifying the early biomarkers for controlling arsenic exposure and T2DM, and for discovering new preventive and curative measures for arsenic-induced T2DM.

## 2. Materials and Methods

### 2.1. Mouse Model for Arsenite Exposure

Eight-week-old male C57BL/6J mice were sourced from SPF Biotechnology Co., Ltd. (Beijing, China) (license No. 1100987757). All the animal experiments and housing conditions were approved by the Laboratory Animal Ethics Committee of Baotou Medical College (approval number No. 002, Baotou Medical College, 2021). The mice were stochastically divided into four groups ($n$ = 12). Sodium arsenite (Sigma, Darmstadt, Germany) was diluted in drinking water to concentrations of 0, 0.5, 5, and 50 ppm, and the mice were allowed to drink the water freely for 12 months. Each mouse was fed with maintenance feed for rats and mice (SPEFO Biotechnology Co., Ltd., Beijing, China), which did not contain arsenic. The water consumption, food intake, and body weight of the mice were recorded weekly. After 12 months of sodium arsenite exposure, the mice were anaesthetised by an intraperitoneal injection of 1% pentobarbital sodium and then euthanised by cervical dislocation, and their livers were collected for further analysis.

### 2.2. Intraperitoneal Glucose Tolerance Tests (IPGTTs) and Insulin Tolerance Tests (ITTs)

The mice were fasted overnight after 12 months of arsenic exposure. The fasting blood glucose in the tail vein was measured using a blood glucose meter (Roche Diagnostics GmbH, Mannheim, Germany). The blood glucose levels were assessed at 15, 30, 60, and 120 min following the administration of a glucose solution (2 g/kg body weight dissolved in saline) via an intraperitoneal injection. The mice were given one day to recover after the IPGTTs. The mice were fasted for 4–6 h before the measurement of the ITTs. Insulin (0.5 IU/kg) was administered via an intraperitoneal injection, followed by blood glucose monitoring at 15, 30, and 60 min post-injection.

### 2.3. Liver Periodic Acid–Schiff (PAS) Staining

The fresh liver tissues were fixed in 4% paraformaldehyde, embedded in paraffin, and cut into 5 μm sections. The sections were dewaxed, rinsed with tap water for 2~3 min, then rinsed twice with distilled water, and placed in an oxidising agent at room temperature (25–30 °C) for 5~10 min. The samples were rinsed twice with distilled water, then put into a PAS staining solution (Solarbio Life Science, Beijing, China) in a dark place at room temperature (25–30 °C) for 10–20 min. The samples were put in a haematoxylin staining solution for 2 min to stain the nucleus. The sections were differentiated with acidic differentiation solution and dehydrated, made transparent, and sealed before visualisation using a microscope.

### 2.4. HE Staining

The fixed tissue samples were washed with running water, dehydrated with gradient alcohol, and embedded. The samples were cut into 3 μm thick paraffin slices and incubated at 65 °C for 4.5 h. The sections were deparaffinised and rehydrated through graded alcohols to water. The sections were then placed in a haematoxylin solution for 3 min, rinsed with running tap water for 5 min, and differentiated in 1% acid alcohol (1% HCl in 70% ethanol) for 10 s. After rinsing with running tap water for 1 min, the sections were placed in a blueing solution for 30 s to 1 min, and then rinsed again with running tap water for 5 min. Next, the sections were stained in an eosin dye solution for 5 min, dehydrated through graded alcohols, and cleared in xylene. Finally, the slides were sealed with a coverslip using a mounting medium, observed under a microscope, and photographed for analysis.

### 2.5. Cell Culture and Treatment

The human hepatocellular carcinoma cell line HepG2 was sourced from Pricella Life Science and Technology Co., Ltd. (Wuhan, China). The cell culture medium was DMEM

(Gibco, Gaithersburg, MD, USA). The complete medium was supplemented with 10% foetal bovine serum (Gibco, Gaithersburg, MD, USA) and 1% antibiotics (100 IU/mL penicillin and 100 μg/mL streptomycin, Beyotime, Shanghai, China). The cells were cultured in a humidified incubator (Thermo Scientific, Waltham, MA, USA) at 37 °C with 5% carbon dioxide. The HepG2 cells were digested with trypsin when they grew to 80–90%, were re-laid evenly in well plates or cell culture dishes, and treated with different concentrations of the sodium arsenite culture solution for 24 h, followed by the addition of 100 nM insulin for 30 min. The cells were collected for subsequent experiments.

### 2.6. Cell Viability Assay

The cell viability was assessed using Cell Counting Kit 8 (CCK-8) reagent (Biosharp, Anhui, China). The cell concentration was determined using a cell counter. The cells (5000 per well) were inoculated into 96-well culture plates. The original medium was discarded after the cells attached to the wall. The cells were then treated with the medium containing different concentrations of sodium arsenite (0, 1, 2, 4, 6, 8, 10, 20, or 30 μM) for 24 h. The CCK-8 reagent (10 μL) was added to each well, and the absorbance was recorded at 450 nm. The cell viability was calculated as a percentage of the absorbance in the control wells.

### 2.7. Cell Transfection

The circ_0000284 inhibitors (si-circ_0000284) and si-circ_NC (si-circ_0000284 negative control) were sourced from IGEBio (Guangzhou, China). The cell transfection was completed using Liposome 2000 reagent (Invitrogen). The cells were inoculated into six-well plates, followed by the addition of the MEM solution containing si-circ_0000284 and the MEM solution with si-NC, mixed with the MEM solution containing the Liposome 2000 reagent, for transfection for 6 h. The cells were then incubated with the sodium arsenite solution for 24 h, and collected for further experiments.

### 2.8. Membrane Protein Extraction and GLUT4 Analysis

A Membrane Protein and Cytoplasmic Protein Extraction Kit (Beyotime, Shanghai, China) was used to extract the membrane proteins and plasma proteins. The HepG2 cells were collected via cell scraping, then centrifuged at 4 °C and 1200 rpm for 5 min. The supernatant was discarded, and the precipitate was retained. Moreover, the liver tissues were cut into pieces. Benzenesulfonyl fluoride (PMSF, Beyotime, Shanghai, China) was added to the cell and tissue samples, then homogenised with a homogeniser, centrifuged at 4 °C and 14,000× $g$ for 30 min. The plasma protein was collected as the supernatant. Membrane Protein Extraction Reagent B was added to the precipitate and centrifuged at 14,000× $g$ and 4 °C for 5 min to collect the membrane protein solution.

The total protein was obtained using a Total Protein extraction kit (Solarbio Life Science, Beijing, China). Protein lysate containing PMSF was added to the petri dish and scraped with a cell scraper after treating the cells according to each experimental protocol. Also, the liver tissue was ground, followed by the addition of protein lysate containing PMSF to prepare the tissue protein lysate. The protein lysates were lysed on ice for 30 min, then centrifuged at 4 °C and 12,000 rpm for 30 min. The supernatant was absorbed into a new centrifuge tube (total protein).

### 2.9. Western Blots

The protein concentration was measured using a BCA kit (APPLYGEN, Beijing, China) after protein extraction. Separation and concentration gels were prepared using an SDS-PAGE gel preparation kit (Solarbio Life Science, Beijing, China), up-sampled for electrophoresis, then transferred to a PVDF membrane. The membrane was blocked with 5% skimmed milk for 2 h and incubated with a primary antibody at 4 °C overnight. The membrane was also incubated with a secondary antibody for 1 h. Finally, the membrane was imaged after treatment with ECL reagent (APPLYGEN, Beijing, China). The primary antibodies for IGF2BP2, GLUT4, PPAR-γ, β-actin, Na/K-ATPase were obtained from Affinity, Abcam, Proteintech, SAB, and Bioss, respectively.

*2.10. RNA Extraction and Quantitative Real-Time PCR (qRT-PCR) Analyses*

The total RNA was extracted by adding 1 mL of TransZol Up reagent (TransGen Biotech, Beijing, China) to each petri dish. The total RNA extracts were reverse transcribed with GoScriptTMReverse Transcription System (Promega, Madison, WI, USA). The levels of circ_0000284 were detected using a PCR kit (Promega, Madison, WI, USA) on a LightCycler96 instrument (Roche, Basel, Switzerland). The data were normalised to β-actin via the $2^{-\Delta\Delta Ct}$ method [32]. The sequences of the specific primers are shown in Table 1.

**Table 1.** Sequences of qRT-PCR primers and siRNAs.

| Genes | F (5′→3′) | R (5′→3′) |
|---|---|---|
| hsa-circ_0000284 | CGGCAGCCTTACAGGGTTAA | GACCAAGACTTGTGAGGCCA |
| mmu-circ_0000284 | TGTTGGIGGATCCTGTTCGC | GACCAAGACTTGTGAGGCCA |
| IGF2BP2 | GTCCTACTCAAGTCCGGCTAC | CATATTCAGCCAACAGCCCAT |
| hsa-β-actin | CAGATGIGGATCAGCAAGCAGGAG | GTCAAGAAAGGGTGTAACGCAACTAAG |
| mmu-β-actin | GGCTGTATTCCCCTCCATCG | CCAGTTGGTAACAATGCCATGT |
| Si-circ_0000284 | GUACUACAGGUAUGGCCUGdTdT | GAGGCCAUACCLGUAGUACdTdT |
| Si-circ_NC | UUCUCCGAACGUGUCACGUTT | ACGUGACACGUUCGGAGAATT |

*2.11. Glycogen and Glucose Consumption Levels*

For the glycogen, the cells were collected, followed by a cell count analysis (5–1 million cells). Glycogen extract (0.75 mL) was added to the collected cells and tissues, centrifuged, and the supernatant was discarded. The glycogen was assessed using a Glycogen Assay Kit (Solarbio, Beijing, China). For the glucose, the cells were collected, followed by a cell count analysis (5–1 million cells). The supernatant (1 mL) was added into boiling water for 10 min, followed by glucose analysis using a glucose assay kit (Solarbio, Beijing, China).

*2.12. Statistical Analysis*

SPSS 26.0 (IBM, Armonk, NY, USA) was used for the statistical analysis of the data, and GraphPad Prism 9.0 (GraphPad Software, San Diego, CA, USA) was used to plot the experimental results. One-way analyses of variance (one-way ANOVAs) were conducted to analyse the variations in the indicators across multiple groups, followed by pairwise comparisons between multiple groups using a Bonferroni correction. Each experiment was performed in at least three biological replicates and the results were expressed as the mean ± SD. Statistical significance was considered for a $p$-value < 0.05.

## 3. Results

*3.1. Chronic Sodium Arsenite Exposure Causes Liver Injury and Hepatic IR in Mice*

The mice were given drinking water containing 0, 0.5, 5, and 50 ppm sodium arsenite for 12 months and subjected to IPGTTs and ITTs. The results show that 5 and 50 ppm sodium arsenite reduced glucose tolerance in mice compared with the control mice, especially in the 50 ppm group (Figure 1A). Moreover, 5 and 50 ppm sodium arsenite significantly increased the glucose levels in the mice after an insulin injection compared with the control mice, thus reducing insulin sensitivity (Figure 1B). The glycogen levels decreased in the liver with increasing doses of sodium arsenite (Figure 1C,D). In addition, the HE staining showed significant liver damage in the high-dose group (Figure 1E). These results suggest that sodium arsenite causes liver injury and hepatic IR in mice.

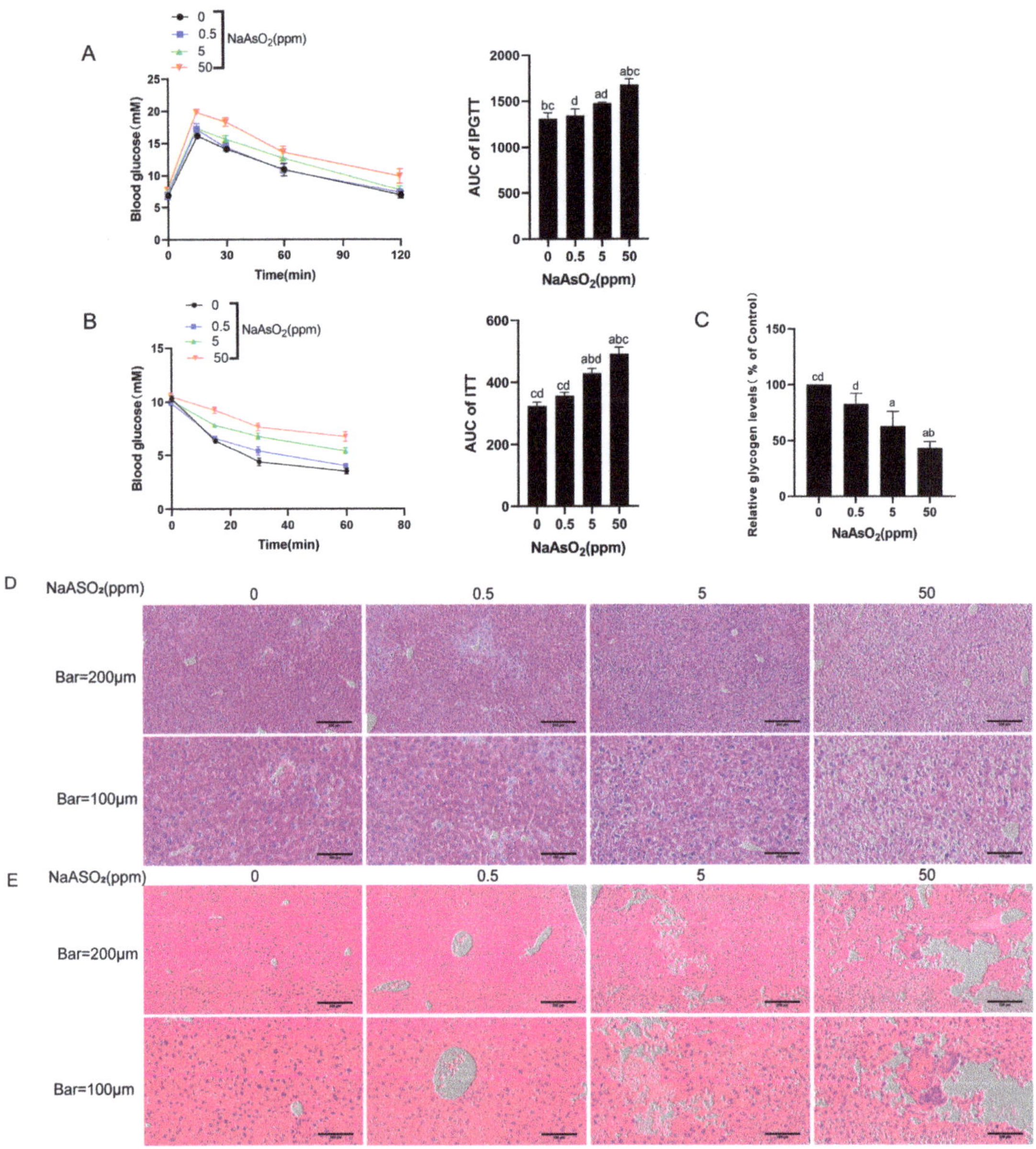


**Figure 1.** Chronic exposure to sodium arsenite causes liver injury and hepatic IR in mice. C57BL/6J mice were allowed to drink water containing 0, 0.5, 5, or 50 ppm sodium arsenite for 12 months. (**A**) IPGTTs showing the blood glucose concentrations at 0, 15, 30, 60, and 120 min in the mice. The area under the curve (AUC) was calculated based on the IPGTTs results. (**B**) ITT assays were performed to determine the blood glucose concentrations of the mice at 0, 15, 30, and 60 min. The AUC

of the ITTs was calculated. (**C**) A glycogen assay kit was used to determine the glycogen concentration in each mouse's liver. (**D**) The detection of hepatic glycogen changes by PAS staining. (**E**) The HE staining images of livers indicating the liver injury level. The data are presented as the mean ± SD, $n = 3$. [a]: $p < 0.05$, compared with the 0 ppm $NaAsO_2$ group; [b]: $p < 0.05$, compared with the 0.5 ppm $NaAsO_2$ group; [c]: $p < 0.05$, compared with the 5 ppm $NaAsO_2$ group; [d]: $p < 0.05$, compared with the 50 ppm $NaAsO_2$ group.

### *3.2. Sodium Arsenite Increases Levels of Circ_0000284 Levels and Decreases IGF2BP2 Levels in Mouse Livers*

The levels of circ_0000284 and IGF2BP2, as well as the protein expression level of IGF2BP2, were evaluated to investigate whether circ_0000284 and IGF2BP2 play a role in arsenite-induced hepatic IR. Furthermore, the circ_0000284 levels were higher in the sodium arsenite-exposed mice than in the controls, especially in the 5 and 50 ppm groups (Figure 2A). Also, the mRNA and protein levels of IGF2BP2 were reduced in the arsenic-exposed mice in a dose–response manner compared with the controls (Figure 2B–D). These findings indicate that sodium arsenite increases circ_0000284 levels and reduces IGF2BP2 levels in mouse livers.

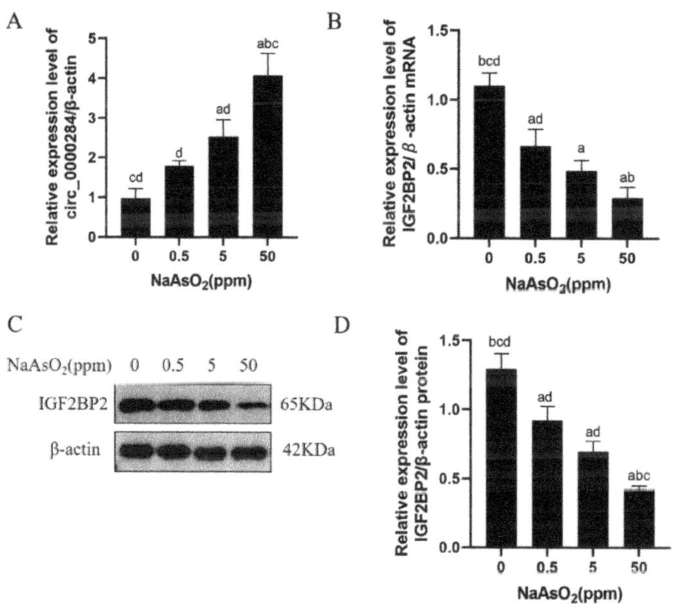


**Figure 2.** Chronic exposure to sodium arsenite induces increased levels of circ_0000284 and decreased levels of IGF2BP2 levels in livers of mice. C57BL/6J mice were allowed to drink water containing 0, 0.5, 5, or 50 ppm sodium arsenite for 12 months. Levels of circ_0000284 (**A**) and IGF2BP2 (**B**) in livers of mice were determined using qRT-PCR assay. (**C**) Western blots of protein bands and (**D**) relative protein levels of IGF2BP2 in livers of mice. Data are presented as mean ± SD, $n = 3$. [a]: $p < 0.05$, compared with 0 ppm $NaAsO_2$ group; [b]: $p < 0.05$, compared with 0.5 ppm $NaAsO_2$ group; [c]: $p < 0.05$, compared with 5 ppm $NaAsO_2$ group; [d]: $p < 0.05$, compared with 50 ppm $NaAsO_2$ group.

### *3.3. Arsenic Exposure Decreases PPAR-γ and Membrane GLUT4 Levels in Mice*

The GLUT4 transporter protein is sequestered in specialised storage vesicles inside a cell under basal conditions. Increased circulating insulin activates an intracellular signalling cascade when glucose levels are elevated, ultimately leading to the translocation of GLUT4 from the storage region to the plasma membrane, thus promoting glucose uptake and maintaining glucose homeostasis [33]. Insulin resistance limits the transportation of GLUT4 transporter proteins to the cell membrane due to the lack of insulin stimulation [34]. The activation of PPAR-γ promotes GLUT4 translocation to the plasma membrane, whereas decreased PPAR-γ expression inhibits GLUT4 translocation to the plasma membrane, affecting cellular glucose homeostasis [35]. Herein, the levels of PPAR-γ and GLUT4 in the cytoplasm and membrane of the mouse livers after exposure to sodium arsenite (0, 0.5, 5, and 50 ppm) were assessed to investigate the roles of altered PPAR-γ expression and GLUT4 translocation in arsenite-induced hepatic insulin resistance. Sodium arsenite decreased the protein levels of PPAR-γ in the mouse livers (Figure 3A,B). Notably, sodium arsenite decreased the membrane protein levels of GLUT4 in the livers in a dose-dependent manner compared with the controls (Figure 3C,D). Moreover, sodium arsenite decreased the ratio of GLUT4 levels in the membrane proteins to cytoplasmic proteins compared with the controls, indicating the inhibition of GLUT4 translocation at the plasma membrane (Figure 3E). These findings suggest that sodium arsenite reduces the level of PPAR-γ expression and blocks the plasma membrane translocation of GLUT4 in hepatocytes.

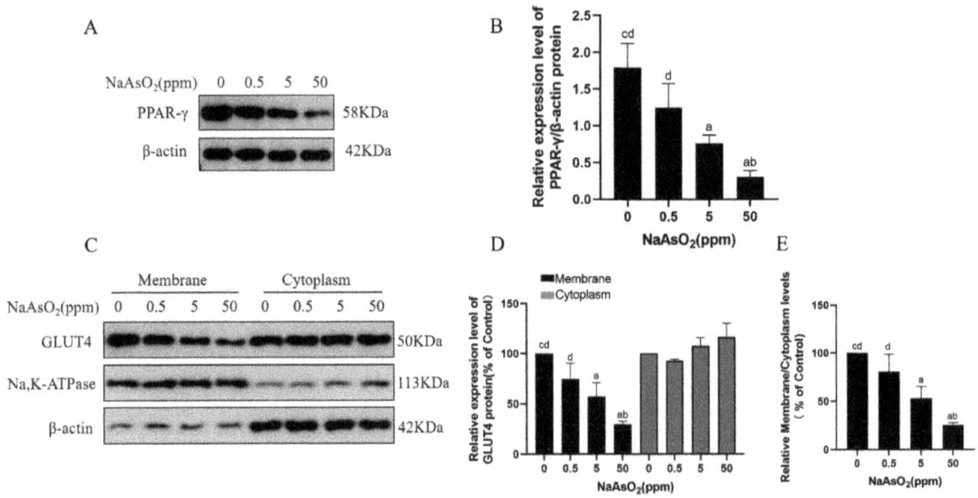


**Figure 3.** Chronic arsenic exposure decreases levels of PPAR-γ and levels of membrane GLUT4 in livers of mice. C57BL/6J mice were allowed to drink water containing 0, 0.5, 5, or 50 ppm sodium arsenite for 12 months. (**A**) Western blots of protein bands and (**B**) relative protein levels of PPAR-γ in livers of mice. (**C**) Western blots of protein bands and (**D**) relative protein levels of GLUT4 in cytoplasm and membrane of mice livers; β-actin served as internal reference for cytoplasm proteins, and Na and K-ATPase as internal references for membrane proteins. (**E**) Ratio of GLUT4 protein levels in membrane to cytoplasm. Data are presented as mean ± SD, $n = 3$. [a]: $p < 0.05$, compared with 0 ppm $NaAsO_2$ group; [b]: $p < 0.05$, compared with 0.5 ppm $NaAsO_2$ group; [c]: $p < 0.05$, compared with 5 ppm $NaAsO_2$ group; [d]: $p < 0.05$, compared with 50 ppm $NaAsO_2$ group.

### 3.4. Sodium Arsenite Decreases Levels of Glucose Consumption and Glycogen in Insulin-Treated HepG2 Cells

In this study, cellular experiments were used to further validate the effects of arsenic exposure on hepatic IR. First, CCK8 experiments were performed to select the appropriate poison dose for the HepG2 cells. Studies have shown that the viability of HepG2 cells does not significantly change at sodium arsenite concentrations ≤ 4 μM, and when the concentration of sodium arsenite is 8 μM, cell viability significantly decreases with statistical significance [23]. The results of this experiment are consistent with those of previous ones. Herein, the cells were treated with 0, 1, 2, 4, 6, 8, 10, 20, or 30 μM sodium arsenite, and the CCK-8 assay showed that the cell viability gradually decreased with an increasing sodium arsenite concentration (Figure 4A). Sodium arsenite < 2 μM did not significantly affect cell viability, while 4 μM sodium arsenite significantly decreased cell viability. The cell viability for 8 μM sodium arsenite decreased to about 70%. It has been shown that the ideal cell status and viability are >60–80% [36]. Therefore, the HepG2 cells were treated with 0, 2, 4, and 8 μM of sodium arsenite in the subsequent experiments. The HepG2 cells were treated with 0, 2, 4, or 8 μM sodium arsenite for 24 h, followed by a 100 nM insulin treatment for 30 min. The results show that the glucose consumption and glycogen levels of the HepG2 cells were lower in the arsenic-exposed cells than in the control cells in a dose-dependent manner (Figure 4B,C). These results suggest that sodium arsenite reduces insulin-dependent glucose consumption and glycogen levels in hepatocytes.

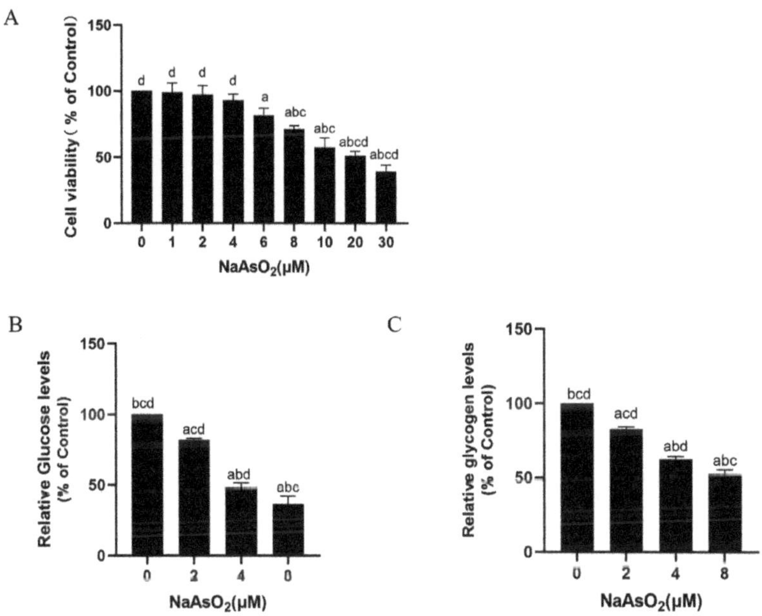


**Figure 4.** Sodium arsenite causes decreased levels of glucose consumption and glycogen in insulin-treated HepG2 cells. HepG2 cells were treated with 0, 1, 2, 4, 8, 10, 20, or 30 μM sodium arsenite for 24 h. (**A**) Cell viability was detected by CCK-8 assay. After HepG2 cells were treated with 0, 2, 4, or 8 μM sodium arsenite for 24 h, they were then treated for 30 min with 100 nM insulin. Glucose consumption (**B**) and glycogen levels (**C**) in HepG2 cells were measured by glucose assay kits and glycogen assay kits. Data are presented as mean ± SD, $n = 3$. [a]: $p < 0.05$, compared with 0 μM $NaAsO_2$ group; [b]: $p < 0.05$, compared with 2 μM $NaAsO_2$ group; [c]: $p < 0.05$, compared with 4 μM $NaAsO_2$ group; [d]: $p < 0.05$, compared with 8 μM $NaAsO_2$ group.

### *3.5. Sodium Arsenite Increases Levels of Circ_0000284 and Decreases Levels of IGF2BP2, PPAR-γ, and Membrane GLUT4 in Insulin-Treated HepG2 Cells*

Similarly, the HepG2 cells were treated with 0, 2, 4, or 8 μM sodium arsenite for 24 h, followed by a 100 nM insulin treatment for 30 min. The levels of circ_0000284 were elevated in the sodium arsenite- and insulin-treated HepG2 cells (Figure 5A). In addition, the protein levels of IGF2BP2 and PPAR-γ were lower in the arsenic-exposed HepG2 cells than in the control cells in a concentration-dependent manner (Figure 5B–D). Compared with the control cells, the membrane protein levels of GLUT4 and the ratio of GLUT4 levels in the membrane proteins to cytoplasmic proteins were reduced, indicating the inhibition of GLUT4 translocation at the plasma membrane (Figure 5E–G). These results suggest that arsenic exposure increases circ_0000284 levels, decreases IGF2BP2 and PPAR-γ expression levels, and blocks the plasma membrane translocation of GLUT4 in hepatocytes.

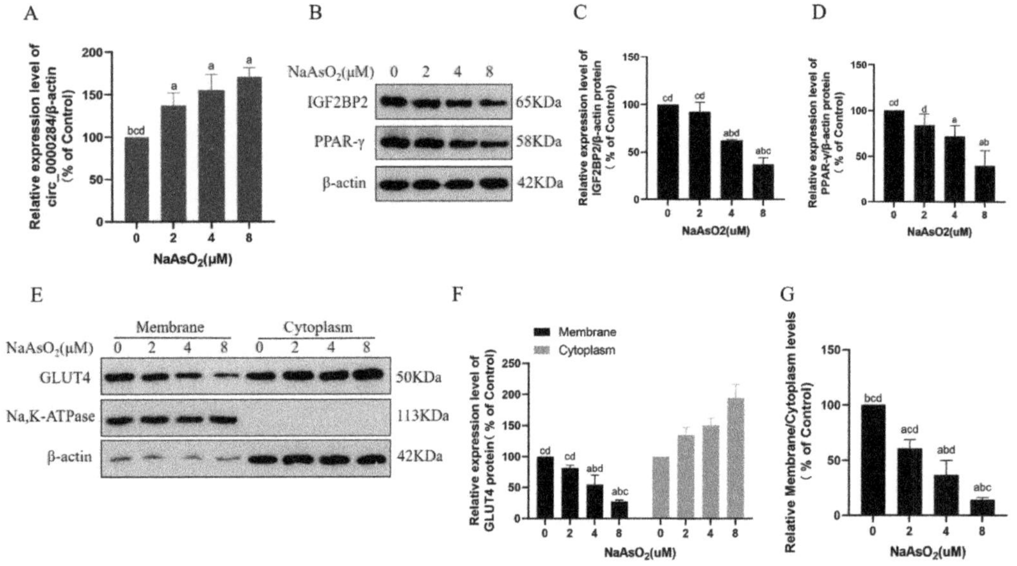


**Figure 5.** Sodium arsenite increases levels of circ_0000284 levels and decreases levels of IGF2BP2, PPAR-γ, and membrane GLUT4 in insulin-treated HepG2 cells. HepG2 cells were treated with 0, 2, 4, or 8 μM sodium arsenite for 24 h, and then treated for 30 min with 100 nM insulin. (**A**) Levels of circ_0000284 were quantified by qRT-PCR. (**B**) Western blots of protein bands and (**C**,**D**) corresponding relative protein levels of IGF2BP2 and PPAR-γ. (**E**) Western blots of protein bands and (**F**) relative protein levels of GLUT4 in cytoplasm and membrane; β-actin served as internal reference for cytoplasm proteins, and Na and K-ATPase as internal references for membrane proteins. (**G**) Ratio of GLUT4 expression levels in membrane proteins to cytoplasm proteins. Data are presented as mean ± SD, $n = 3$. [a]: $p < 0.05$, compared with 0 μM $NaAsO_2$ group; [b]: $p < 0.05$, compared with 2 μM $NaAsO_2$ group; [c]: $p < 0.05$, compared with 4 μM $NaAsO_2$ group; [d]: $p < 0.05$, compared with 8 μM $NaAsO_2$ group.

### *3.6. Inhibition of Circ_0000284 Blocks Sodium Arsenite-Induced Increases in Circ_0000284 Levels and Decreases in Glucose Consumption and Glycogen Levels in Insulin-Treated HepG2 Cells*

The glucose consumption and glycogen levels were examined after the HepG2 cells were transfected with 0 or 50 nM si-circ_0000284 or si-circ_NC for 6 h to determine the role of circ_0000284 in hepatic IR in HepG2 cells exposed to arsenite. Notably, the cells were treated with 0 or 8 μM sodium arsenite for 24 h, followed by a 100 nM insulin treatment for 30 min. The downregulation of circ_0000284 levels by si-circ_0000284 reversed the sodium arsenite-induced effect on the circ_0000284 levels, glucose consumption, and glycogen levels in the insulin-stimulated HepG2 cells (Figure 6), indicating that circ_0000284 is involved in arsenite-induced IR in hepatocytes.

### *3.7. Inhibition of Circ_0000284 Blocks Sodium Arsenite-Induced Decreases in IGF2BP2, PPAR-γ, and Membrane GLUT4 Levels in Insulin-Treated HepG2 Cells*

The effects of circ_0000284 on sodium arsenite-induced decreases in the levels of IGF2BP2, PPAR-γ, and membrane GLUT4 in insulin-treated HepG2 cells were examined to further investigate the mechanisms of circ_0000284 in hepatic IR in HepG2 cells exposed to sodium arsenite. HepG2 cells were cultured in a medium containing arsenite (0 or 8 μM) for 24 h after transfection with si-circ_0000284 or si-circ_NC, followed by an insulin (100 nM) treatment for 30 min. The results show that circ_0000284 downregulation after treatment with si-circ_0000284 alleviated the arsenite-induced decrease in the protein levels of PPAR-γ and IGF2BP2 (Figure 7A–C). Furthermore, the circ_0000284 inhibition blocked the decrease in GLUT4 levels at the membrane in the arsenic-induced HepG2 cells (Figure 7D–F). These findings suggest that circ_0000284 inhibitors can reverse the reduction in IGF2BP2 and PPAR-γ expression levels and the blockade of the plasma membrane translocation of GLUT4 in hepatocytes exposed to arsenic.

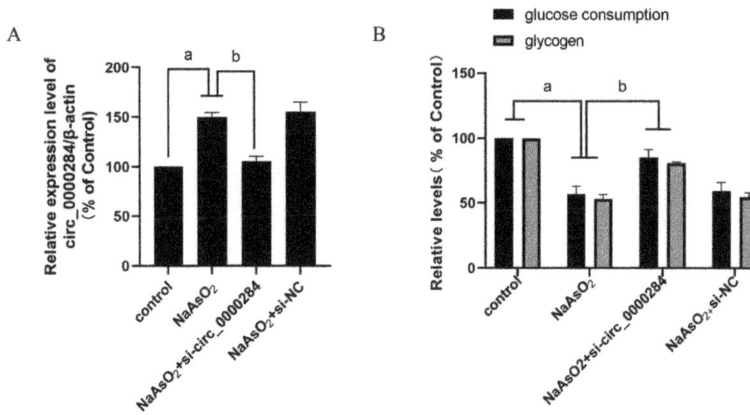

**Figure 6.** Inhibition of circ_0000284 blocks sodium arsenite-induced increases in circ_0000284 levels and decreases in glucose consumption and glycogen levels in insulin-treated HepG2 cells. HepG2 cells were transfected with 0 or 50 nM si-circ_0000284 or si-circ_NC for 6 h, followed by treatment with 0 or 8 μM sodium arsenite for 24 h, respectively, and then treated for 30 min with 100 nM insulin. (**A**) Levels of circ_0000284 in HepG2 cells were detected by qRT-PCR assay. (**B**) Glucose consumption and glycogen levels in HepG2 cells were measured by glucose assay kits and glycogen assay kits. Data are presented as mean ± SD, $n = 3$. [a]: $p < 0.05$, compared with HepG2 cells without arsenite treatment; [b]: $p < 0.05$, compared with si circ_0000284-treated HepG2 cells.

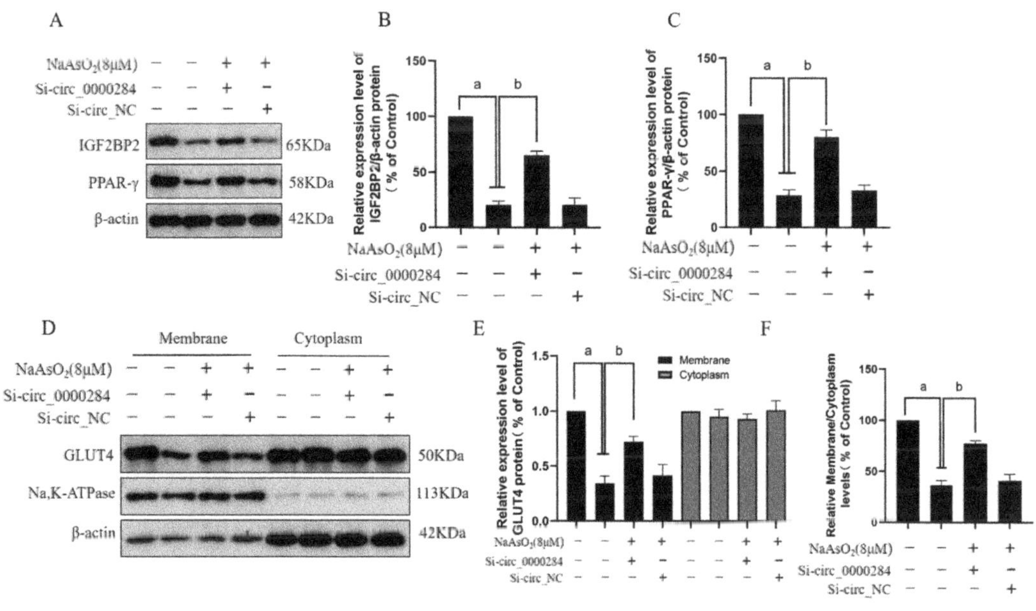

**Figure 7.** Inhibition of circ_0000284 blocks sodium arsenite-induced decreases in IGF2BP2, PPAR-γ, and membrane GLUT4 levels in insulin-treated HepG2 cells. After HepG2 cells were transfected with

0 or 50 nM si-circ_0000284 or si-circ_NC for 6 h, and then with 0 or 8 μM sodium arsenite for 24 h, respectively, they were then treated for 30 min with 100 nM insulin. (**A**) Western blots of protein bands and (**B**,**C**) corresponding relative protein levels of IGF2BP2 and PPAR-γ. (**D**) Western blots of protein bands and (**E**) corresponding relative protein levels of GLUT4 in cytoplasm and membrane; β-actin served as internal reference for cytoplasm proteins, and Na and K-ATPase served as internal references for membrane proteins. (**F**) Ratio of GLUT4 expression levels in membrane proteins to cytoplasm proteins. Data are presented as mean ± SD, $n = 3$. [a]: $p < 0.05$, compared with HepG2 cells without arsenite treatment; [b]: $p < 0.05$, compared with si-circ_0000284-treated HepG2 cells.

## 4. Discussion

Currently, several high-arsenic areas exist in all countries around the world, and arsenic exposure from drinking water can cause severe health problems in humans. Long-term arsenic exposure can induce liver fibrosis, nonalcoholic fatty liver disease, diabetes, and other diseases [37–39]. Arsenic exposure has been linked to T2DM, and T2DM is correlated with IR and insufficient insulin secretion [40–42]. The liver is the main target organ of arsenic metabolism. In recent years, an increasing number of studies have demonstrated that arsenic exposure may trigger hepatic IR, reduce the sensitivity of liver cells to insulin, hinder the uptake of glucose by liver cells, affect liver glycogen synthesis, and elevate blood sugar levels, which increase the risk of diabetes [43]. We found that arsenic exposure decreased the glycogen content and reduced the glucose consumption in HepG2 cells, inducing liver damage in mice, as well as impaired glucose tolerance and insulin sensitivity, leading to hepatic insulin resistance. However, the molecular mechanism leading to arsenic-induced hepatic IR is not well understood. In this study, arsenic exposure models of mice and HepG2 cells were established to explore the epigenetic mechanism of arsenic-induced hepatic IR.

In recent years, the role of ncRNA in the progression of diabetes following arsenic exposure has been extensively investigated in vivo [44]. Arsenic exposure can alter the expression of various proteins by affecting changes in ncRNA, causing IR [10]. However, the role of circRNAs in IR induced by arsenic exposure is not fully understood. Circ_0000284 can regulate apoptosis, proliferation, migration, and angiogenesis, as well as influence the development of cardiovascular diseases [45]. Circ_0000284 may also promote the proliferation of hepatobiliary carcinoma and breast cancer cells [14,46]. In this study, we showed that circ_0000284 expression was elevated in hepatic IR induced by arsenic exposure. This is consistent with the results obtained from the clinical experiments of Su et al. that, through a circRNA chip analysis of the peripheral blood of T2DM patients and a control group, revealed that the expression level of circ_0000284 in the T2DM group was significantly higher than that in the control group [47]. These results indicate that circ_0000284 is involved in the occurrence of hepatic IR induced by arsenic exposure.

CircRNAs have been implicated in the regulation of β cell function, IR, adipocyte function, inflammation, and oxidative stress by interacting with RBP [13]. IGF2BP2, as an RBP regulating multiple biological processes, is a T2DM-related molecule that regulates cellular metabolism in a variety of cell types. The expression of IGF2BP2 has been linked to liver fibrosis, T2DM, and cancer [21,48]. Furthermore, Greenwald found that the reduced activity of the IGF2BP2 homolog, Imp2, in mouse islets, impaired islet chromatin accessibility and glucose-stimulated insulin secretion [49]. Here, we show that IGF2BP2 serves as the downstream target of circ_0000284 through gene prediction tools. The results of this study show that with increasing levels of arsenic exposure, the expression level of circ_0000284 in liver cells increases, while the expression level of IGF2BP2 decreases, leading to liver IR. Furthermore, the silencing of circ_0000284 in hepatocytes results in the upregulation of the expression of IGF2BP2.

PPAR-γ is a ligand-activated nuclear transcription factor associated with adipose differentiation, obesity, and insulin resistance. PPAR-γ can affect glucose uptake in IR-mediated tissues and maintain glucose homeostasis [50]. Increased PPAR-γ expression is associated with improved insulin sensitivity and reduced insulin resistance [51]. In bone marrow-derived macrophages (BMDMs), IGF2BP2 can bind to fragments of PPAR-$\gamma$ mRNA, thereby enhancing its stability [52]. In the liver tissues of WT mice, PPAR-$\gamma$ mRNA is enriched in IGF2BP2 immunosuppression samples, and IGF2BP2 mediates the post-transcriptional regulation of PPAR-$\gamma$ in the liver [53]. The deletion of IGF2BP2 is linked to a marked reduction in PPAR-$\gamma$ mRNA levels [19]. In our study, as the level of arsenic exposure increased, the expression level of IGF2BP2 in the liver cells decreased, and the expression level of PPAR-$\gamma$ also decreased. Consequently, we have established a correlation between IGF2BP2 and PPAR-$\gamma$. And, after knocking down circ_0000284 in the hepatocytes, the expression level of IGF2BP2 increased, and the level of PPAR-$\gamma$ also increased. These findings indicate that circ_0000284 regulates IGF2BP2/PPAR-$\gamma$ expression, influencing liver insulin resistance following exposure to arsenic.

GLUT4 serves as a pivotal regulator of the overall glucose balance within the body. Insulin reduces blood glucose levels by inhibiting hepatic glucose production and stimulating glucose uptake in tissues through GLUT4 [54]. Insulin binds to the receptors on the cell membrane, triggering a cascade of intracellular signalling events that result in the translocation of GLUT4 to the cell surface. This mechanism facilitates the absorption and transport of glucose into cells, maintaining glucose homeostasis. The aberrant expression of GLUT4 affects glucose homeostasis [55]. Research has demonstrated that the activation of PPAR-$\gamma$ by insulin modulates GLUT4 translocation and lowers cellular glucose levels [56]. Furthermore, a diet high in sugar can trigger insulin resistance by decreasing the protein expression of PPAR-$\gamma$ and GLUT4 within liver tissue, thereby disrupting glucose homeostasis [28]. While PPAR-$\gamma$'s role in arsenic-induced hepatic IR and its regulation of GLUT4 expression requires further investigation, our study confirms a dose-dependent decrease in PPAR-$\gamma$ expression in hepatocytes exposed to arsenic. Simultaneously, the presence of GLUT4 in the cell membrane is decreased, suggesting GLUT4 translocation. The downregulation of circ_0000284 counteracts this effect. These findings suggest that circ_0000284 inhibits the translocation of GLUT4 to the plasma membrane of hepatocytes by modulating the IGF2BP2/PPAR-$\gamma$ pathway, facilitating hepatic insulin resistance induced by arsenic exposure.

This study still has the following limitations. Firstly, we only studied the role of circ_0000284 in arsenic-induced insulin resistance in HepG2 cells, and there was a lack of an inhibitor group in vivo, which is a flaw of our study. In our next study, we will construct an animal model with the knockdown of circ_0000284 to further confirm its role in arsenite-induced hepatic insulin resistance. Secondly, we did not initially test for arsenic levels in the livers, which represents a lapse in our experimental design. Moving forward, we will measure the arsenic content in the liver tissues of mice.

## 5. Conclusions

In summary, arsenic exposure increases circ_0000284 levels in mouse livers and insulin-treated hepatocytes. Arsenic exposure affects insulin-dependent glucose consumption and glycogen accumulation by altering the expression level of circ_0000284 in hepatocytes, and affecting the expression of IGF2BP2, PPAR-$\gamma$, and GLUT4 in membrane proteins. These results indicate that circ_0000284 is involved in arsenite-induced hepatic IR through blocking the plasma membrane translocation of GLUT4 in hepatocytes via IGF2BP2/PPAR-$\gamma$. This study provides a scientific basis for finding early biomarkers for the control of arsenic exposure, offering insights into identifying the biomarkers for T2DM and for the prevention and treatment of arsenic poisoning.

**Author Contributions:** Writing—Original Draft Preparation, S.X.; Data Curation, Z.H.; Conceptualisation, Y.W.; Software, Z.W.; Methodology, T.M. and S.W.; Validation, S.X. and Q.Z.; Formal Analysis, S.X.; Investigation, S.X.; Resources, L.W.; Writing—Review and Editing, L.W. and X.W.; Supervision, S.W. and T.M.; Funding Acquisition and Project Administration, L.W. All authors have read and agreed to the published version of the manuscript.

**Funding:** This research was funded by the Natural Science Foundation of China (82060605) and the Natural Science Foundation Project of Inner Mongolia Autonomous Region (2024LHMS08008).

**Institutional Review Board Statement:** This study was conducted according to the guidelines of the Declaration of Helsinki, and all animal experiments and housing conditions were approved by the Laboratory Animal Ethics Committee of Baotou Medical College (approval number No, 002, Baotou Medical College, 2021).

**Informed Consent Statement:** Not applicable.

**Data Availability Statement:** The data that support the findings of this study are available from the corresponding author upon reasonable request.

**Acknowledgments:** This work was supported by the Natural Science Foundation of China (82060605) and the Natural Science Foundation Project of Inner Mongolia Autonomous Region (2024LHMS08008). We would also like to thank everyone who worked so hard on this whole experiment.

**Conflicts of Interest:** The authors declare no conflicts of interest.

## References

1. Ahmad, I.; Suhail, M.; Ahmad, A.; Alhosin, M.; Tabrez, S. Interlinking of diabetes mellitus and cancer: An overview. *Cell Biochem. Funct.* **2023**, *41*, 506–516. [CrossRef] [PubMed]
2. Wu, Z.; Jin, T.; Weng, J. A thorough analysis of diabetes research in China from 1995 to 2015: Current scenario and future scope. *Sci. China Life Sci.* **2019**, *62*, 46–62, Erratum in *Sci. China Life Sci.* **2023**, *66*, 2958. [CrossRef] [PubMed]
3. Petersen, M.C.; Vatner, D.F.; Shulman, G.I. Regulation of hepatic glucose metabolism in health and disease. *Nat. Rev. Endocrinol.* **2017**, *13*, 572–587. [CrossRef] [PubMed]
4. Garelick, H.; Jones, H.; Dybowska, A.; Valsami-Jones, E. Arsenic pollution sources. *Rev. Environ. Contam. Toxicol.* **2008**, *197*, 17–60. [PubMed]
5. Frisbie, S.H.; Mitchell, E.J. Arsenic in drinking water: An analysis of global drinking water regulations and recommendations for updates to protect public health. *PLoS ONE* **2022**, *17*, e0263505. [CrossRef]
6. Martínez-Castillo, M.; García-Montalvo, E.A.; Arellano-Mendoza, M.G.; Sánchez-Peña, L.D.C.; Soria Jasso, L.E.; Izquierdo-Vega, J.A.; Valenzuela, O.L.; Hernández-Zavala, A. Arsenic exposure and non-carcinogenic health effects. *Hum. Exp. Toxicol.* **2021**, *40*, S826–S850. [CrossRef]
7. Rahaman, M.S.; Rahman, M.M.; Mise, N.; Sikder, M.T.; Ichihara, G.; Uddin, M.K.; Kurasaki, M.; Ichihara, S. Environmental arsenic exposure and its contribution to human diseases, toxicity mechanism and management. *Environ. Pollut.* **2021**, *289*, 117940. [CrossRef]
8. Shakya, A.; Dodson, M.; Artiola, J.F.; Ramirez-Andreotta, M.; Root, R.A.; Ding, X.; Chorover, J.; Maier, R.M. Arsenic in Drinking Water and Diabetes. *Water* **2023**, *15*, 1751. [CrossRef]
9. Kirkley, A.G.; Carmean, C.M.; Ruiz, D.; Ye, H.; Regnier, S.M.; Poudel, A.; Hara, M.; Kamau, W.; Johnson, D.N.; Roberts, A.A.; et al. Arsenic exposure induces glucose intolerance and alters global energy metabolism. *Am. J. Physiol. Regul. Integr. Comp. Physiol.* **2018**, *314*, R294–R303. [CrossRef]
10. Li, W.; Wu, L.; Sun, Q.; Yang, Q.; Xue, J.; Shi, M.; Tang, H.; Zhang, J.; Liu, Q. MicroRNA-191 blocking the translocation of GLUT4 is involved in arsenite-induced hepatic insulin resistance through inhibiting the IRS1/AKT pathway. *Ecotoxicol. Environ. Saf.* **2021**, *215*, 112130. [CrossRef]
11. Paul, D.S.; Hernández-Zavala, A.; Walton, F.S.; Adair, B.M.; Dědina, J.; Matoušek, T.; Stýblo, M. Examination of the effects of arsenic on glucose homeostasis in cell culture and animal studies: Development of a mouse model for arsenic-induced diabetes. *Toxicol. Appl. Pharmacol.* **2007**, *222*, 305–314. [CrossRef] [PubMed]
12. Waghe, P.; Sarath, T.S.; Gupta, P.; Kutty, H.S.; Kandasamy, K.; Mishra, S.K.; Sarkar, S.N. Subchronic arsenic exposure through drinking water alters vascular redox homeostasis and affects physical health in rats. *Biol. Trace Elem. Res.* **2014**, *162*, 234–241. [CrossRef] [PubMed]
13. Li, Z.; Ren, Y.; Lv, Z.; Li, M.; Li, Y.; Fan, X.; Xiong, Y.; Qian, L. Decrypting the circular RNAs does a favor for us: Understanding, diagnosing and treating diabetes mellitus and its complications. *Biomed. Pharmacother.* **2023**, *168*, 115744. [CrossRef] [PubMed]
14. Sun, J.; Feng, M.; Zou, H.; Mao, Y.; Yu, W. Circ_0000284 facilitates the growth, metastasis and glycolysis of intrahepatic cholangiocarcinoma through miR-152-3p-mediated PDK1 expression. *Histol. Histopathol.* **2023**, *38*, 1129–1143.
15. Cai, H.; Jiang, Z.; Yang, X.; Lin, J.; Cai, Q.; Li, X. Circular RNA HIPK3 contributes to hyperglycemia and insulin homeostasis by sponging miR-192-5p and upregulating transcription factor forkhead box O1. *Endocr. J.* **2020**, *67*, 397–408. [CrossRef]
16. Christiansen, J.; Kolte, A.M.; Hansen Tv Nielsen, F.C. IGF2 mRNA-binding protein 2: Biological function and putative role in type 2 diabetes. *J. Mol. Endocrinol.* **2009**, *43*, 187–195. [CrossRef]
17. Ji, J.; Li, C.; Wang, J.; Wang, L.; Huang, H.; Li, Y.; Fang, J. Hsa_circ_0001756 promotes ovarian cancer progression through regulating IGF2BP2-mediated RAB5A expression and the EGFR/MAPK signaling pathway. *Cell Cycle* **2022**, *21*, 685–696. [CrossRef]

18. Dai, N. The Diverse Functions of IMP2/IGF2BP2 in Metabolism. *Trends Endocrinol. Metab.* **2020**, *31*, 670–679. [CrossRef]
19. Regué, L.; Minichiello, L.; Avruch, J.; Dai, N. Liver-specific deletion of IGF2 mRNA binding protein-2/IMP2 reduces hepatic fatty acid oxidation and increases hepatic triglyceride accumulation. *J. Biol. Chem.* **2019**, *294*, 11944–11951. [CrossRef]
20. Cao, J.; Yan, W.; Ma, X.; Huang, H.; Yan, H. Insulin-like Growth Factor 2 mRNA-Binding Protein 2—A Potential Link Between Type 2 Diabetes Mellitus and Cancer. *J. Clin. Endocrinol. Metab.* **2021**, *106*, 2807–2818. [CrossRef]
21. Chen, H.; Tan, H.; Wan, J.; Zeng, Y.; Wang, J.; Wang, H.; Lu, X. PPAR-γ signaling in nonalcoholic fatty liver disease: Pathogenesis and therapeutic targets. *Pharmacol. Ther.* **2023**, *245*, 108391. [CrossRef] [PubMed]
22. Ge, Z.; Zhang, P.; Hong, T.; Tang, S.; Meng, R.; Bi, Y.; Zhu, D. Erythropoietin alleviates hepatic insulin resistance via PPARγ-dependent AKT activation. *Sci. Rep.* **2015**, *5*, 17878. [CrossRef] [PubMed]
23. Gao, N.; Yao, X.; Jiang, L.; Yang, L.; Qiu, T.; Wang, Z.; Pei, P.; Yang, G.; Liu, X.; Sun, X. Taurine improves low-level inorganic arsenic-induced insulin resistance by activating PPARγ-mTORC2 signalling and inhibiting hepatic autophagy. *J. Cell. Physiol.* **2019**, *234*, 5143–5152. [CrossRef] [PubMed]
24. Swain, S.K.; Dash, U.C.; Kanhar, S.; Sahoo, A.K. Network pharmacology-based elucidation of bioactive compounds and experimental exploration of antidiabetic mechanisms of *Hydrolea zeylanica*. *Cell. Signal.* **2024**, *114*, 110999. [CrossRef] [PubMed]
25. Odongo, K.; Abe, A.; Kawasaki, R.; Kawabata, K.; Ashida, H. Two Prenylated Chalcones, 4-Hydroxyderricin, and Xanthoangelol Prevent Postprandial Hyperglycemia by Promoting GLUT4 Translocation via the LKB1/AMPK Signaling Pathway in Skeletal Muscle Cells. *Mol. Nutr. Food Res.* **2024**, *68*, e2300538. [CrossRef] [PubMed]
26. Kurabayashi, A.; Furihata, K.; Iwashita, W.; Tanaka, C.; Fukuhara, H.; Inoue, K.; Furihata, M.; Kakinuma, Y. Murine remote ischemic preconditioning upregulates preferentially hepatic glucose transporter-4 via its plasma membrane translocation, leading to accumulating glycogen in the liver. *Life Sci.* **2022**, *290*, 120261. [CrossRef]
27. Miao, L.; Zhang, X.; Zhang, H.; Cheong, M.S.; Chen, X.; Farag, M.A.; Cheang, W.S.; Xiao, J. Baicalin ameliorates insulin resistance and regulates hepatic glucose metabolism via activating insulin signaling pathway in obese pre-diabetic mice. *Phytomedicine* **2024**, *124*, 155296. [CrossRef] [PubMed]
28. Zhu, Y.; Engmann, M.; Medina, D.; Han, X.; Das, P.; Bartke, A.; Ellsworth, B.S.; Yuan, R. Metformin treatment of juvenile mice alters aging-related developmental and metabolic phenotypes in sex-dependent and sex-independent manners. *Geroscience* **2024**, *46*, 3197–3218. [CrossRef] [PubMed] [PubMed Central]
29. Oyebode, O.A.; Erukainure, O.L.; Chuturgoon, A.A.; Ghazi, T.; Naidoo, P.; Chukwuma, C.I.; Islam, M.S. *Bridelia ferruginea* Benth. (*Euphorbiaceae*) mitigates oxidative imbalance and lipotoxicity, with concomitant modulation of insulin signaling pathways via GLUT4 upregulation in hepatic tissues of diabetic rats. *J. Ethnopharmacol.* **2022**, *284*, 114816. [CrossRef]
30. Chadt, A.; Al-Hasani, H. Glucose transporters in adipose tissue, liver, and skeletal muscle in metabolic health and disease. *Pflug. Arch.* **2020**, *472*, 1273–1298. [CrossRef]
31. Balakrishnan, B.B.; Krishnasamy, K.; Mayakrishnan, V.; Selvaraj, A. Moringa concanensis Nimmo extracts ameliorates hyperglycemia-mediated oxidative stress and upregulates PPARγ and GLUT4 gene expression in liver and pancreas of streptozotocin-nicotinamide induced diabetic rats. *Biomed. Pharmacother.* **2019**, *112*, 108688. [CrossRef] [PubMed]
32. Zhang, J.; Li, J.; Xiong, Y.; Li, R. Circ_0000284 upregulates RHPN2 to facilitate pancreatic cancer proliferation, metastasis, and angiogenesis through sponging miR-1179. *J. Biochem. Mol. Toxicol.* **2023**, *37*, e23274. [CrossRef] [PubMed]
33. Watson, R.T.; Pessin, J.E. Intracellular organization of insulin signaling and GLUT4 translocation. *Recent Prog. Horm. Res.* **2001**, *56*, 175–193. [CrossRef] [PubMed]
34. Irudayaraj, S.S.; Stalin, A.; Sunil, C.; Duraipandiyan, V.; Al-Dhabi, N.A.; Ignacimuthu, S. Antioxidant, antilipidemic and antidiabetic effects of ficusin with their effects on GLUT4 translocation and PPARγ expression in type 2 diabetic rats. *Chem. Biol. Interact.* **2016**, *256*, 85–93. [CrossRef] [PubMed]
35. Giacoman-Martínez, A.; Alarcón-Aguilar, F.J.; Zamilpa, A.; Huang, F.; Romero-Nava, R.; Román-Ramos, R.; Almanza-Pérez, J.C. α-Amyrin induces GLUT4 translocation mediated by AMPK and PPARδ/γ in C2C12 myoblasts. *Can. J. Physiol. Pharmacol.* **2021**, *99*, 935–942. [CrossRef]
36. Wang, P.; Yao, Q.; Zhu, D.; Yang, X.; Chen, Q.; Lu, Q.; Liu, A. Resveratrol protects against deoxynivalenol-induced ferroptosis in HepG2 cells. *Toxicology* **2023**, *494*, 153589. [CrossRef] [PubMed]
37. Wu, M.; Sun, J.; Wang, L.; Wang, P.; Xiao, T.; Wang, S.; Liu, Q. The lncRNA HOTAIR via miR-17-5p is involved in arsenite-induced hepatic fibrosis through regulation of Th17 cell differentiation. *J. Hazard. Mater.* **2023**, *443 Pt B*, 130276. [CrossRef] [PubMed]
38. Sun, J.; Wu, M.; Wang, L.; Wang, P.; Xiao, T.; Wang, S.; Liu, Q. miRNA-21, which disrupts metabolic reprogramming to facilitate CD4+ T cell polarization toward the Th2 phenotype, accelerates arsenite-induced hepatic fibrosis. *Ecotoxicol. Environ. Saf.* **2022**, *248*, 114321. [CrossRef] [PubMed]
39. Lai, C.; Chen, L.; Zhong, X.; Tian, X.; Zhang, B.; Li, H.; Zhang, G.; Wang, L.; Sun, Y.; Guo, L. Long-term arsenic exposure decreases mice body weight and liver lipid droplets. *Environ. Int.* **2024**, *192*, 109025. [CrossRef] [PubMed]
40. Spaur, M.; Galvez-Fernandez, M.; Chen, Q.; Lombard, M.A.; Bostick, B.C.; Factor-Litvak, P.; Fretts, A.M.; Shea, S.J.; Navas-Acien, A.; Nigra, A.E. Association of Water Arsenic with Incident Diabetes in U.S. Adults: The Multi-Ethnic Study of Atherosclerosis and the Strong Heart Study. *Diabetes Care* **2024**, *47*, 1143–1151. [CrossRef]
41. Ndisang, J.F.; Vannacci, A.; Rastogi, S. Insulin Resistance, Type 1 and Type 2 Diabetes, and Related Complications 2017. *J. Diabetes Res.* **2017**, *2017*, 1478294. [CrossRef] [PubMed]

42. Fan, C.; Zhan, Z.; Zhang, X.; Lou, Q.; Guo, N.; Su, M.; Gao, Y.; Qin, M.; Wu, L.; Huang, W.; et al. Research for type 2 diabetes mellitus in endemic arsenism areas in central China: Role of low level of arsenic exposure and KEAP1 rs11545829 polymorphism. *Arch. Toxicol.* **2022**, *96*, 1673–1683. [CrossRef] [PubMed]
43. Gerich, J.E. Contributions of insulin-resistance and insulin-secretory defects to the pathogenesis of type 2 diabetes mellitus. *Mayo Clin. Proc.* **2003**, *78*, 447–456. [CrossRef] [PubMed]
44. Sira, J.; Zhang, X.; Gao, L.; Wabo, T.M.; Li, J.; Akiti, C.; Zhang, W.; Sun, D. Effects of Inorganic Arsenic on Type 2 Diabetes Mellitus In Vivo: The Roles and Mechanisms of miRNAs. *Biol. Trace Elem. Res.* **2024**, *202*, 111–121. [CrossRef]
45. Chen, M.; Cai, Y.; Guo, J.; Gong, Y.; Xu, X.; Lin, Y.; Hu, Y.; Wen, Y.; Yang, L.; Li, H.; et al. Circ_0000284: A risk factor and potential biomarker for prehypertension and hypertension. *Hypertens. Res.* **2023**, *46*, 720–729. [CrossRef]
46. Qi, L.; Sun, B.; Yang, B.; Lu, S. circHIPK3 (hsa_circ_0000284) Promotes Proliferation, Migration and Invasion of Breast Cancer Cells via miR-326. *OncoTargets Ther.* **2021**, *14*, 3671–3685. [CrossRef]
47. Su, M.; Yu, T.; Yu, Y.; Cheng, Q.; Zheng, Y.; Liao, R.; Zeng, Z. hsa-miR-607, lncRNA TUG1 and hsa_circ_0071106 can be combined as biomarkers in type 2 diabetes mellitus. *Exp. Biol. Med.* **2022**, *247*, 1609–1618. [CrossRef] [PubMed] [PubMed Central]
48. Zhou, Y.; Yan, J.; Huang, H.; Liu, L.; Ren, L.; Hu, J.; Jiang, X.; Zheng, Y.; Xu, L.; Zhong, F.; et al. The m6A reader IGF2BP2 regulates glycolytic metabolism and mediates histone lactylation to enhance hepatic stellate cell activation and liver fibrosis. *Cell Death Dis.* **2024**, *15*, 189. [CrossRef] [PubMed] [PubMed Central]
49. Greenwald, W.W.; Chiou, J.; Yan, J.; Qiu, Y.; Dai, N.; Wang, A.; Nariai, N.; Aylward, A.; Han, J.Y.; Kadakia, N.; et al. Pancreatic islet chromatin accessibility and conformation reveals distal enhancer networks of type 2 diabetes risk. *Nat. Commun.* **2019**, *10*, 2078. [CrossRef]
50. Vasu, G.; Sundaram, R.; Muthu, K. Chebulagic acid attenuates HFD/streptozotocin induced impaired glucose metabolism and insulin resistance via up regulations of PPAR γ and GLUT 4 in type 2 diabetic rats. *Toxicol. Mech. Methods* **2022**, *32*, 159–170. [CrossRef]
51. Qu, X.; Guan, P.; Xu, L.; Liu, B.; Li, M.; Xu, Z.; Huang, X.; Han, L. Riligustilide alleviates hepatic insulin resistance and gluconeogenesis in T2DM mice through multitarget actions. *Phytother. Res.* **2022**, *36*, 462–474. [CrossRef] [PubMed]
52. Wang, X.; Ji, Y.; Feng, P.; Liu, R.; Li, G.; Zheng, J.; Xue, Y.; Wei, Y.; Ji, C.; Chen, D.; et al. The m6A Reader IGF2BP2 Regulates Macrophage Phenotypic Activation and Inflammatory Diseases by Stabilizing TSC1 and PPARγ. *Adv. Sci.* **2021**, *8*, 2100209. [CrossRef] [PubMed]
53. Jiang, Y.; Peng, J.; Song, J.; He, J.; Jiang, M.; Wang, J.; Ma, L.; Wang, Y.; Lin, M.; Wu, H.; et al. Loss of Hilnc prevents diet-induced hepatic steatosis through binding of IGF2BP2. *Nat. Metab.* **2021**, *3*, 1569–1584. [CrossRef] [PubMed]
54. Ramalingam, S.; Packirisamy, M.; Karuppiah, M.; Vasu, G.; Gopalakrishnan, R.; Gothandam, K.; Thiruppathi, M. Effect of β-sitosterol on glucose homeostasis by sensitization of insulin resistance via enhanced protein expression of PPRγ and glucose transporter 4 in high fat diet and streptozotocin-induced diabetic rats. *Cytotechnology* **2020**, *72*, 357–366. [CrossRef]
55. Wang, J.; Wu, T.; Fang, L.; Liu, C.; Liu, X.; Li, H.; Shi, J.; Li, M.; Min, W. Peptides from walnut (Juglans mandshurica Maxim.) protect hepatic HepG2 cells from high glucose-induced insulin resistance and oxidative stress. *Food Funct.* **2020**, *11*, 8112–8121. [CrossRef]
56. Armoni, M.; Harel, C.; Karnieli, E. Transcriptional regulation of the GLUT4 gene: From PPAR-gamma and FOXO1 to FFA and inflammation. *Trends Endocrinol. Metab.* **2007**, *18*, 100–107. [CrossRef]

toxics

MDPI

Communication

# Uranium and Radium in Groundwater and Incidence of Colorectal Cancer in Georgia Counties, USA: An Ecologic Study

Taylor Rooney [1,2], Lissa Soares [3], Tesleem Babalola [3], Alex Kensington [1], Jennie Williams [2,3] and Jaymie R. Meliker [3,*]

1 Department of Undergraduate Biology, Stony Brook University, Stony Brook, NY 11794, USA
2 Increasing Diversity in Undergraduate Cancer Biology, Education, and Research (INDUCER) Program, Stony Brook University, Stony Brook, NY 11794, USA
3 Program in Public Health, Department of Family, Population and Preventive Medicine, Stony Brook University, HSC L3, Rm 071, Stony Brook, NY 11794, USA
* Correspondence: jaymie.meliker@stonybrook.edu

**Abstract:** Colorectal cancer (CRC) is the third most commonly occurring cancer in the United States, with higher incidence rates among Black populations. Groundwater concentrations of natural radionuclides uranium and radium have seldom been investigated in relation to CRC despite their known carcinogenicity. We investigate spatial patterns of CRC by race, and in relation to groundwater concentrations of uranium and radium, testing the hypothesis that uranium and radium in groundwater might differentially contribute to incident CRC in Black and White populations in counties of Georgia, USA. Black populations showed a higher incidence of CRC than White populations; the median incident rate difference was 9.23 cases per 100,000 (95% CI: 2.14, 19.40). Spatial cluster analysis showed high incidence clusters of CRC in similar regions for Black and White populations. Linear regression indicated there are, on average, 1–2 additional cases of colorectal cancer in counties with higher levels of radium in their groundwater, irrespective of race. Uranium was not associated with CRC. This ecologic study suggests that radium in groundwater may be linked with increased incidence of CRC, although it did not explain higher CRC incidence rates in Black populations. Further studies are needed to verify this association given the inherent limitations in the ecologic study design and the crude exposure assessment.

**Keywords:** radionuclides; colorectal cancer; radium; uranium; spatial analysis

## 1. Introduction

Colorectal cancer (CRC) is the third most commonly occurring cancer among men and the second most commonly occurring cancer among women in the United States [1,2]. In the state of Georgia, the age-adjusted incidence rate of CRC was 40.4 per 100,000 people in 2015–2019, with 41.9 new cases for every 100,000 Black individuals and 37.0 new cases for every 100,000 White individuals [3].

After accounting for known risk factors, many cases of CRC remain unexplained. Environmental carcinogens uranium and radium [4] can induce the promotion of cancer [5] and might be linked with CRC, as has been observed with other drinking water contaminants [6]. Drinking water is an important source of exposure to uranium and radium [4,7]. The mean radium-226 contents of diets in 11 cities in the United States were estimated to be 0.52 to 0.73 pCi/kg of food consumed [8]; drinking water is considered a more pronounced source of exposure in many regions of the US [7]. Uranium levels in drinking water vary widely, with a mean population-weighted average of 0.8 pCi/L in the US [4]. Uranium emits alpha particles that are absorbed by the human body to lead to harmful effects such as DNA damage, genetic mutations, abnormalities in chromosomes, or abnormal activity throughout the process of mitosis and cellular proliferation [5]. Uranium's chemical properties, and not its radiological properties, however, are most relevant for disease risk at concentrations of exposure relevant to the general population [7]. Radium emits gamma radiation that can be absorbed by the body [4]. Radium is a radioactive metal that occurs naturally, similarly to uranium, and is produced from the degradation of uranium and thorium [4].

Studies have begun to investigate the relationship between uranium and CRC. In an ecologic epidemiologic study in South Carolina, census tracts with higher concentrations of uranium showed higher rates of colorectal cancer comparing the highest quartile of groundwater uranium concentrations (0.39–64.03 μg/L) to those in the lowest exposure quartile (<0.05 μg/L) [9]. Trend tests also showed an increase in the standardized incidence ratio (SIR) for uranium in census tracts with a high proportion (>38%) of Black residents ($\beta = 0.09$, $p = 0.06$), suggesting that these radionuclides might explain some of the racial disparities in CRC incidence. In another ecologic study in Germany, there was no association reported between uranium in drinking water in men or women and CRC [10]. We could not find any epidemiologic studies of radium and risk of CRC; however, one ecologic study pointed to elevated risks associated with well water use, which was correlated with radon and uranium in soil, among other factors [11]. Additional studies are needed to clarify the relationship between exposure to radionuclides and CRC, and their role in racial disparities of CRC.

Herein, we investigate the relationship between uranium and radium in groundwater and CRC incidence at the county level in Georgia, USA, one of the few regions in the USA with a large population of Black residents and elevated concentrations of uranium and radium in the groundwater. We investigate spatial patterns of CRC by race, and in relation to groundwater concentrations of uranium and radium, testing the hypothesis that uranium and radium in groundwater might differentially contribute to incident CRC in Black and White populations in Georgia.

## 2. Materials and Methods

This is an ecologic study of colorectal cancer and radionuclides in groundwater at the county level in Georgia, USA.

### 2.1. Datasets

Datasets publicly available online and supplied by the Georgia Cancer Registry were accessed for colorectal cancer incidence rates in Georgia, 1999–2008 (http://cancer-rates.info/ga/, accessed on 1 January 2023). Incident cases by sex and race were downloaded along with age-adjusted population for each sex and race group, using year 2000 as the standard. Data were organized into nine different groupings: all cases; all males; all females; all Black individuals; all White individuals; White males; White females; Black males; and Black females.

Drinking water uranium and radium concentrations at the county level were reported by the US Geological Survey (USGS) in 2003 [12]. Uranium concentrations were categorized in two ways: as above or below 27 pCi/L, which is equivalent to the maximum contaminant limit (MCL) in drinking water set by the US Environmental Protection Agency (EPA); and above or below 270 pCi/L, a value 10 times the MCL. The combined radium-226 and -228 isotopes were categorized as above or below 5 pCi/L, the USEPA drinking water MCL. Counties were coded based on the presence of at least one sample that exceeds predefined cutoff values. There were 628 uranium analytical results, including 192 resulting in concentrations higher than 27 pCi/L and 7 counties with at least one sample of uranium concentration higher than 270 pCi/L [12]. Of the 955 total results of combined radium-226 and -228, 476 had concentrations greater than 5 pCi/L [12].

Covariates at the county level were also downloaded from year 2000 US census data [13]. These include: median household income (HHI), and rural or urban classification [14]. We also were able to download county risk factor rankings from countyhealthrankings.org; the earliest data available were from 2010. Each county receives a score based on many factors including smoking, obesity, alcohol use, physical activity, community resources, access to care, among others; 2 counties were missing data. As a sensitivity analysis, we also adjusted for this county risk factor ranking.

### 2.2. Spatial Clustering Analysis

Spatial cluster analyses were run in SaTScan version 10.1 (Calverton, MD, USA) to look for areas of high or low rates of incident CRC. The nine different race–sex groupings of the population were investigated separately. Cancer cases, population at risk, and geographic coordinate centroids of each county were imported into SaTScan. Each Poisson cluster model was set to display a maximum spatial search window of 10% of the population at risk. We only report high-rate clusters with at least 2 cases and a relative risk value greater than or equal to 1.5. Low-rate clusters were restricted to a relative risk value less than or equal to 0.67. Spatial analysis was run using 999 replications to generate the statistical distribution for calculating $p$-values. Circular clusters were allowed to overlap neighboring circular clusters so long as cluster centers did not overlap. The resulting cluster maps were exported using an HTML file for Google Maps.

### 2.3. Spatial Regression Analysis

In GeoDa 1.20.0.22 (Chicago, IL, USA), an ordinary least-squares regression was calculated at the county level between the dependent variable, log of colorectal cancer cases, and the independent variables radium or uranium and age-adjusted population size. There were two different measures of elevated uranium, one measure of elevated radium, and nine different sex–race groupings of the population resulting in 27 different regression models. In addition, to control for potential confounding, we included HHI and urban/rural classification as covariates in fully adjusted models. As a regression diagnostic assessing independence of observations and potential heteroskedasticity, spatial autocorrelation in the residuals was assessed by calculating a Moran's I coefficient using Queen's contiguity of nearest neighbors with an order of one. If spatial autocorrelation was present ($p < 0.05$), then Lagrange Multiplier spatial diagnostics were applied to determine whether to run a spatial lag or spatial error regression model to account for the spatial dependence in the observations [15].

## 3. Results

### 3.1. Descriptive Findings

Counties with uranium greater than 27 pCi/L were found in the northern third of Georgia, with a sprinkling of counties with greater than 270 pCi/L throughout the state (Figure 1). Counties with elevated radium-226 and -228 were distributed broadly across the state of Georgia (Figure 1). Out of the different race–sex groupings, Black males showed elevated incidence rates of CRC in the most counties (Figure 2). Males, in general, displayed higher rates of CRC incidence than females and Black populations showed higher incidence than White populations (Figure 2). The Black–White incident rate ratio has a median value of 1.20 (95% CI:1.04, 1.40), while the Black–White incident rate difference has a median value of 9.23 cases per 100,000 (95% CI: 2.14, 19.40) (Table 1).

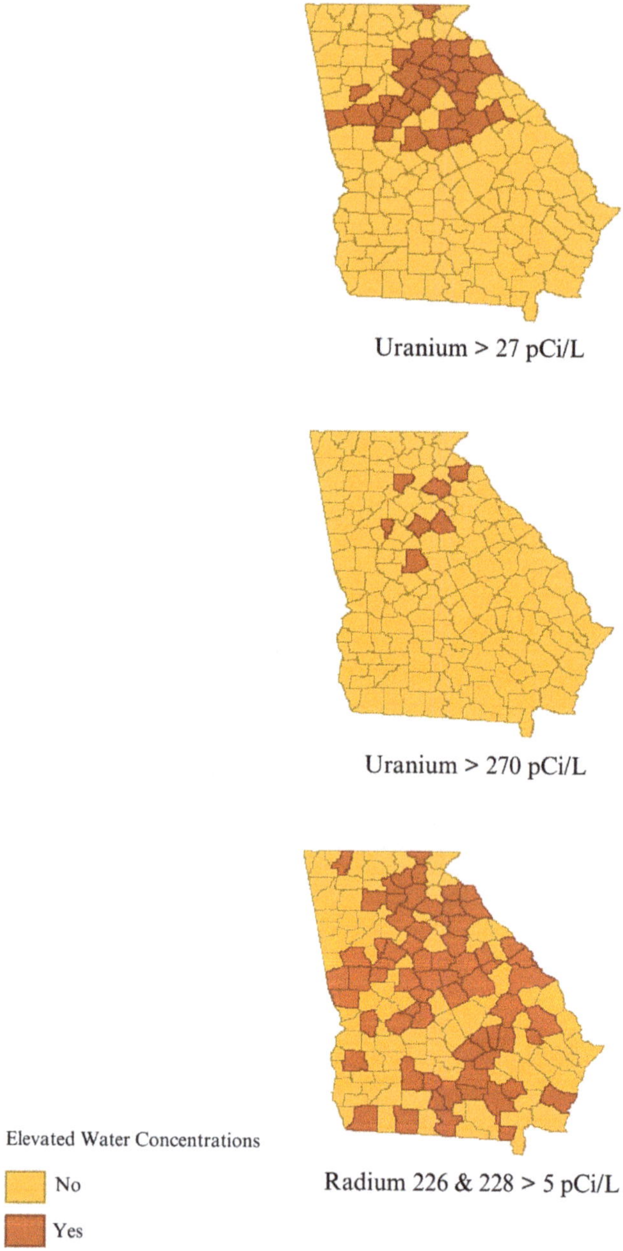


**Figure 1.** Georgia counties with at least one sample of uranium or radium-226 and -228 above concentration indicated.

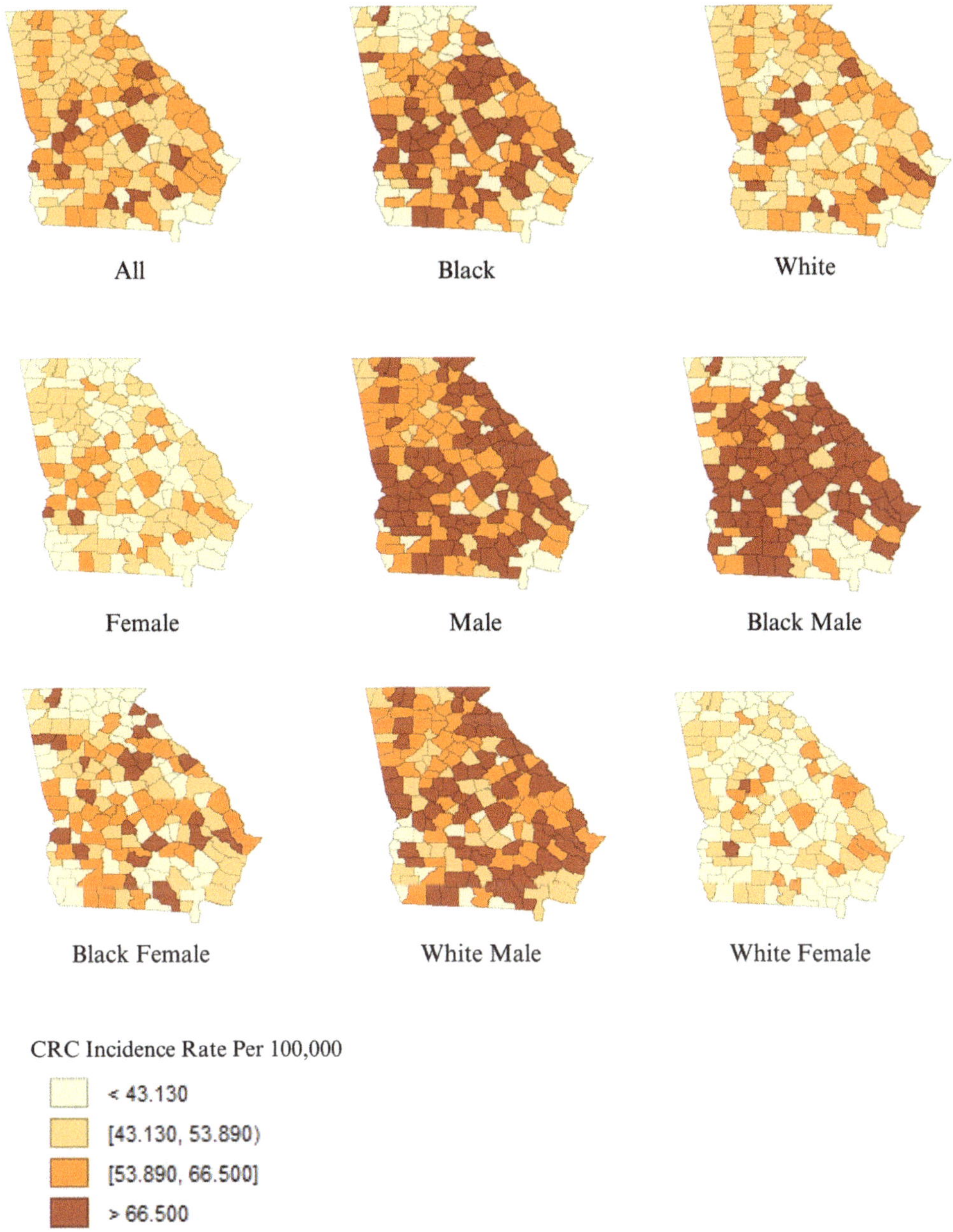


**Figure 2.** Age-adjusted CRC incidence rate per 100,000 individuals across counties in Georgia, by sex–race groupings of the population.

**Table 1.** Characteristics of the population.

| | Med, IQR | No. of Counties |
|---|---|---|
| No. of cases/county | 122 (61–224) | 159 |
| Age-adjusted population at risk/county | 227,000 (113,000–4,400,000) | 159 |
| Black–White incident rate ratio | 1.20 (1.04–1.40) | 159 |
| Black: White–incident rate difference * | 9.23 (2.14–19.40) | 159 |
| County HHI | 31,950 (27,873–38,782)1 | 159 |
| Water samples exceed uranium > 27 pCi/L | | 31 |
| Water samples exceed uranium > 270 pCi/L | | 7 |
| Water samples exceed radium > 5 pCi/L | | 66 |
| Urban counties | | 51 |

* per 100,000 people; HHI = household income.

### 3.2. *Spatial Clusters of CRC Incidence*

Spatial cluster analysis showed high incidence clusters of CRC in the northeastern and southwestern counties of Georgia, and between the cities of Atlanta and Augusta for the total population and the White population (Figure 3A,B). The Black population showed high incidence spatial clusters in the same areas, as well as between the cities of Columbus and Augusta, Georgia. Clusters of lower incidence occurred only for the Black population, near Atlanta and just south of Savannah, Georgia (Figure 3C).

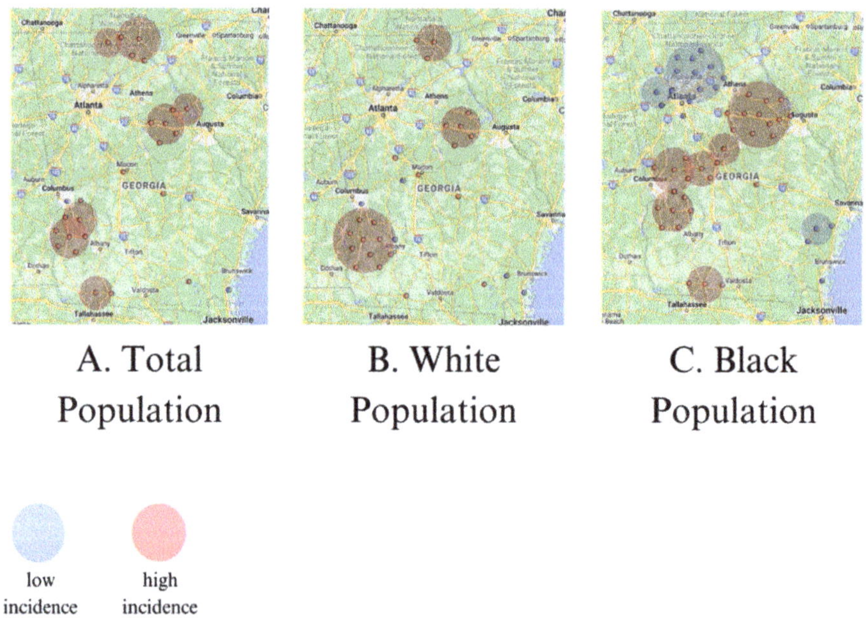


**Figure 3.** Clusters of low and high incidence of CRC per 100,000 in Georgia.

### 3.3. *Linear Regression between Radionuclides and CRC Incidence*

Linear regression analyses at the county level revealed an association between radium in groundwater and incident cases of colorectal cancer, adjusted for population, HHI, and urban/rural classification (Table 2). This association was present in all the different race–sex categories. After adjusting for the population size in each county, the beta coefficients across the race–sex groupings, when exponentiated to account for the log transformation of the dependent variable, indicate there are, on average, 1–2 additional cases of colorectal cancer in counties with higher levels of radium in their groundwater. Uranium in groundwater was not associated with colorectal cancer. Spatial diagnostics indicated spatial autocorrelation was present in some of the models, and we adjusted using spatial error models as indicated by the diagnostics and results were not meaningfully different. Similarly, models only adjusted for population size, but not HHI and urban/rural classification, produced similar results, as did models adjusted for a 2010 county risk factor ranking.

**Table 2.** Association between uranium, radium, and incidence of colorectal cancer (CRC) at the county level in Georgia, 1999–2008.

| | Radium > 5 pCi/L | | Uranium > 27 pCi/L | | Uranium > 270 pCi/L | |
|---|---|---|---|---|---|---|
| | β | *p*-Value | B | *p*-Value | β | *p*-Value |
| All cases * | 0.27 | 0.004 | 0.12 | 0.33 | 0.13 | 0.52 |
| Black population * | 0.18 | 0.006 | 0.08 | 0.49 | −0.14 | 0.35 |
| White population * | 0.13 | 0.003 | 0.07 | 0.32 | 0.03 | 0.78 |
| Males | 0.12 | 0.004 | 0.06 | 0.34 | 0.06 | 0.59 |
| Females | 0.12 | 0.007 | 0.04 | 0.55 | 0.08 | 0.45 |
| Black males * | 0.20 | 0.005 | 0.14 | 0.23 | −0.12 | 0.46 |
| Black females * | 0.15 | 0.002 | 0.07 | 0.42 | 0.03 | 0.80 |
| White males * | 0.18 | 0.02 | 0.01 | 0.96 | −0.21 | 0.23 |
| White females * | 0.15 | 0.003 | 0.05 | 0.54 | 0.04 | 0.75 |

Adjusted for population size, HHI, and urban/rural classification; * Spatial error term was included, as indicated by regression diagnostics in Geoda.

## 4. Discussion

We identified clusters of elevated rates of CRC in the northeastern and southwestern counties of Georgia, and between the cities of Atlanta and Augusta. The areas of elevated risk were generally similar for the total population, White population, and Black population, with additional areas of heightened risks for Black populations between the cities of Columbus and Augusta. Counties with elevated concentrations of uranium in groundwater were mainly seen in the northern third of Georgia, and were not associated with elevated CRC incidence rates in the total population nor any of the subpopulations considered. Areas with elevated concentrations of radium-226 and -228 in groundwater were distributed across the state and were associated with elevated CRC incidence in the total population and all subpopulations of males, females, White populations, and Black populations. Even though we observed higher rates of CRC among males and Black populations, as expected in the US population [3], radium did not explain the racial and gender disparities as the strength of the association with CRC was comparable in the different subpopulations (Table 2).

Age-adjusted CRC incidence rates have been falling for White men and women since the late 1970s, but the decreases began later and moved more slowly for Black men and women [16]. Before 1980, CRC incidence and mortality rates were lower in Black populations than in White populations [16], indicating it is unlikely that the disparity in CRC incidence is the result of biological factors. Differences in socioeconomic status and the resulting differential access to screening are likely important factors [17] but do not explain all of the disparities [18], indicating the need to identify additional causes of the CRC disparities. Gut microbiota and the lifestyle choice of the foods one eats can contribute to disparities in CRC incidence [19]; we also hypothesized that differential exposure to the radiologic drinking water contaminants uranium and radium could play a role. Uranium was not associated with CRC, while radium was associated with CRC in the total population, and among subpopulations of White and Black individuals. The strength of the association between radium and CRC incidence was similar among all groups studied, suggesting radium is not explaining racial disparities in CRC; the search for additional explanatory factors continues.

Radiation has long been linked with CRC. Exposure to ionizing radiation in the workplace [20,21] and among atomic bomb survivors [22] has been linked with excess incidence of CRC. Evidence linking radiologic groundwater contaminants to CRC is more tenuous. One ecologic study linked uranium in groundwater to a higher incidence of CRC [9], but another ecologic study reported no association [10], similar to our findings. To the best of our knowledge, ours is the first study to investigate radium in groundwater as a possible risk factor for CRC. In our ecologic study, we report a positive association, but limitations inherent to ecologic studies must be considered.

This ecologic study is limited by the fact that we do not know whether cases of CRC were due to drinking or were otherwise exposed to groundwater rich in radium or uranium. While we have detailed data on colorectal cancer incidence over a decade with power to assess racial disparities in CRC incidence, our assessment of county-level exposure to uranium or radium relies on a sparsely sampled dataset provided by the USGS, which does not include average levels of uranium or radium but rather only lists counties as having measurements above or below a pre-defined value [12]. These data also do not provide any information about changes in concentrations of radium or uranium over the 1999–2008 period of case ascertainment, nor during earlier periods. Cancer incident data and groundwater radionuclide data were not available at a smaller geographic unit than the county. We do not know whether associations or clusters identified here would have persisted had we relied on data in smaller geographic units. Furthermore, counties reported to be rich in either of these groundwater contaminants may be associated with another variable which could confound the associations studied here. We adjusted for county-level census data from 2000 and for county health rankings available for 2010; unfortunately, earlier county health data were not available and our adjustment for county-level covariates may still leave the possibility of residual confounding. Therefore, this ecologic epidemiologic study should be considered a first glance at the link between radium and CRC incidence which needs to be verified with stronger epidemiologic studies that address potential confounding variables, and better assess individual-level exposure.

## 5. Conclusions

This ecologic study shines a spotlight on radium in groundwater as a possible risk factor for CRC incidence. Further studies are needed to verify this association given the inherent limitations in the ecologic study design and the crude exposure assessment.

**Author Contributions:** Conceptualization, T.R. and J.R.M.; methodology, T.R. and J.R.M.; formal analysis, T.R. and J.R.M.; resources, T.R. and J.R.M.; data curation, T.R.; writing—original draft preparation, T.R. and J.R.M.; writing—review and editing, L.S., T.B., A.K. and J.W.; visualization, T.R. and J.R.M.; supervision, L.S., T.B. and J.R.M.; project administration, L.S., T.B., A.K. and J.R.M.; funding acquisition, J.W. All authors have read and agreed to the published version of the manuscript.

**Funding:** The time and effort of individuals to conduct this research was supported by NIH R01AR081125 and R25CA214272.

**Institutional Review Board Statement:** Not applicable.

**Informed Consent Statement:** Not applicable.

**Data Availability Statement:** County-level data on cancer cases, population at risk, uranium and radium, and key covariates will be available in DRYAD. Meliker, Jaymie (Forthcoming 2024). Georgia county-level datasets [Dataset]. Dryad. https://doi.org/10.5061/dryad.b5mkkwhnz.

**Conflicts of Interest:** The authors declare no conflicts of interest.

## References

1. Alzahrani, S.M.; Al Doghaither, H.A.; Al-Ghafari, A.B. General insight into cancer: An overview of colorectal cancer (Review). *Mol. Clin. Oncol.* **2021**, *15*, 271. [CrossRef] [PubMed]
2. Sawicki, T.; Ruszkowska, M.; Danielewicz, A.; Niedźwiedzka, E.; Arłukowicz, T.; Przybyłowicz, K.E. A Review of Colorectal Cancer in Terms of Epidemiology, Risk Factors, Development, Symptoms and Diagnosis. *Cancers* **2021**, *13*, 2025. [CrossRef] [PubMed]

3. CDC. USCS Data Visualizations. Gis.cdc.gov. June 2021. Available online: https://gis.cdc.gov/Cancer/USCS/#/AtAGlance/ (accessed on 15 July 2024).
4. Agency for Toxic Substances and Disease Registry (ATSDR). *Toxicological Profile for Uranium*; USDHHS: Atlanta, GA, USA, 2013.
5. Kim, S.B.; Bozeman, R.G.; Kaisani, A.; Kim, W.; Zhang, L.; Richardson, J.A.; Wright, W.E.; Shay, J.W. Radiation promotes colorectal cancer initiation and progression by inducing senescence-associated inflammatory responses. *Oncogene* **2016**, *35*, 3365–3375. [CrossRef] [PubMed]
6. Villanueva, C.M.; Espinosa, A.; Gracia-Lavedan, E.; Vlaanderen, J.; Vermeulen, R.; Molina, A.J.; Amiano, P.; Gómez-Acebo, I.; Castaño-Vinyals, G.; Vineis, P.; et al. Exposure to widespread drinking water chemicals, blood inflammation markers, and colorectal cancer. *Environ. Int.* **2021**, *157*, 106873. [CrossRef] [PubMed]
7. Agency for Toxic Substances and Disease Registry (ATSDR). *Toxicological Profile for Radium*; US Public Health Service & USEPA: Atlanta, GA, USA, 1990.
8. Eisenbud, M. Natural radioactivity. In *Environmental Radioactivity*; Academic Press: New York, NY, USA, 1973; pp. 159–174.
9. Wagner, S.E.; Burch, J.B.; Bottai, M.; Puett, R.; Porter, D.; Bolick-Aldrich, S.; Temples, T.; Wilkerson, R.C.; Vena, J.E.; Hébert, J.R. Groundwater uranium and cancer incidence in South Carolina. *Cancer Causes Control* **2011**, *22*, 41–50. [CrossRef] [PubMed]
10. Radespiel-Tröger, M.; Meyer, M. Association between drinking water uranium content and cancer risk in Bavaria, Germany. *Int. Arch. Occup. Environ. Health* **2013**, *86*, 767–776. [CrossRef] [PubMed]
11. Schwartz, G.G.; Klug, M.G.; Rundquist, B.C. An exploration of colorectal cancer incidence rates in North Dakota, USA, via structural equation modeling. *Int. J. Color. Dis.* **2019**, *34*, 1571–1576. [CrossRef] [PubMed]
12. Albertson, P.N. Naturally occurring radionuclides in Georgia water supplies: Implications for community water systems. In Proceedings of the 2003 Georgia Water Resources Conference, Athens, GA, USA, 23–24 April 2003; Hatcher, K.J., Ed.;
13. United States Census. Profile of Selected Economic Characteristics: 2000. DP3. 2024. Available online: https://data.census.gov/table/DECENNIALDPSF32000.DP3?q=2000%20georgia%20county%20median%20household%20income&g=040XX00US13$0500000 (accessed on 15 July 2024).
14. Georgia Department of Community Health. Georgia Rural Counties Map. 2021. Available online: https://dch.georgia.gov/divisionsoffices/state-office-rural-health/sorh-maps-georgia (accessed on 15 July 2024).
15. Anselin, L. Exploring Spatial Data with GeoDa: A Workbook. 2005. Available online: https://geodacenter.github.io/documentation.html (accessed on 15 July 2024).
16. American Cancer Society. Colorectal Cancer Facts & Figures 2008–2010. Atlanta, GA. 2008. Available online: www.cancer.org/content/dam/cancer-org/research/cancer-facts-and-statistics/colorectal-cancer-facts-and-figures/colorectal-cancer-facts-and-figures-2008-2010.pdf (accessed on 15 July 2024).
17. DeLancey, J.O.; Thun, M.J.; Jemal, A.; Ward, E.M. Recent trends in Black-White disparities in cancer mortality. *Cancer Epidemiol. Biomark. Prev.* **2008**, *17*, 2908–2912. [CrossRef] [PubMed]
18. Lansdorp-Vogelaar, I.; Kuntz, K.M.; Knudsen, A.B.; van Ballegooijen, M.; Zauber, A.G.; Jemal, A. Contribution of screening and survival differences to racial disparities in colorectal cancer rates. *Cancer Epidemiol. Biomark. Prev.* **2012**, *21*, 728–736. [CrossRef] [PubMed]
19. Carson, T.L.; Byrd, D.A.; Smith, K.S.; Carter, D.; Gomez, M.; Abaskaron, M.; Little, R.B.; Holmes, S.T.; van Der Pol, W.J.; Lefkowitz, E.J.; et al. A case-control study of the association between the gut microbiota and colorectal cancer: Exploring the roles of diet, stress, and race. *Gut Pathog.* **2024**, *16*, 13. [CrossRef] [PubMed]
20. Boice, J.D.; Cohen, S.S.; Mumma, M.T.; Dupree Ellis, E.; Eckerman, K.F.; Leggett, R.W.; Boecker, B.B.; Brill, A.B.; Henderson, B.E. Mortality among radiation workers at Rocketdyne (Atomics International), 1948–1999. *Radiat. Res.* **2006**, *166 Pt 1*, 98–115. [CrossRef] [PubMed]
21. Lashner, B.A.; Epstein, S.S. Industrial risk factors for colorectal cancer. *Int. J. Health Serv.* **1990**, *20*, 459–483. [CrossRef] [PubMed]
22. Sugiyama, H.; Misumi, M.; Brenner, A.; Grant, E.J.; Sakata, R.; Sadakane, A.; Utada, M.; Preston, D.L.; Mabuchi, K.; Ozasa, K. Radiation risk of incident colorectal cancer by anatomical site among atomic bomb survivors: 1958–2009. *Int. J. Cancer* **2020**, *146*, 635–645. [CrossRef] [PubMed]

MDPI AG
Grosspeteranlage 5
4052 Basel
Switzerland
Tel.: +41 61 683 77 34

*Toxics* Editorial Office
E-mail: toxics@mdpi.com
www.mdpi.com/journal/toxics

www.ingramcontent.com/pod-product-compliance
Lightning Source LLC
Chambersburg PA
CBHW061616210926
51850CB00009B/2337